Edited by
Sterling Clarren,
Amy Salmon, and
Egon Jonsson

Prevention of Fetal Alcohol
Spectrum Disorder FASD

Titles of the series "Health Care and Disease Management"

Riley, E.P., Clarren, S., Weinberg, J., Jonsson, E. (eds.)

Fetal Alcohol Spectrum Disorder

Management and Policy Perspectives of FASD

2011
978-3-527-32839-0

Martin, W., Suchowersky, O., Kovacs Burns, K., Jonsson, E. (eds.)

Parkinson Disease

A Health Policy Perspective

2010
ISBN: 978-3-527-32779-9

Rapoport, J., Jacobs, P., Jonsson, E. (eds.)

Cost Containment and Efficiency in National Health Systems

A Global Comparison

2009
ISBN: 978-3-527-32110-0

Rashiq, S., Schopflocher, D., Taenzer, P., Jonsson, E. (eds.)

Chronic Pain

A Health Policy Perspective

2008
ISBN: 978-3-527-32382-1

Lu, M., Jonsson, E. (eds.)

Financing Health Care

New Ideas for a Changing Society

2008
ISBN: 978-3-527-32027-1

Related Titles

Riley, E.P., Clarren, S., Weinberg, J., Jonsson, E. (eds.)

Fetal Alcohol Spectrum Disorder

Management and Policy Perspectives of FASD

2011
978-3-527-32839-0

Miller, N.S., Gold, M.S. (eds.)

Addictive Disorders in Medical Populations

2010
ISBN: 978-0-470-74033-0

Mitcheson, L., Maslin, J., Meynen, T., Morrison, T., Hill, R., Wanigaratne, S., Padesky, C.A. (Foreword by)

Applied Cognitive and Behavioural Approaches to the Treatment of Addiction: A Practical Treatment Guide

2010
ISBN: 978-0-470-51062-9

Edited by Sterling Clarren, Amy Salmon, and Egon Jonsson

Prevention of Fetal Alcohol Spectrum Disorder FASD

Who is responsible?

⊛WILEY-BLACKWELL

The Editors

Prof. Sterling Clarren
University of British Columbia
Faculty of Medicine
L408–4480 Oak Street
Vancouver, BC V6H 3V4
Canada

Dr. Amy Salmon
University of British Columbia
Faculty of Medicine
E202–4500 Oak Street
Vancouver, BC V6H 3N1
Canada

Prof. Dr. Egon Jonsson
University of Calgary
Department of Public
Health Sciences
CEO Institute of Health
Economics
1200 10405 Jasper Avenue
Edmonton, AB T5J 3N4
Canada

Series Editor

Prof. Dr. Egon Jonsson
University of Calgary
Department of Public
Health Sciences
Institute of Health Economics
1200 10405 Jasper Avenue
Edmonton, AB T5J 3N4
Canada

Cover
Oil painting on canvas by
Egon Jonsson

Library of Congress Card No.: applied for

British Library Cataloguing-in-Publication Data
A catalogue record for this book is available from the British Library.

Bibliographic information published by the Deutsche Nationalbibliothek
The Deutsche Nationalbibliothek lists this publication in the Deutsche Nationalbibliografie; detailed bibliographic data are available on the Internet at <http://dnb.d-nb.de>.

© 2011 Wiley-VCH Verlag & Co. KGaA, Boschstr. 12, 69469 Weinheim, Germany

Wiley-Blackwell is an imprint of John Wiley & Sons, formed by the merger of Wiley's global Scientific, Technical, and Medical business with Blackwell Publishing.

Typesetting   Toppan Best-set Premedia Limited, Hong Kong
Printing and Binding   betz-druck GmbH, Darmstadt
Cover Design   Adam-Design, Weinheim

Printed in the Federal Republic of Germany
Printed on acid-free paper

ISBN Print: 978-3-527-32997-7

ISBN oBook: 978-3-527-63548-1
ISBN ePDF: 978-3-527-63550-4
ISBN ePub: 978-3-527-63549-8
ISBN Mobi: 978-3-527-63551-1

ISSN: 1864-9947

Contents

**3   A Systematic Review of the Effectiveness of Prevention Approaches for
        Fetal Alcohol Spectrum Disorder   99**
        Maria Ospina, Carmen Moga, Liz Dennett, and Christa Harstall

Preface

Research has well established that alcohol consumption during pregnancy may cause serious and irreversible brain damage to the fetus. Nobody would think of giving alcohol to a toddler; nevertheless, at least one in every 100 babies is born with a lifelong disorder resulting from the effects of fetal alcohol exposure. Fetal alcohol spectrum disorder – or FASD – is devastating for both the individual and the family, and its prevention is considered to be a high public health priority in many jurisdictions.

This book reviews evidence from research on the effectiveness of various strategies for the prevention of FASD. Considerable doubt continues to be raised about the effectiveness of some of the most commonly used prevention strategies, such as public media campaigns and printed information about the harm of alcohol use during pregnancy, as well as prenatal programs that educate pregnant women about the risks of drinking but do not address the root causes of drinking. There is, however, evidence that intensive interventions and other types of targeted support for high-risk mothers are both effective and cost-effective.

Every year, thousands of children are born with permanent brain injury resulting from exposure to alcohol during gestation. The response to that should be a forceful, determined, and sustainable effort to prevent this situation from occurring. It seems reasonable to suggest, therefore, that current approaches to prevention of FASD need to be reconsidered, and that a reallocation of resources to strategies that have a proven effectiveness should become a priority. Moreover, concerted efforts must be given to the development of new strategies for preventing this disorder.

But, who will take responsibility for FASD prevention? FASD falls across many areas of potential responsibility. It does not have a home in any particular specialty of medicine – its implications are shared by ministries of health, education, children, and social services. To some extent, it also concerns departments and institutions responsible for correctional services, since individuals with FASD seems to be disproportionately represented among those in conflict with the justice system.

We argue that provincial, national, and international bodies need to work together to develop the multisectoral strategies required for the effective prevention of FASD. Moreover, we believe that the World Health Organization, in collaboration with member states, should take the initiative in formulating priorities in research and policy development for the prevention of FASD–in addition to its more general global strategy to reduce harmful use of alcohol.

Vancouver and Edmonton, February 2011

Sterling Clarren
Amy Salmon
Egon Jonsson

Note from the editors: This is the second of two books on FASD produced by the Institute of Health Economics in Edmonton, Canada, and published by Wiley-Blackwell. The first book, which focuses on FASD in a policy and management perspective, also contains several chapters that relate to the prevention of FASD (see *Fetal Alcohol Spectrum Disorder: Management and Policy Perspectives of FASD*, by Riley, E.P., Clarren, S., Weinberg, J., and Jonsson, E., Wiley-Blackwell, 2011, ISBN 978-3-527-32839-0).

List of Contributors

Lola Baydala
University of Alberta
Faculty of Medicine and Dentistry
Department of Pediatrics
87 Avenue
Edmonton
Alberta T5R 4H5
Canada

June Bergman
University of Alberta
Faculty of Medicine and Dentistry
Department of Pediatrics
87 Avenue
Edmonton
Alberta T5R 4H5
Canada

Sterling Clarren
Canada Northwest FASD Research
Network
L 408–4480 Oak Street
Vancouver
British Columbia V6H 3V4
Canada

Liz Dennett
University of Calgary
Institute of Health Economics
1200 10405 Jasper Avenue
Edmonton
Alberta T5J 3N4
Canada

Christa Harstall
University of Calgary
Institute of Health Economics
1200 10405 Jasper Avenue
Edmonton
Alberta T5J 3N4
Canada

Egon Jonsson
University of Calgary
Department of Public
Health Sciences
Executive Director & CEO
Institute of Health Economics
1200 10405 Jasper Avenue
Edmonton
Alberta T5J 3N4
Canada

Carmen Moga
University of Calgary
Institute of Health Economics
1200 10405 Jasper Avenue
Edmonton
Alberta T5J 3N4
Canada

Maria Ospina
Institute of Health Economics
1200 10405 Jasper Avenue
Edmonton
Alberta T5J 3N4
Canada

Amy Salmon
University of British Columbia
Faculty of Medicine
School of Population and Public
Health, and Canada Northwest FASD
Research Network
E202–4500 Oak Street
Vancouver
British Columbia V6H 3N1
Canada

Robin Thurmeier
University of Calgary
University of Regina
Faculty of Business Administration
1918 Cairns Avenue
Saskatoon
Saskatchewan S7J 1T4
Canada

Nancy Whitney
University of Washington
King County Parent-Child Assistance
Program
Psychiatry and Behavioral Sciences
650 S. Orcas Street 103
Seattle WA 98108
USA

1
Introduction

Sterling Clarren, Amy Salmon, and Egon Jonsson

This book is about the prevention of a disability that does not need to exist: fetal alcohol spectrum disorder (FASD). Alcohol use during pregnancy is the direct cause of this disability, which the baby must live with for the rest of its life. The damage caused to the brain of the fetus by exposure to alcohol is irreparable. Who is responsible for this?

For almost 40 years, FASD has been said to be entirely preventable, and ever since the cause of the disorder was established, women who drink while they are pregnant have been made to feel fully responsible for perpetuating this "entirely preventable" condition. But, the more we learn about FASD and the challenges to its prevention, the more we realize that investing only pregnant women with the responsibility for FASD prevention is misguided, ineffective, and punitive. Yet, if the responsibility for FASD prevention does not lie only with women who drink when they are pregnant, who else is responsible?

That question is not as easy to answer as it may seem, since there are many reasons for alcohol use during pregnancy. Men who are violent at home, who abuse alcohol themselves and who encourage or demand their pregnant partner to drink with them are responsible for the syndrome. The social determinants of health, such as poverty, poor housing, poor nutrition, along with other complicating social circumstances, may also be implicated in the alcohol use that causes FASD. Healthcare and social service providers who fail not only to ask pregnant women about their alcohol use but also to provide meaningful support to women at risk, may be seen as responsible. Governments who do not adequately fund the programs, services, and infrastructure necessary for providers to reach families who are struggling also hold responsibility for FASD.

Pregnant women who drink are, of course, also responsible. Some women drink before they know that they are pregnant; some may believe that only heavy drinking will endanger their baby, and that consuming a moderate amount of alcohol is harmless; some may drink in conformance with cultural norms and beliefs. It is well known from several scientific studies that many women drink during their pregnancy simply to cope with their difficult living circumstances and relationships—to lessen their fear, anxiety, depression, and loneliness.

Prevention of Fetal Alcohol Spectrum Disorder FASD: Who is Responsible?, First Edition. Edited by Sterling Clarren, Amy Salmon, Egon Jonsson.
© 2011 Wiley-VCH Verlag GmbH & Co. KGaA. Published 2011 by Wiley-VCH Verlag GmbH & Co. KGaA.

Not only women, but also their male partners, their social support networks, and society at large are responsible for FASD, and must also be held responsible for its prevention. At least one in every 100 babies born has to live with this permanent disability. In Canada alone, with a population of 33 million, there are about 300 000 individuals living with this injury. If the same incidence holds for the United States, with its population of 307 million, there are about three million people in that country forever incapacitated by having been exposed to alcohol during their most vulnerable time in life – their first nine months. In Europe, with a population of more than 500 million, there may be as many as five million people living with this preventable syndrome.

When thousands of babies are born every year with permanent brain injury of known cause, the response to that ought to be a forceful, determined, concerted, compassionate, sustainable and effective effort to prevent such an occurrence.

1.1
The Content of This Book

This book presents findings from research on different strategies to prevent FASD. Although prevention of this syndrome is challenging, promising results have been obtained from many studies, demonstrating that certain prevention programs are effective in reducing alcohol use during pregnancy.

Chapters 2 and 3, which form the core of the book, are systematic reviews of a large number of studies on the prevention of FASD that have been published in the scientific literature. Chapter 2 also includes a review of the effectiveness of different strategies for diagnosis and treatment, which also are relevant in FASD prevention. Maria Ospina and colleagues have examined the strength of the evidence in each of the studies, and have found some prevention strategies that have clearly been shown to work. But, perhaps more importantly, they have also identified other programs that may not be effective.

It seems self-evident that ineffective strategies for prevention should not be used. However, the reviews show, for example, that widely used and comparatively expensive strategies – such as alcohol-related warning messages, alcohol bans, and some other social marketing strategies implemented on a massive scale – have a limited effectiveness. They do not seem to increase knowledge of FASD, nor to change attitudes toward alcohol use during pregnancy.

On the other hand, focused multimedia education programs aimed at youth in school settings show some evidence of effectiveness, as do health education programs directed at women of childbearing age and pregnant women. Some screening programs for the prenatal use of alcohol have proven effective in identifying high-risk women, and there is strong evidence of the effectiveness of several types of intervention in reducing alcohol use during pregnancy.

The most important finding from the systematic reviews may be that comparatively few FASD-prevention programs have been evaluated. Moreover, among those that have been assessed, only a small fraction have employed a rigorous scientific methodology. The authors argue for more evaluation and for research into the broader social and systemic causes of alcohol use during pregnancy. They also point to the importance of promoting strategies for which there is empirical evidence of effectiveness.

Chapter 4 includes five presentations made at a consensus development conference on FASD. Lola Baydala, from the University of Alberta, presents strong evidence for school-based substance use-prevention programs and, in particular, for the Life Skills Training program initially developed at Cornell University. That program has been shown to be highly effective with students from different geographic regions and with different socioeconomic, racial, and ethnic backgrounds.

Robin Thurmeier from the Saskatchewan Prevention Institute reviews the evaluations of Canadian primary prevention campaigns for FASD. This review is based on an inventory of FASD primary prevention resources, which included campaigns such as "Be Safe; This is Our Baby"; "Alcohol and Pregnancy"; "Born Free"; "Mother Kangaroo"; and "With Child, Without Alcohol." Some of these programs have been found to have had a high impact on the awareness of what FASD is, and that it is linked to alcohol use during pregnancy. However, little is known about how effective these campaigns are in promoting behavioral change. Robin concludes that a behavioral change model needs to be employed to guide the creation of materials and interventions, and she offers "Protection Motivation Theory" as one potential theoretical framework for guiding future prevention campaigns.

June Bergman, from the University of Calgary, discusses the role of primary healthcare in the prevention of FASD, and points out that primary care not only addresses a large majority of personal healthcare needs but also has numerous other dimensions. These include prevention and attention to the social determinants of health, as well as creating community capacity as needed. For example, primary care physicians could be more involved in screening for alcohol use during pregnancy; however, June points out that there are currently a number of barriers to that, such as lack of time and training, shortages of resources, and lack of access to the services of trained counselors when alcohol use is identified.

Nancy Whitney, from the University of Washington, discusses mentoring programs for mothers at risk and, specifically, the Parent–Child Assistance Program (PCAP), which is an intensive three-year home visitation program. The PCAP originated in Washington State some 20 years ago, and has since been replicated all over the United States. The program is tailor-made for each woman, many of whom live in poverty and with domestic violence and untreated mental health problems. The aim is to motivate these women to stop drinking before and during pregnancy, and to help those women who cannot stop drinking to avoid becoming pregnant by using family planning. Several assessments of the program have demonstrated that most women in the PCAP go from chaos to stability, become sober, live in permanent housing, become less dependent on social welfare, and use family planning. The program also seems highly cost-effective. The author recommends this type of intensive case-management program aimed at the highest-risk mothers in the community, along with the support of specialized addiction treatment centers that welcome the women and their children. Unfortunately, such programs continue to be few in number, and are under enormous pressure to meet demands for their services.

Amy Salmon, from University of British Columbia, reminds us of our common assumption that healthy women have healthy babies, and underlines the importance of looking beyond biological factors and genetic endowment to support good health in women. She stresses the need to focus on the social determinants of health in the prevention of FASD. This requires attention to income and social status, social support networks, education, employment and working conditions, social environments, personal health practices, healthy child development, culture, and gender – all of which are unevenly supported in different jurisdictions. Findings from research have shown that those women who give birth to children with FASD are also most likely to have their own health and well-being compromised by addictions, depression, anxiety, high stress levels, and experiences of violence, trauma, grief, and loss. Clearly, the messages in FASD prevention must not build on shame and blame, which stigmatizes, discriminates and isolates women from exactly the kinds of care that they need. Increasing the system capacity for effective FASD prevention, focused on the root causes of alcohol use during pregnancy, requires a full recognition of women's health issues in its broadest sense.

1.2
What is FASD?

The notion that alcohol consumption during pregnancy might be harmful to a developing fetus has been occasionally considered since antiquity. Seminal studies conducted in France and in the United States during the late 1960s and early 1970s brought a more concerted attention to the possibility. In both places, physicians detected a specific, recognizable pattern of physical traits that were consistent in some children who had been exposed to alcohol during gestation. David W. Smith and his group called this syndrome "fetal alcohol syndrome" (FAS) [1], even though they were not sure that alcohol was the true etiologic agent. Nevertheless, they were convinced that the syndrome's prevention included the elimination of alcohol from the embryo–fetal milieu. FAS was soon defined to include structural brain damage (or, at least, clinical evidence of significant brain dysfunction), a typical set of specific minor facial anomalies, and slower prenatal and/or postnatal growth. There was also evidence of problems in other organs, such as the skeleton, kidneys and heart, although these were considered to be associative rather than necessary for defining the syndrome.

Over time, the results of studies conducted with animals have proved that alcohol is indeed capable of producing embryonic and fetal damage (teratogenic). These studies have also shown that the mechanisms of teratogenesis are complex and multifaceted, so that a simple medical approach to blocking a pathway and reducing harm has not been forthcoming. The original human observations have also been confirmed, that the most common impact of fetal alcohol exposure is found in the brain. Those children who were first described with FAS had obvious brain problems typified by severe structural malformations, significantly smaller heads than normal for their age and gender (microcephalus), neurologic problems such as seizures or cerebral palsy, and intellectual handicap. However, these severe manifestations of alcohol's effect were found over time to be only the most extreme examples, not the most common. It is now understood that alcohol primarily alters the microscopic structure and the neurochemistry of the brain, and that this can lead to global, diffuse problems with memory, executive function, social communication, complex learning tasks, attention and other processing dysfunctions.

Affected individuals have different degrees of challenge within and among functions. Among those children initially identified, tests of intellectual quotient (IQ) were frequently within the normal range. However, clinical findings from all measures would sum to a final common pathway of poor adaptive function in society, school and at home that could not be explained by any single deficit alone. The patterns and severity of the functional components were the same in children exposed to alcohol who had the facial and/or growth abnormalities, and those who did not. This led ultimately to the term "fetal alcohol spectrum disorder" (FASD), which was meant to include those with FAS and all those exposed to alcohol who demonstrated the neurobehavioral deficits without the more easily identifiable physical signs. The term FASD was meant to de-emphasize the importance of the physical findings in making a diagnosis, and to re-emphasize the "hidden" nature of this neurodevelopmental condition.

1.3
How Common is FASD?

The incidence and prevalence of FASD is poorly established because of the limited ability to detect the condition. This is itself a multifaceted problem. First, there is no full agreement on what term should be used to describe the level of brain structural abnormality found in FASD. Should this be called "prenatal brain damage," "prenatal traumatic brain injury," "diffuse brain dysfunction," "adaptive brain functional disorder," or something else? Without a uniformly recognized term and then a clear definition of severity, it has been difficult to propose or define a functional severity score that could appropriately be used to define who has been affected to the point of a disability. To date, the recognition of brain differences has been through a broad battery of cognition and performance measures that are not usually sensitive and therefore predictive of dysfunction until children are over four years of age (unless the patient has a more severe intellectual handicap as a component). This type of diagnosis is generally possible only through the work of specialized multidisciplinary teams that are in very short supply. Indeed, probably fewer than 2000 diagnoses can be made annually in all of Canada.

The study of newborns can detect babies with FAS based on growth abnormalities, the facial features, and the most severe forms of prenatal brain injury. Active case-finding studies conducted primarily during the 1970s and early 1980s found that the features of the full syndrome and a confirmed history of gestational alcohol exposure occurred in 1 to 3 per 1000 live births in the United States and

Europe [2]. Later studies suggested that the population of those with FASD might be 1 in 100 individuals, or more, depending on the levels of brain dysfunction and physical findings required by the researchers and the level of proof needed to establish the history of gestational alcohol exposure.

At the present time, there is no evidence that the rate of FASD has changed in Canada during the past two decades; nor do we know the rate at which individuals with FASD emigrate from and immigrate to other countries through adoption or immigration, nor if those with FASD have a higher death rate. However, assuming that 1 in 100 is a valid estimate of FASD prevalence, over 330 000 people in Canada have this condition right now. Far fewer than 20 000 of them have had a full FASD evaluation in a clinic that routinely uses the Canadian Guidelines for FASD Diagnosis. In fact, diagnostic capacity cannot keep pace with new cases, let alone deal with the backlog of older children, youth, and adults. While more active surveillance and case finding could be carried out at this time, the clinical capacity to make final diagnoses is the limiting factor in establishing the true prevalence of this condition in Canada, and elsewhere.

1.4
What is the Economic Burden of FASD?

The economic burden of FASD is substantial by any measure. The total cost of the disorder in Canada in 2009 has been conservatively estimated at CAD7.6 billion, based on a prevalence of nine cases per 1000 births. This amount includes the cost of medical care, education, social and correctional services, as well as out-of-pocket costs and indirect costs due to caregivers' productivity losses. The direct cost of FASD in Canada for healthcare alone was CAD2.1 billion in 2009 (Table 1.1).

1.4.1
Annual Cost Per Person with FASD

While the annual cost of healthcare for a person with FASD is estimated at CAD6860 (Table 1.2), the annual total of all direct and indirect costs is about CAD25 000 per person. The total lifetime cost of services per person with FASD in Canada was CAD1.8 million in 2009.

Table 1.1 Cost of FASD in Canada, 2009.

Total annual direct and indirect costs	CAD7.6 billion
Total annual direct costs[a]	CAD4.9 billion
Total annual direct cost of healthcare for people with FASD	CAD2.1 billion

a) Includes the cost of healthcare and educational and social services, but excludes out-of-pocket costs and the cost of correctional services. Source: From Refs [3, 4] (adjusted to include all ages).

Table 1.2 Annual costs per person with FASD, aged 0–53 years, in Canada 2009.

Cost item	CAD
Medical	6860
Education	5443
Social services	4217
Out-of-pocket	2912
Total direct costs	19432
Indirect cost	1481
Total direct and indirect costs	20912
Adjusted for severity of disability, age	22393
Adjusted for estimated cost of correctional services	25000

Source: From Refs [3, 5–7].

Table 1.3 Annual direct cost of selected diseases and FASD in Canada in 2009[a].

Cost item	Annual cost (CAD)
Direct healthcare costs of respiratory diseases	4.8 billion
Direct healthcare costs of all forms of cancer	4.7 billion
Direct healthcare costs of FASD	2.1 billion

a)   Includes cost of hospitalization, physicians, and drugs for each item.
Source: From Ref. [8] (discounted to 2009).

Table 1.4 Direct annual cost of selected diseases and of FASD in Alberta, 2009.

Cost item	Annual cost (CAD)
Direct cost of healthcare of cardiovascular diseases (CVD)	773.8 million
Direct cost of healthcare of FASD	229.8 million
Direct cost of healthcare of type 2 diabetes	155.1 million
Direct cost of lung cancer	121.6 million

Source: From Ref. [8] (discounted to 2009).

1.4.2
Comparing Costs

A comparison of the costs associated with FASD and those associated with other conditions and types of care at the macroeconomic level, helps to shed light on the economic magnitude of FASD. In order to put the cost of FASD into perspective, Tables 1.3 and 1.4 show the cost of FASD in relation to the costs of various forms of healthcare, selected on the basis of available data.

The total direct yearly cost of healthcare for FASD is almost half of the equivalent cost of all forms of cancer (Table 1.3). However, healthcare for FASD (CAD2.1 billion) is significantly more costly than, for example, the yearly cost of breast cancer and colon cancer, which are CAD380 million and CAD449 million, respectively. In fact, FASD requires more than twice the resources for healthcare alone as these two forms of cancer combined.

Another comparison at the macro level shows that the annual cost of FASD is significant also in relation to the cost of drugs. In the Canadian province of Alberta, for example, the total direct and indirect cost of FASD was CAD520 million in 2009, an amount equivalent to 25–30% of the cost of all pharmaceuticals used in the province that year [9]. The provincial healthcare costs of cardiovascular diseases, FASD, type 2 diabetes, and lung cancer are shown in Table 1.4.

1.4.3
Cost of Prevention versus Cost of Inaction

There are many competing priorities in healthcare, as in other sectors of society. Whilst it is common to place a higher priority in public policy on health conditions that have significant economic implications, the relative neglect of FASD shows that this is not always the case. While some countries or individual provinces do make considerable investments in FASD prevention, it is not known precisely how much any jurisdiction spends on FASD prevention; neither is it known precisely what the results of those investments have been.

In Canada, the provincial and territorial funding provided for all areas of activity in FASD (including, but not limited to, prevention) amounted to CAD26.8 million in 2007. Although funding may have increased in Canada during the past few years, it remains far short of the estimated CAD125.6 million required annually ([10], discounted) to ensure that all women receive the level of support necessary to assist them in abstaining from alcohol use during pregnancy. Conversely, the theoretical maximum cost savings of preventing FASD in Canada, which is equivalent to the total incremental cost of FASD, is approximately CAD2.6 billion annually.

What does it cost to leave FASD without prevention? The answer to this question is, to a certain extent, illuminated above. It can be further demonstrated by, for example, comparing the economic benefit of preventing one case of FASD with the cost of certain specific interventions in healthcare. For such a comparison, it is important to make use of the lifetime incremental cost per person with FASD, which is the added cost attributable to FASD alone, over and above the cost of healthcare, educational, social and correctional services for the general population. The lifetime incremental cost of one case of FASD is CAD742 000 in Canada (at 2009 cost levels). This figure may be regarded as the theoretical maximum that could be spent on preventing one case of FASD. Looked at another way, it is the revenue that becomes available for other purposes when one case of FASD is prevented, or the opportunity cost for leaving FASD without prevention. The benefit of preventing one single case of FASD would amount to, for example, the

Table 1.5 Opportunity cost of preventing *one case of FASD* in Canada in 2009.

Procedure	Average cost (CAD)[a]	Number of procedures that could be performed by preventing one case of FASD
Repair of inguinal hernia	4938	150
Appendectomy	5505	135
Cesarean section	5303	140
Hysterectomy	6317	117
Cholecystectomy	6985	106
Discectomy	7601	98
Knee replacement	10903	68
Hip replacement total and ⋯al	13182	56
Coronary artery bypass	24966	30

⋯ to perform 135 appendecto-
⋯ (Table 1.5).

⋯ the costs of FASD,
⋯ut this disorder.
⋯vention of
⋯le

⋯th

⋯d, years o⋯ ⋯er of
⋯s intervened, ⋯ ⋯therwise
⋯orted. In a so-call⋯ ⋯tility
⋯sis, the cost per qual⋯⋯, ⋯djusted years
⋯es saved is calculated.

landscape for over 100 years. Indeed, they represent a relatively inexpensive and uncontroversial means of showing that some policy attention is being paid to health inequities [12, 13]. To date, the FASD-prevention activities most commonly undertaken by governments in Canada have been those aimed at changing an individual woman's alcohol use during pregnancy. For the most part, this has taken the form of primary prevention campaigns intended to increase public awareness of the risk posed by prenatal alcohol exposure, and urging pregnant women to abstain from drinking [14].

In Canada, most pregnant women whose pre-pregnancy drinking falls into "low-risk" patterns abstain from alcohol for the duration of their pregnancy. According to the most recent Canadian data, 11–15% of women consumed alcohol during their last pregnancy [15, 16]. In some countries, it is reportedly widely believed that drinking during pregnancy is good for the fetus. For example, a survey conducted in 1998 under the auspices of the Australia National Drug Strategy reported that 73.1% of pregnant women had consumed alcohol recently, and 17% of all pregnant respondents reported drinking at least three standard drinks when they drank [17]. A recent UK study [18] reported that, among the 83% of mothers who consumed alcohol prior to pregnancy, 54% continued to drink while they were pregnant.

Overall, both the incidence and prevalence of alcohol use in pregnancy seem to be changing. Most of this change is due to the fact that those women whose drinking patterns were low-risk to begin with are now abstaining completely. In Canada, although an overwhelming majority of women (98%) are aware that there is a link between alcohol use during pregnancy and harm to the fetus, a large fraction of women (62% in 2006) believe that a small amount of alcohol use during pregnancy is safe [19]. Confusion over the safety of small amounts of alcohol is evident in the conflicting guidance provided by health professionals and professional bodies. While Health Canada Report 2009 [20], the US Surgeon General [21], the Royal Australian and New Zealand College of Obstetricians and Gynaecologists [19], and the British Medical Association [22] have all taken a cautionary approach in advising women to abstain from alcohol completely while they are pregnant, others – such as the British Royal College of Obstetricians and Gynaecologists [23] – counsel that "… it remains the case that there is no evidence of harm from low levels of alcohol consumption, defined as no more than one or two units of alcohol once or twice a week." Moreover, rates of episodic high-volume and high-frequency drinking (often referred to as "binge drinking") among pregnant women and nonpregnant women of childbearing age have remained relatively stable [16, 21]. It is these drinking patterns that are most closely associated with the likelihood of having a child with FASD [24–26].

Primary prevention campaigns tend to be aimed either directly at women, or at those who might be in a position to influence a woman's alcohol use (such as partners, family members, friends, or the broader community). Such campaigns have been in existence since the mid-1970s; indeed, over 350 direct-messaging campaigns have been used in northwestern Canada alone since 2000 [27]. The presentations vary greatly from "soft" recommendations for having a healthy baby to negative ads warning about the lifelong problems faced by children affected by alcohol. Awareness-raising materials that depict male partners, friends and family rarely provide direct suggestions on how these concerned persons might effectively help a woman to stop drinking, and no evaluations of the utility or success of these indirect messaging campaigns have yet been found. More often, the visual image is that of a lone pregnant woman or, in an attempt to make the message more universal, sometimes the focus is on the pregnant torso. However, such images may reinforce notions that FASD prevention is confined to the womb of an individual woman, thus negating the role of social, political, and economic conditions that so profoundly shape a woman's risk for having a child with FASD.

While these direct-messaging campaigns are extensive and expensive, few research data have been published that has evaluated their effectiveness in changing the behavior of pregnant women and their supporters. In fact, the materials raise many new questions:

- What harm may come from showing such messages to pregnant women, who might then worry about the potential injury to which their fetus has already been exposed?

- What is needed to ensure that primary prevention campaigns are effective across different communities, age groups, or economic or social circumstances?

- How can primary prevention campaigns avoid "blaming and shaming" women who drink while pregnant?

- Since drinking is legal and socially condoned, what written warnings would be most effective in helping women know when and how to stop?

- How can primary prevention campaigns account for relative risk?

In summary, both general and focused public awareness campaigns advising women of the harm of the gestational use of alcohol are common. Yet, remarkably few campaigns have been evaluated (see Chapters 2 and 3), and therefore little is known about their impacts. Without serious and sustained efforts to understand this social marking experiment, improvements will not be possible. Epidemiological research on the prevalence of drinking during pregnancy indicates that while public education campaigns seem to have increased the awareness of FASD—and, by extension, have encouraged abstinence among those women whose drinking patterns place them at lowest risk—these campaigns alone have not been sufficient to support women in the highest-risk groups to abstain from alcohol during their pregnancies [2].

1.5.2
Screening for Prenatal Alcohol Exposure in Obstetric Settings

At present, two forms of screening for prenatal alcohol use are employed in obstetric settings: biomarkers (in the form of meconium testing; see below) and maternal self-reports of alcohol use using direct or indirect questioning (which may involve the use of standardized screening instruments).

1.5.2.1 Meconium Testing

Meconium testing involves screening samples of a newborn's first stool for the presence of fatty acid ethyl esters (FAEEs), which confirm exposure to alcohol during the last two trimesters of fetal development. Some advocates have suggested that a targeted implementation of meconium screening may be useful. For example, a recent study in a high-risk obstetric unit indicated that infants born in this unit had a 12-fold higher risk of screening positive for second- and third-trimester alcohol exposure than infants born in the general population of the referring community [28]. However, while an FAEE-positive screen can provide an indication that a woman was drinking alcohol during her pregnancy, a number of concerns regarding meconium testing as a tool for prevention and intervention in FASD exist. First, the predictive value of FAEE-positive meconium with regard to neurodevelopmental delays has not yet been established [29]; thus, in the absence of other evidence of compromised fetal development or neurobehavioral symptoms, an FAEE-positive screen itself cannot confirm that an infant has been negatively affected by prenatal alcohol exposure. Moreover, screening for alcohol (and other drug) use is different from all other types of newborn screening. In most cases, diagnostic tests reveal information that is not known to the patient or anyone else. In this case, the mother knows that she consumed alcohol in volume, and has decided not to reveal that information voluntarily. This may be because substance use during pregnancy is often interpreted as a form of abuse or neglect, which may trigger the apprehension of the infant by child welfare authorities [30]. Therefore, the implementation of meconium screening may have an unintended consequence of discouraging high-risk women from accessing obstetric care for fear of losing their children to foster care.

1.5.2.2 Maternal Self-Reporting

Evidence suggests that women accurately and willingly describe their prenatal substance use when asked, provided that safety is assured. An accurate identification and assessment of alcohol-related pregnancy risk factors can be enhanced through the use of reliable screening tools [24]. Indeed, Chang [31] argues that the routine use of screening questionnaires in clinical practice may reduce the stigma associated with asking women about their alcohol use, and result in a more accurate and consistent evaluation (see also Ref. [32]). At present, there is no consensus in Canada on which standardized screening tools to use: each province and territory, healthcare organization, and healthcare provider uses a variety of formal and informal screening tools [33]. However, previous systematic reviews have demonstrated that using *any* standardized screening tool tends to make it more likely that pregnant women will disclose their alcohol use than when "standard care" practices are followed (which typically involve no direct questioning on alcohol use at all) [32]. While there are often concerns that fear, stigma, and shame can influence women to under-report their alcohol use, studies have shown that

"... there is no systematic tendency for women generally to understate the amount they drink during pregnancy" [34]; indeed, antenatal maternal reports of high-risk alcohol use tend to predict infant neurodevelopmental delay better than do postpartum maternal self-reports, most likely due to compromised recall [34]. Accurate maternal self-reporting can be improved by offering strong assurances of confidentiality,[2)] conducting the screening in a community setting, inviting women to complete a printed questionnaire rather than to undergo direct questioning, using more than one alcohol-consumption measure, and wording the questions clearly [35].

However, at least in maternity care settings, it appears that women are not asked as frequently as they should be. In addition, there are inconsistent processes across Canada for recording alcohol use in a woman's medical chart, and for transferring this information to the child's health records [33]. In 2007, only three Canadian provinces (British Columbia. Yukon, and Newfoundland) included questions in their prenatal records inquiring about pre-pregnancy alcohol use. Only two provinces (which use the same reporting form) included prompts to elicit additional information regarding women's usual, pre-pregnancy alcohol consumption patterns (such as average amount of alcohol consumed per drinking session) [36]. Given that Pregnancy Risk Assessment Monitoring System (PRAMS) data show high rates of unplanned pregnancies – especially among young women who are the most likely to drink in binge patterns – this represents a missed opportunity for providing education, counseling, and referral for women who may be experiencing a pregnancy complicated by alcohol use.

1.5.3
Selective Prevention

Most selective prevention approaches to FASD combine some form of brief intervention and motivational interviewing. This approach has been best studied among women aged 18 to 44 years, who do not meet the criteria for alcohol dependency or a substance-use disorder, and among younger women who drink in binge patterns (i.e., Refs [35, 37]). For example, a randomized controlled trial (Project CHOICES) conducted in six community-based settings in the United States found that women who received a brief motivational intervention, consisting of four counseling sessions and a contraception consultation delivered over 14 weeks, significantly reduced their risk of having an alcohol-exposed pregnancy (as measured by decreased risky drinking and/or effective use of contraception) compared to women who received information only [24, 38].

---

2) It is important to note that research on maternal self-reporting has tended to involve studies with an experimental design, in which researchers were able to assure the women participating that their responses would be treated as confidential and would not be forwarded to their treating physician. This, in itself, may have mitigated the woman's fear of possible negative reprisals resulting from her disclosure, but would significantly limit the generalizability of these findings to the clinical setting [24].

Although, the efficacy of paired brief intervention and motivational interviewing approaches in reducing alcohol-exposed pregnancies has not been extensively researched in Canadian settings, a range of initiatives has drawn on these findings to provide FASD-prevention supports to women. In British Columbia, Healthy Choices in Pregnancy (a component of the provincial government's healthy living initiative that included FASD-prevention targets) provided training to healthcare and related service providers to incorporate brief intervention and motivational interviewing into coordinated, informed, respectful responses to substance-using pregnant women.[3] Similarly, the Alberta Alcohol and Drug Abuse Commission's Enhanced Services for Women has incorporated both motivational interviewing and brief intervention techniques into a wide range of resources to encourage the identification and referral of pregnant women with substance-use problems.

1.5.4
Indicated Prevention

It is now abundantly clear that women who give birth to children with FASD are most often those whose own health and well-being are also significantly compromised. The lives of birth mothers of children diagnosed with FASD are frequently imbued with violence, isolation, poverty, mental ill health (including diagnosed psychiatric conditions, very high stress levels, and trauma), addictions, and lack of supportive health and social care before, during, and after their pregnancy [10, 39, 40]. Undoubtedly, the complexity of these issues demands a timely and coordinated approach to care that addresses social determinants of women's health.

Despite increasing acknowledgment that isolation and a lack of social support are common among pregnant women and mothers with substance-use problems, women who are most vulnerable to having a child with FASD often have difficulty accessing timely and supportive services for addictions treatment [41]; for parenting support [40, 42]; and support for issues related to violence and trauma [43]. While public health messaging campaigns exhort pregnant women to identify their drinking as problematic, and to seek professional help if they cannot stop drinking on their own, health systems and services are often unprepared to provide help when women seek it. More often than not, pregnant women facing concurrent problems with violence, mental health, and addictions will be shuffled between uncoordinated systems of care with competing and contradictory service mandates and access criteria. To illustrate this, women presenting to addictions services are often told that they need to get treatment for their mental health issues before they can enter addictions treatment, while mental health services often require abstinence from alcohol and (nonprescribed) drugs before women can be admitted into their care. Likewise, transition houses and other services for women experiencing violence have often been unprepared to provide service to women with untreated mental-health and substance-use problems [44, 45].

---

3) See www.hcip-bc.org for more information.

Thus, women who seek help often find themselves bounced around and between systems of care, until they are bounced out of them entirely [46].

While multiple barriers to care continue to exist, evidence is also accumulating that interventions to increase social support for pregnant women and new mothers by addressing social determinants of women's health can improve outcomes for mothers and children, and also reduce the likelihood of future substance-exposed pregnancies [32, 47–51]. For example, mentoring programs built upon the Parent–Child Assistance Program (PCAP) model (see Chapter 4) offer women who have had a previous substance-exposed pregnancy practical assistance with meeting their basic needs for food, housing, transportation, childcare, advocacy, and parenting skills/teaching. Once engaged in a supportive relationship with their PCAP mentor (many of whom are women with their own experiences of being pregnant and/or parenting with an addiction), women may begin to request birth control, mental healthcare, addictions treatment, employment readiness training, or help in fleeing from a violent relationship. PCAP mentors are able to help make referrals and facilitate the needed interventions. The program has demonstrated success in reducing alcohol-exposed pregnancies [49] and has been replicated in many communities in Canada. Currently, there are as many as 40–50 programs in western Canada alone working with high-risk women in this way.

The findings from programs such as PCAP have shown that efforts to prevent FASD must extend beyond a singular focus on alcohol use in pregnancy. Research is increasingly demonstrating the complex roles of social determinants of health in mediating the outcomes of alcohol-exposed pregnancies for women and their children. For example, Bingol *et al.* [52] were among those to document the effect of socioeconomic status in the development of FAS. In a population-based sample of women who admitted to drinking three or more alcoholic beverages per week during pregnancy, 71% of low-income women gave birth to children who were diagnosed with FAS by school age, whereas only 4.5% of women of higher socioeconomic status had children diagnosed with FAS. This study identified nutritional status during pregnancy (which is directly related to poverty) as the key variable accounting for these disparate outcomes (see also Ref. [53]). Elsewhere, the teratogenic effects of alcohol have been shown to be compounded by maternal smoking, stress, and exposure to environmental toxins [54].

Focusing only on alcohol (and other drug) use may limit the effectiveness of prevention efforts, particularly among the most marginalized women, by eclipsing opportunities for addressing factors beyond an individual woman's control that influence the likelihood of having a child with FASD. While FASD, by definition, occurs only in individuals exposed prenatally to alcohol, researchers, clinicians, and other front-line service providers are increasingly recognizing that equally important in mediating outcomes of such pregnancies are considerations such as whether a pregnant woman has access to good nutrition, pre- and post-natal medical care, safe and stable housing, support from partners, family, and friends, and other factors that help her to care for herself and her child(ren) [55]. These observations suggest an urgent need for ways to consider FASD prevention that extend beyond an individualized "alcohol awareness" approach to acknowledge the conditions in which women negotiate and experience the complexities of sub-stance use, pregnancy, and mothering.

Research to define and examine the roles of social determinants of women's health in mediating the risk and protective factors for FASD is still in its infancy, as are strategies for embedding timely, respectful, and appropriate FASD prevention into systems that might serve women and children for other initial, linked needs. Studies demonstrating the effectiveness of this approach are urgently needed in order to assist governments to develop policy and funding frameworks that can enhance these collaborative approaches. Regardless of the circumstances in which they become pregnant, give birth to, and raise their children, mothers in contemporary western societies are still invested with the primary responsibility of ensuring that their children achieve an optimal level of health and well-being. When mothers are unable to do so, they become objects of derision, particularly if this outcome is understood to be the result of "poor choices" rather than of circumstances beyond their control [56]. Although they are common, shame-and-blame approaches to FASD prevention have been repeatedly shown as ineffective at reducing drinking among women at highest risk of having a child with FASD, and have resulted in many missed opportunities for providing supportive care [39, 40, 57].

1.6
FASD Prevention in Aboriginal Communities

FASD has been described as a "crisis situation" among Aboriginal peoples in Canada, among whom both the incidence and prevalence of FASD are believed to be much higher than in the general population ([58, 59]; see also Ref. [60]). Data derived from individual First Nation communities in Canada suggest that the incidence in these locales varies from 25 per 1000 [61] to 190 per 1000 [62]. However, these data were collected in response to concern from community leaders that FASD incidence appeared to be high, in order to demonstrate unmet needs that would garner support for implementing intervention and prevention activities. No representative data on FASD incidence or prevalence are available from Canadian Aboriginal communities in which FASD has not been locally identified as a priority issue. Moreover, there are presently no population-level data available showing the extent to which Aboriginal women in Canada drink (or abstain) during pregnancy, or exhibit patterns of alcohol use that are (or are not) distinct from other of those of other Canadian women. There is also a lack of data describing how Aboriginal women's alcohol use varies by age, income or education level, employment status, place of residence, cultural affiliation, or any other factors which have been shown to differentiate alcohol use patterns in other populations [63].

FASD prevention efforts undertaken in First Nations communities must account for the specific cultural, historic, political, and social contexts in which pregnant women drink [59, 60]. Accordingly, these prevention initiatives often take different forms, from "mainstream" approaches to prevention. The incidences and experiences of FASD in Aboriginal communities are mediated by the contemporary legacies of state-sponsored activities designed to dismantle Aboriginal cultures, languages, spiritualities, families, and social and political institutions. In particular, the intergenerational impacts of residential schooling policies, forced relocations, and other government policies which resulted in trauma, violence, and disrupted family structures have been identified as among the most salient "root causes" of FASD among indigenous people [59, 60]. Thus, efforts undertaken at the community level to support cultural revitalization and strengthen families have provided a foundation on which to build programming aimed at improving the health and well-being of Aboriginal women, children, families, and communities, which incorporate specific initiatives to prevent FASD.

1.7
Main obstacles to Preventing FASD

Efforts undertaken at all levels of prevention activity have yielded substantive increases in public awareness of the importance of avoiding alcohol use in pregnancy, and of the challenges faced by children with FASD. These are clearly important developments to be celebrated. However, a consequence of these efforts has also been to construct FASD in the public (and political) imagination as a *children's* health issue. This has inspired reductionist approaches to FASD prevention as primarily a problem of maternal ignorance and/or malfeasance. In other words, the task of preventing FASD has come to be understood by many as an effort to improve children's health by intervening with their mothers, to ensure that women who drink are aware that they are "hurting their babies," and to "protect" those babies whose mothers continue to knowingly put them at risk. Moreover, in Canada, there remains a salient belief that FASD is a problem that is particularly attributable to specific groups identifiable by race (i.e., Aboriginal peoples) and class (i.e., women living in poverty). These beliefs about who is "at risk" for FASD may encourage inappropriate intervention in some cases (in which an individual woman or specific community is wrongly identified as being "at risk"), and lack of intervention in others where "no risk" is believed to be present. In so doing, opportunities have been missed to understand that FASD and its prevention are directly related to women's health status, and to act to reduce FASD prevalence at a population level by improving social, economic, and political contexts which give rise to problematic substance use among women and compromise maternal and child health [64].

Beliefs about who is "responsible" for preventing FASD, and who is "at risk" have also constrained the availability and distribution of resources to support prevention initiatives, with many groups remaining underserved. Among the barriers to preventing FASD at the population level has been the difficulty and discomfort experienced by health professionals when asked to discuss alcohol use with pregnant women. For example, a 2002 survey of physicians and midwives in

Canada conducted by Tough *et al.* [65] found that, while 94% of providers had knowledge about FASD and its causes, only 45% frequently discussed alcohol or other drug use, or addiction history, with women of childbearing age, and only 54% felt prepared to care for pregnant women who had substance-use problems. Here, a primary concern cited by care providers was a lack of confidence that they could make an appropriate referral to specialist services, indicating a lack of strong cohesion between primary care, maternity care, and addictions services, as well as a potential belief among those outside of the addictions field that maternal substance use and FASD are not among the required competencies for their field. This may also reflect a well-documented concern among maternity care providers that they are becoming overwhelmed by a perception of increasing expectations that they screen women for a range of issues (such as smoking and intimate partner violence), without having access to additional resources to provide appropriate supports to those who screen positive [66].

1.8
Challenges in Measuring Effectiveness of FASD Prevention Initiatives

One reason that so much basic work still needs to be done seems to be related to a failure of FASD to be incorporated into the general cloth of medical work, or easily addressed and accommodated in systems like education, social services, mental health, justice, and so on. To improve that situation, we need solid research to evaluate what we are doing; we need to determine how it might be done better; and we need to implement change where and when it is most needed.

Effective, integrated policy responses are clearly and urgently needed to prevent FASD and to improve the outcomes for those affected. This gives rise to a critical question: What evidence is needed by policymakers to garner sufficient political will for supporting FASD prevention?

Much of the activity being undertaken to prevent FASD is happening at the community level, in small, frequently under-funded and over-extended programs. Overall, there has been a lack of funding and support for designing and implementing projects at the community level that are tied explicitly to evaluation. Often, when an evaluation of prevention initiatives occurs, it will be in an opportunistic fashion, because a program provider happens to have resources that can be earmarked for evaluation, or because a partnership evolves between a researcher and a service provider which is successful in attracting research funds to examine a specific set of outcomes for clients. In some cases, program funders actively discourage evaluation by excluding evaluation activities from funding agreements, or by restricting the collection of data within programs.

When such evaluations are conducted, a key challenge lies in identifying evaluation methods, outcome measures, and indicators of "success" that are appropriate for research undertaken in programs that are delivered in community settings. This is particularly true for intensive intervention services that are focused broadly on preventing FASD through acting on the social determinants of women's health. In such programs, the traditional medical model for outcome research, which holds blinded, controlled trials as the "gold standard" for evidence, does not fit well, and may in fact be highly problematic on ethical and humanitarian grounds. How, for example, could the randomization of high-risk, marginalized, alcohol-dependent pregnant women into a "usual care" arm of a trial of a comprehensive support program be justified when "usual care" often results in irreversible, lifetime disadvantage for both mother and child? How could the assignment of participants to a control or intervention condition be double-blinded under these circumstances?

The end outcome in FASD prevention would be a reduction in the number of babies born with FASD. However, due to the difficulty of diagnosing FASD (particularly the neurodevelopmental aspects of this condition that are not found on physical examination at or near birth), it may not be possible to determine such an outcome until long after birth. Another methodological challenge in assessing the effectiveness of FASD prevention is that the benefits of preventive programs may accrue gradually over time, and therefore may not appear to be significant in the short term. Prevention programs that require behavioral, social, and cultural changes are thus forced to focus on intermediate outcomes of different types, measured by both quantitative and qualitative techniques. Such outcomes may include increases in knowledge about the effects of alcohol use in pregnancy, increases in self-reports of intention to abstain from alcohol in future pregnancies, decreases in binge drinking, increases in the effective use of contraceptives, or improvements in conditions that increase the risk for developing alcohol-related problems, such as stress, depression, or social isolation. Such outcome measures are common in studies of primary and indicated prevention interventions, and are amenable to study using experimental designs with short-term follow-up and comparisons of pre- and post-intervention measures. This problem could be solved by the findings obtained from well-designed longitudinal studies. However, the funding for such studies is typically difficult to secure, particularly in the Canadian research context where research grants normally extend for no more than five years. Thus, no results from such studies are available to date.

Although, high-quality data from qualitative studies may provide useful insights into these issues (for example, by documenting women's changing relationships with health and social care providers that decrease barriers to care, or by illuminating social contexts in which women negotiate issues surrounding alcohol use in pregnancy), such data are rarely included for consideration in systematic reviews, and most systematic review methodologies lack the criteria to allow for accurately assessing the strength of evidence generated through the analysis of qualitative data. These data would, however, be difficult to use in an expression of the cost–effectiveness or cost–benefit of an FASD-prevention program.

1.9
Who is Responsible for the Prevention of FASD?

FASD prevention is simple in theory: if pregnant women abstain from alcohol, their children will not develop FASD. In practice, however, FASD prevention is nearly unparalleled in its complexity, requiring not only changes in beliefs and culture but also major political interventions that address the inequalities and social determinants of women's and children's health.

In resource-constrained environments where health, social service, and educational systems must constantly seek ways to reduce costs and to cut back on the delivery of expensive and time-consuming services, mother-blaming discourses may be more readily invoked to offer a rationale for shifting responsibility away from governments and systems and onto individual women and their families. As a result, individual women have been stigmatized, shamed, blamed and, in some contexts, also prosecuted when they are unable on their own to reduce their alcohol use in response to public health warnings or brief interventions. These mother-blaming discourses have resulted in public opinions and policy responses that artificially separate women's alcohol use from the broader social, economic, and political conditions in which they live [57]. These beliefs about FASD as a disability caused to children by the actions of their mothers have also frequently served to marginalize mothers raising children with FASD, who often hear that "the problem is at home" when they attempt to advocate for additional supports for their child.

An important obstacle for the prevention of diseases and disorders in general – and the prevention of FASD in particular – is the fact that effective prevention usually requires attention to the social determinants for health. Although this might be well known among different professions in healthcare, there is no particular mandate, responsibility or financial incentive, nor are there enough resources allocated to approaching these effectively from the health sector perspective at any level of intervention.

As shown above, FASD is accompanied by considerable costs and opportunities lost, in particular for health services, although the overall economic implications of FASD are visible also in educational, social, and correctional services. The provincial governments in Canada seem to deal with FASD mainly through their departments of children and youth and their departments of health. The health implications of FASD are most likely given the same priority as any other condition when acute healthcare is needed. Educational and social support may also be provided to the same extent as other needs in these fields. Consequently, data must be collected systematically to demonstrate the support needs of pregnant women, mothers, families, and people living with FASD: this could also demonstrate gaps in service provision that could subsequently render governments accountable for ensuring that such needs are met

Problems of the complexity of FASD prevention require a long-term commitment to improvement and change. Although it is usually thought that government will provide this commitment, because of competing interests a consistent government response to any problem with adequate funding and incremental policy improvement will require ongoing advocacy. In the medical fields, this advocacy usually involves a partnership between professional groups who work with the condition, and patients and families. In the case of FASD advocacy, both groups are hard to find.

Who, in medicine, is "in charge" of FASD? Should it be the professional organizations that represent pediatrics, obstetrics, genetics, neurology, psychiatry, addictions treatment and/or family practice? They all play a role, but none has taken up the mantle of speaking for the condition as a whole, let alone for its prevention. Can any of them do so? Who, too, should speak for the legal, psychological, social, and educational intervention aspects? Since no one has volunteered, perhaps the job needs to be assigned, but who would–or could–do that? When a condition does not fall squarely into a field that is ready to catch it, the condition is dropped. That may not be unique to FASD, but it has happened to FASD.

Where, too, is the parent group? The social stigma associated with giving birth to a child with FASD has unfairly made it difficult for birth mothers who may still have active alcohol-dependency issues to advocate for their children. But where are the fathers, the mothers now in recovery, the extended families and adoptive parents? As individuals they arrive in the clinic deeply concerned about their children, frustrated at the lack of services and the poor coordination of services that do exist. Individuals have effectively represented themselves and their families. Some degree of organization has been tried (e.g., the National Organization of Fetal Alcohol Syndrome [NOFAS]), but a politically vibrant family-driven voice has not emerged. Neither have disability-rights organizations run by people with disabilities incorporated the concerns of people with FASD meaningfully and systematically into their social justice work.

FASD also falls within and between every ministry in government that deals with people: health, mental health, social services, education, justice, and so on. No single ministry has taken the lead on FASD, nor has been asked to do so. The structure of government and funding works against conditions that require such vast inter-ministerial cooperation and coordination.

The "natural experiment" conducted since this condition was first identified 40 years ago has made it apparent that the systems will not become organized, as they need to be organized spontaneously. However, this extensive, expensive, and devastating condition should not be held captive to organizational structures that work well for so many issues, but not for FASD.

Clearly, in Canada a conference should be called as soon as possible, bringing together professional leadership, family advocates, and government representatives with the aim of establishing a leadership approach for the long run.

References

1 Clarren, S. and Smith, D.W. (1978) The fetal alcohol syndrome. *N. Engl. J. Med.*, **298** (19), 1063–1067.

2 Centers for Disease Control (2002) FAS: Alaska, Arizona, Colorado, and New York 1995–1997. *MMWR Morb. Mortal. Wkly Rep.*, **514**, 433–435.

3 Thanh, N.X., Jonsson, E., Dennett, L., and Jacobs, P. (2010) Costs of fetal alcohol spectrum disorder, in *Fetal Alcohol Spectrum Disorder FASD; Management and Policy Perspectives* (eds E. Riley, *et al.*), Wiley-VCH Verlag GmbH, Weinheim.

4 Thanh, N.X. and Jonsson, E. (2009) Costs of fetal alcohol spectrum disorder in Alberta, Canada. *Can. J. Clin. Pharmacol.*, **16**, e80–e90.

5 Fuchs, D., Burnside, L., De Riviere, L., Brownell, M., Marchenski, S., Mudry, A., and Dahl, M. (2009) *Economic Impact of Children in Care with FASD and Parental Alcohol Issues Phase 2: Costs and Service Utilization of Health Care, Special Education, and Child Care*, Centre of Excellence for Child Welfare, Ottawa, Available at: http://www.cecw-cepb.ca/sites/default/files/publications/en/FASD_Economic_Impact_Phase2.pdf.

6 Stade, B., Ali, A., Bennett, D., Campbell, D., Johnston, M., Lens, C., Tran, S., and Koren, G. (2009) The burden of prenatal exposure to alcohol: revised measurement of cost. *Can. J. Clin. Pharmacol.*, **16** (1), e91–e102.

7 Stade, B., Ungar, W.J., Stevens, B., Beyene, J., and Koren, G. (2006) The burden of prenatal exposure to alcohol: measurement of cost. *J. FAS Int.*, **4**, e5.

8 Patra, J., Popova, S., Rehm, J., Bondy, S., Flint, R., and Giesbrecht, N. (2007) *Economic Cost of Chronic Disease in Canada 1995–2003*, Ontario Chronic Disease Prevention Alliance and Ontario Public Health Association.

9 Alberta Health and Wellness (2009) *Annual Report 2009*, Edmonton, Alberta, Available at: http://www.health.alberta.ca/documents/Annual-Report-10.pdf (accessed August 2010).

10 Astley, S., Bailey, D., Talbot, C., and Clarren, S. (2000) Fetal Alcohol Syndrome primary prevention through diagnosis: I. Identification of high risk birth mothers through the diagnosis of their children and II. A comprehensive profile of 80 birth mothers of children with FAS. *Alcohol*, **35** (5), 499–519.

11 Koechlin, F., Lorenzoni, L., and Schreyer, P. (2010) OECD Health Working Paper No 53: Comparing price levels of hospital services across countries: Results of a pilot study. OECD, Paris.

12 Arnup, K. (1994) *Education for Motherhood: Advice for Mothers in Twentieth- Century Canada*, University of Toronto Press, Toronto.

13 Salmon, A. (2011) Aboriginal mothering, FASD prevention, and the contestations of neoliberal citizenship, in *Alcohol, Tobacco, and Obesity: Morality, Mortality,* *and the New Public Health* (eds K. Bell, D. McNaughton, and A. Salmon), Routledge, London.

14 Deshpande, S., Basil, M., Basford, L., Thorpe, K., Piquette-Tomei, N., Droessler, J., Cardwell, K., Williams, R.J., and Bureau, A. (2005) Promoting alcohol abstinence among pregnant women: potential social change strategies. *Health Mark. Q*, **23** (2), 45–67.

15 Environics Research Group (2006) *Alcohol Use During Pregnancy and Awareness of Fetal Alcohol Syndrome and Fetal Alcohol Spectrum Disorder: Results of A National Survey*, Public Health Agency of Canada, Ottawa.

16 Poole, N. and Dell, C.A. (2005) *Girls, Women, and Substance Use*, Canadian Centre on Substance Abuse and BC Centre of Excellence for Women's Health, Ottawa and Vancouver.

17 Adhikari, P. and Summerill, A. (2000) *1998 National Drug Strategy Household Survey: Detailed Findings*. Australian Institute of Health and Welfare, Canberra.

18 Bollin, K., Grant, C., Hamlyn, B., and Thornton, A. (2007) *Infant feeding survey 2005*. The Information Centre, Leeds.

19 Royal Australian and New Zealand College of Obstetricians and Gynaecologists (2008) *College Statement: Alcohol in Pregnancy*, RANWCOG, East Melbourne.

20 Health Canada Report (2009) Available at: www.hc-sc.gc.ca (accessed May 2010).

21 US Surgeon General (2005) *Surgeon General's Advisory on Alcohol Use in Pregnancy*, Office of the US Surgeon General, Washington.

22 British Medical Association (2007) *Fetal Alcohol Spectrum Disorders*, BMA, London.

23 Royal College of Obstetricians and Gynaecologists (2006) *RCOG Statement No.5: Alcohol Consumption and the Outcomes of Pregnancy*, RCOG, London.

24 Floyd, R.L., Sobell, M., Velasquez, M.M., Ingersoll, K., Nettleman, M., Sobell, L., *et al.* (2007) Preventing alcohol-exposed pregnancies: a randomized controlled trial. *Am. J. Prev. Med.*, **32** (1), 1–10.

25 May, P.A., Gossage, J.P., White-Country, M., Goodhart, K., Decoteau, S., Trujillo,

P.M., Kalberg, W.O., Viljoen, D.L., and Hoyme, H.E. (2004) Alcohol consumption and other maternal risk factors for fetal alcohol syndrome among three distinct samples of women before, during, and after pregnancy: the risk is relative. *Am. J. Med. Genet.*, **127C** (1), 10–20.

26 Maier, S.E. and West, J.R. (2001) Drinking patterns and alcohol related birth defects. *Alcohol Res. Health*, **25** (3), 168–174F.

27 Cismaru, M., Deshpande, S., Thurmeier, R., Lavack, A.M., and Agrey, N. (2010) Preventing Fetal Alcohol Syndrome Spectrum Disorders: the role of Protection Motivation Theory. *Health Mark. Q.*, **27** (1), 66–85.

28 Goh, Y.I., Hutson, J.R., Lum, L., Roukema, H., Gareri, J., Lynr., H., and Koren, G. (2010) Rates of fetal alcohol exposure among newborns in a high-risk obstetric unit. *Alcohol*, **44** (7-8), 629–634.

29 Zelner, I., Shor, S., Gareri, J., Lynn, H., Roukema, H., Lum, L., Eisinga, K., Nulman, I., and Koren, G. (2010) Universal screening for prenatal alcohol exposure: a progress report of a pilot study in the region of Grey Bruce, Ontario. *Ther. Drug Monit.*, **32** (3), 305–310.

30 Marcellus, L. (2007) Is meconium screening appropriate for universal use? Science and ethics say no. *Adv. Neonatal Care*, **7** (4), 207–214.

31 Chang, G. (2001) Alcohol-screening instruments for pregnant women. *Alcohol Res. Health*, **25** (3), 204–210.

32 Parkes, T., Poole, N., Salmon, A., Greaves, L., and Urquhart, C. (2008) *Double Exposure: A Better Practices Review on Alcohol Interventions during Pregnancy*, British Columbia Centre of Excellence for Women's Health, Vancouver.

33 Sarkar, M., Burnett, M., Carrière, S., Cox, L.V., Dell, C.A., Gammon, H., Geller, B., Graves, L., Koren, G., Lee, L., Mousmanis, D.M.P., Schuurmans, N., Senikas, V., Soucy, D., and Wood, R. (2009) Screening and recording of alcohol use among women of child-bearing age and pregnant women (2009). *Can. J. Clin. Pharmacol.*, **16** (1), e242–e263.

34 Jacobson, S.W., Chiodo, L.M., Sokol, R.J., and Jacobson, J.L. (2002) Validity of maternal report of prenatal alcohol, cocaine, and smoking in relation to neurobehaviorial outcome. *Pediatrics*, **109** (5), 815–825.

35 O'Connor, M.J. and Whaley, S.E. (2007) Brief intervention for alcohol use by pregnant women. *Am. J. Public Health*, **97** (2), 252–258.

36 Premji, S. and Semenic, S.S. (2009) Do Canadian prenatal record forms integrate evidence-based guidelines for the diagnosis of a FASD? *Can. J. Public Health*, **100** (4), 274–280.

37 Manwell, L.B., Fleming, M.F., Mundt, M.P., Stauffacher, E.A., and Barry, K.L. (2000) Treatment of problem alcohol use in women of childbearing age: results of a brief intervention trial. *Alcohol. Clin. Exp. Res.*, **24** (10), 1517–1524.

38 The Project CHOICES Intervention Research Group (2003) Reducing the risk of alcohol-exposed pregnancies: a study of a motivational intervention in community settings. *Pediatrics*, **111**, 1131–1135.

39 Salmon, A. (2007) Adaptation and decolonization: the role of "culturally appropriate" health education in the prevention of fetal alcohol syndrome. *Can. J. Native Educ.*, **30** (2), 257–274.

40 Badry, D. (2007) Birth mothers of children with fetal alcohol syndrome, in *Social Justice in Context*, vol. 3, 2007–2008 (eds M.J. Jackson, M.J. Pickard, and E.W. Bawner), Carolyn Freeze Baynes Institute for Social Justice, Greenville, pp. 88–108.

41 United Nations Office on Drugs and Crime (2004) *Substance Abuse Treatment and Care for Women: Case Studies and Lessons Learned*, The United Nations Office on Drugs and Crime, Vienna.

42 Salmon, A. (2007) Dis/abling states, dis/abling citizenship: young Aboriginal mothers, substantive citizenship, and the medicalization of FAS/FAE. *J. Crit. Educ. Policy*, **5** (2), 112–123.

43 Moses, D.J., Reed, B.G., Mazelis, R., and D'Ambrosio, B. (2003) *Creating Services for Women with Co-Occurring Disorders*, Substance Abuse and Mental Health Services Administration and

Centre for Mental Health Services, Alexandria.

44 Godard, L., Cory, J., and Abi-Jaoude, A. (2008) *Summary Report of Building Bridges: Linking Woman Abuse, Substance Use and Mental Ill Health*, BC Women's Hospital and Health Centre, Vancouver.

45 Morrissey, J.P., Ellis, A.R., Gatz, M., Amaro, H., Reed, B.G., Savage, A., Finkelstein, N., Mazelis, R., Brown, V., Jackson, E.W., and Banks, S. (2005) Outcomes for women with co-occurring disorders and trauma: program and person-level effects. *J. Subst. Abuse Treat.*, **28** (2), 121–133.

46 Salmon, A. and Clarren, S. (2010) *FASD Research in Primary, Secondary, and Tertiary Prevention: Building the Next Generation of Policy Responses. Fetal Alcohol Spectrum Disorders - Management and Policy Considerations* (eds E. Riley, S. Clarren, J. Weinberg, and E. Jonsson) Wiley-VCH GmbH, Weinheim.

47 Motz, M., Leslie, M., Pepler, D.J., Moore, T.E., and Freeman, P.A. (2006) Breaking the cycle: measures of progress 1995–2005. *J. FAS Int. Special Suppl.*, **4** (e22). Available at: http://www.motherisk.org/JFAS_documents/BTC_JFAS_ReportFINAL.pdf.

48 Poole, N. (2000) *Evaluation Report of the Sheway Project for High Risk Pregnant and Parenting Women*, British Columbia Centre of Excellence for Women's Health, Vancouver.

49 Grant, T.M., Ernst, C.C., Streissguth, A., and Stark, K. (2005) Preventing alcohol and drug exposed births in Washington State: intervention findings from three parent-child assistance program sites. *Am. J. Drug Alcohol Abuse*, **31** (3), 471–490.

50 Creamer, S. and McMurtrie, C. (1998) Special needs of pregnant and parenting women in recovery: a move toward a more woman-centered approach. *Women's Health Issues*, **8** (4), 239–245.

51 Sweeney, P., Schwartz, R., Mattis, N., and Vohr, B. (2000) The effect of integrating substance abuse treatment with prenatal care on birth outcome. *J. Perinatol.*, **4**, 19–24.

52 Bingol, N., Schuster, C., Fuchs, M., Iosub, S., Turner, G., Stone, R.K., and

Gromisch, D.S. (1987) The influences of socioeconomic factors on the occurrence of fetal alcohol syndrome. *Adv. Alcohol Subst. Abuse*, **6** (4), 105–118.

53 George, A. (2001) The effects of prenatal exposure to alcohol, tobacco, and other risks on children's health, behaviour, and academic abilities. Unpublished PhD dissertation. University of British Columbia, Vancouver, British Columbia, Canada.

54 Abel, E.A. (1995) Maternal risk factors in fetal alcohol syndrome: provocative and permissive influences. *Neurotoxicol. Teratol.*, **17** (4), 445–462.

55 Sun, A.-P. (2004) Principles for practice with substance-abusing pregnant women: a framework based on the five social work intervention roles. *Soc. Work*, **49** (3), 383–394.

56 Bell, K., McNaughton, D., and Salmon, A. (2009) Medicine, morality, and mothering: public health discourses on fetal alcohol exposure, smoking around children, and childhood overnutrition. *Crit. Public Health*, **19** (2), 155–170.

57 Armstrong, E.M. (2003) *Conceiving Risk, Bearing Responsibility: Fetal Alcohol Syndrome and the Diagnosis of Moral Disorder*, The John Hopkins University Press, Baltimore and London.

58 Tait, C.L. (2000) *A Study of the Service Needs of Pregnant Addicted Women in Manitoba*, Manitoba Health, Winnipeg.

59 Tait, C.L. (2003) *Fetal Alcohol Syndrome Among Canadian Aboriginal Peoples: Review and Analysis of the Intergenerational Links to Residential Schools*, The Aboriginal Healing Foundation, Ottawa.

60 Van Bibber, M. (1997) *It Takes a Community: A Resource Manual for Community-Based Prevention of FAS and FAE*, Health Canada, Ottawa.

61 Asante, K.O. and Nelms-Matzke, J. (1985) *Survey of Children With Chronic Handicaps and Fetal Alcohol Syndrome in the Yukon and Northwest of British Columbia*, Health and Welfare Canada, Ottawa.

62 Robinson, G.C., Conry, J.L., and Conry, R.F. (1987) Clinical profile and prevalence of fetal alcohol syndrome in an isolated community in British Columbia. *Can. Med. Assoc. J.*, **137** (3), 203–207.

63 Adlaf, E.M., Begin, P., and Sawka, E. (eds) (2005) *Canadian Addictions Survey (CAS): A National Survey of Canadians' Use of Alcohol and Other Drugs*, Canadian Centre on Substance Abuse, Ottawa.

64 Clarren, S. and Salmon, A. (2010) Prevention of fetal alcohol spectrum disorder: Proposal for a comprehensive approach. *Expert Rev. Obstet. Gynaecol.*, **5** (1), 23–30.

65 Tough, S.C., Clarke, M.E., Hicks, M., and Clarren, S.K. (2005) Attitudes and approaches of Canadian providers to preconception counselling and the prevention of fetal alcohol spectrum disorders. *J. FAS Int.*, **3e2**, 1–16.

66 Kennedy, C., Finkelstein, N., Hutchins, E., and Mahoney, J. (2004) Improving screening for alcohol use during pregnancy: The Massachusetts ASAP Program. *Matern. Child Health J.*, **8** (3), 137–147.

2

An Overview of Systematic Reviews on the Prevention, Diagnosis, and Treatment of Fetal Alcohol Spectrum Disorder

Maria Ospina, Carmen Moga, Liz Dennett, and Christa Harstall

Summary

The prevention, identification and treatment of fetal alcohol spectrum disorder (FASD) are public health priorities. Success in these areas would not only improve the outcomes for affected individuals and their families, but also would benefit the health system and society at large. It is impossible to work effectively in FASD prevention, diagnosis, and treatment without the support of a strong evidence base and knowledge with which to guide clinical practice and policy decisions. Clinicians and policy makers need to know what evidence is available, and which questions have not yet been addressed. Systematic reviews are considered to be the best method for identifying and evaluating the available evidence. However, it is not known whether such reviews in areas of FASD prevention, diagnosis and treatment have been conducted according to a structured methodological approach to ensure the control of systematic errors in the review process. An evaluation of these systematic reviews will allow for greater confidence in their results and conclusions.

Objectives

This overview of systematic reviews aims to provide an up-to-date synthesis of the evidence on the best practices for the prevention, diagnosis, and treatment of FASD.

Results

Eight reports of systematic reviews met the selection criteria. One of the reports was considered to be three systematic reviews, because it included data for all three questions of the overview. Therefore, a total of 10 systematic reviews was included in the overview of prevention, diagnosis, and treatment strategies for

(Continued)

Prevention of Fetal Alcohol Spectrum Disorder FASD: Who is Responsible?, First Edition. Edited by Sterling Clarren, Amy Salmon, Egon Jonsson.
© 2011 Wiley-VCH Verlag GmbH & Co. KGaA. Published 2011 by Wiley-VCH Verlag GmbH & Co. KGaA.

FASD. Six reviews addressed questions related to the effectiveness of prevention approaches in reducing prenatal alcohol use and preventing the occurrence of FASD. One systematic review evaluated evidence pertaining to the accuracy of postnatal screening and diagnostic tools in identifying individuals who may have FASD. Three systematic reviews assessed evidence on the effectiveness of therapeutic interventions for children and youth with FASD. Four of the reviews were produced in Canada: three reviews related to the prevention of prenatal alcohol use and FASD occurrence, and one review to treatment strategies for children and youth with FASD.

Systematic Reviews on the Effectiveness of Prevention Approaches for FASD

General Characteristics: Prevention interventions that were considered in the six systematic reviews on prevention approaches varied widely in their characteristics and purpose. They included home visits during pregnancy and/or after birth (one review), psychological and educational interventions for reducing prenatal alcohol use (two reviews), and any strategy aimed at reducing prenatal alcohol use and the incidence of FASD (three reviews). Two systematic reviews also assessed the effectiveness of alcohol screening during pregnancy. Only one of the six systematic reviews conducted a meta-analysis of primary studies, which evaluated the effectiveness of a preventive intervention in reducing alcohol consumption during pregnancy. The other five reviews conducted a narrative synthesis of the results from primary studies on prevention of FASD and prenatal alcohol use.

The systematic reviews included a median of 22 primary studies per review. Only two systematic reviews (one on the effectiveness of home visits and the other on the effectiveness of psycho-educational prevention interventions) based their conclusions on evidence provided by randomized controlled trials (RCTs) exclusively. All of the other systematic reviews expanded their evidence base to include studies with a variety of methodological designs: controlled clinical trials; CCTs); observational analytical studies; and studies with no control groups.

Methodological Quality: The methodological quality of the systematic reviews on the prevention of FASD and prenatal alcohol use was rated moderate to high on the Assessment of Multiple Systematic Reviews (AMSTAR) (median AMSTAR score: 8.5/11). Three reviews were considered of high quality (AMSTAR scores 9–11), two reviews were rated moderate in quality (AMSTAR scores 5–8), and one review was considered of low quality (AMSTAR score ≤4).

Evidence on the Effectiveness of Prevention Approaches for FASD

- One high-quality systematic review provided evidence of moderate quality on the effectiveness of home visits during or after pregnancy to women with an alcohol-use problem. The results were inconsistent across the studies, and did not allow for the formulation of clear conclusions regarding the effectiveness of the intervention.

- Two moderate-quality systematic reviews provided evidence of moderate quality that prenatal alcohol screening is an efficient strategy for identifying prenatal alcohol use.

- One moderate-quality systematic review identified evidence of low quality on the effectiveness of primary, secondary, and tertiary prevention approaches. The results of the individual studies in the review did not allow for the formulation of clear conclusions regarding the benefits of these approaches.

- One high-quality systematic review identified low-quality evidence on the effectiveness of universal and indicated prevention approaches. The evidence did not allow for the formulation of clear conclusions regarding the benefits of these approaches. The review found evidence of moderate quality that selective prevention approaches are effective in reducing alcohol use in pregnant women and other women of childbearing age.

- Two systematic reviews, one of moderate quality and one of high quality, identified evidence of low quality that brief interventions (including motivational interviews) can help to reduce the risk of alcohol-exposed pregnancy among women of childbearing age.

- One moderate-quality systematic review identified moderate-quality evidence that intensive interventions are successful in reducing alcohol use during pregnancy.

- Two systematic reviews, one of low quality and one of high quality, reported evidence on the effectiveness of education and counseling. This evidence was of low quality and did not allow for the formulation of clear conclusions regarding the benefits of these interventions.

- The evidence reported in one high-quality systematic review on the effectiveness of cognitive behavioral self-help intervention was limited, and did not show that the intervention was effective in reducing alcohol use during pregnancy.

Systematic Reviews on the Diagnosis of FASD

General Characteristics: One systematic review addressed questions related to the effectiveness of postnatal screening tools for identifying individuals who should undergo a full diagnostic evaluation for FASD, and the accuracy of tools used to diagnose FASD. The systematic review did not find primary research or systematic reviews on the effectiveness of postnatal screening and FASD diagnostic tools. Therefore, a narrative synthesis of clinical practice guidelines for diagnosing FASD was conducted.

(Continued)

Methodological Quality: The methodological quality of the systematic review on postnatal screening and diagnosis of FASD was rated as moderate (AMSTAR score: 8/11).

Evidence on the Effectiveness of Diagnostic Approaches to FASD

No primary studies have evaluated the efficacy of tools or classification systems used to diagnose FASD. The diagnostic guidelines and criteria identified in the systematic review were based on the opinion of a panel of clinicians. Therefore, they represent the lowest level of evidence available to inform decisions on the most effective diagnostic options for FASD.

Systematic Reviews on Treatment Approaches for FASD

General Characteristics: The three systematic reviews on treatment approaches to FASD examined a broad spectrum of interventions, such as pharmacological treatments, behavioral interventions, speech therapy, occupational therapy, physiotherapy and psychosocial, and educational interventions. None of the systematic reviews conducted a meta-analysis of primary studies; rather, they conducted a narrative synthesis of findings from primary or secondary sources of evidence.

The reviews included a median number of six studies per review. One systematic review incorporated data from other systematic reviews and clinical practice guidelines into the evidence summary on the effectiveness of treatment approaches for FASD. The two other reviews based their conclusions on evidence provided by RCTs, CCTs, and before-and-after studies.

Methodological Quality: The methodological quality of the systematic reviews on therapeutic approaches to FASD was rated moderate (median AMSTAR score: 8/11).

Evidence on the Effectiveness of Therapeutic Approaches for FASD

- Three moderate-quality systematic reviews summarized moderate-quality evidence from studies on the effectiveness of cognitive control therapy for individuals with FASD. The results were inconsistent across the studies and did not allow for the formulation of clear conclusions regarding the benefits of this intervention.

- Evidence from three moderate-quality systematic reviews on the effectiveness of psychostimulant medications for individuals with FASD and ADHD showed inconsistent results across the studies. No clear conclusions can be made regarding the benefits of this intervention.

- One moderate-quality systematic review reported moderate-quality evidence that interventions focused on basic literacy skills, math skills, social skills and communication, and interventions aimed at increasing the child's safety, can be effective in treating certain cognitive and social disabilities secondary to FASD.

• One moderate-quality systematic review reported moderate-quality evidence that the effectiveness of behavioral interventions for FASD is unclear. No clear conclusions can be made regarding the benefits of this intervention.

• Moderate-quality evidence from one moderate-quality systematic review did not show a clear benefit from teacher-modeling strategies as a treatment option for FASD.

Conclusions

The development, evaluation, and dissemination of evidence-based preventive interventions, diagnostic tools, and therapeutic interventions for FASD and prenatal alcohol use have lagged significantly since the disorder was identified during the 1970s. Encouragingly, some evidence has accumulated regarding the effectiveness of screening tools for prenatal alcohol use; of certain prevention approaches, such as brief and intensive interventions to reduce prenatal alcohol use; and of therapeutic options aimed at reducing the cognitive and social disabilities experienced by individuals with FASD. It is important to increase efforts to expand the evidence base to better inform policy and healthcare decisions regarding the prevention and diagnosis of FASD and the treatment options for individuals with FASD and their families.

Methodology

Comprehensive searches of biomedical electronic databases were conducted for the period from 2004 to March 2010. The search strategy comprised both controlled vocabulary and key words. Internet searches via Google and Google Scholar were supplemented with hand searches of the reference lists in the articles retrieved in the search. The authors of reviews were contacted to identify other potentially relevant reviews. Gray literature searches were conducted to identify literature reviews from nontraditional sources, including proceedings from relevant scientific meetings, government documents, theses and dissertations, and ongoing reviews. The search was limited to reviews published in English.

Two reviewers independently applied a set of inclusion and exclusion criteria to select the reviews and assessed their methodological quality. Data were extracted by one reviewer and verified independently by a second reviewer. A narrative synthesis of review results was undertaken.

2.1
Introduction

Fetal alcohol spectrum disorder (FASD) is a descriptive term that refers to a group of disorders characterized by physical, mental, behavioral, and learning disabilities that can endure a lifetime and are associated with prenatal alcohol exposure [1]. FASD is often – but not always – characterized by prenatal and postnatal impairments, such as growth retardation, a unique cluster of facial anomalies, and a variety of neurological, cognitive and behavioral disorders [2]. Four diagnostic categories (Figure 2.1) have been described within the continuum of FASD, from most severe to less severe: fetal alcohol syndrome (FAS); partial FAS (pFAS); alcohol-related neurodevelopmental disorders (ARND); and alcohol-related birth defects (ARBD) [3, 4].

The prevalence of all disorders in the continuum of FASD has been estimated at 2–4% in the general population [5]. Investigators using passive methods of surveillance have estimated the incidence of FASD at one in 100 live births in the general population of the United States [5]. Active surveillance studies are likely to identify a higher incidence of FASD (i.e., one in 25 and one in 50 live births) [5]. Variation in FASD rates results from differences in the populations being studied, in case definitions, and in the methods used to identify cases. It has been suggested that the true prevalence of FASD in a general population has not been established anywhere [6] due to an insufficiency of the multidisciplinary capacity and resources required to recognize and diagnose these conditions in a reliable manner.

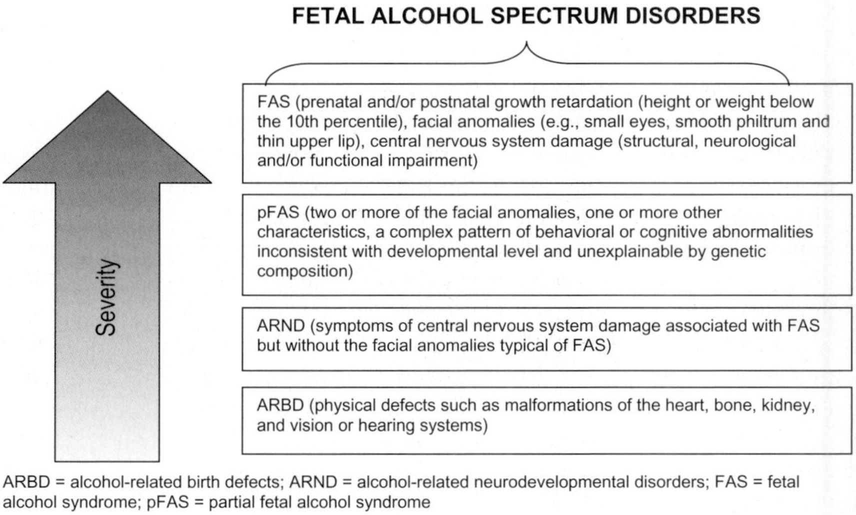

FETAL ALCOHOL SPECTRUM DISORDERS

FAS (prenatal and/or postnatal growth retardation (height or weight below the 10th percentile), facial anomalies (e.g., small eyes, smooth philtrum and thin upper lip), central nervous system damage (structural, neurological and/or functional impairment)

pFAS (two or more of the facial anomalies, one or more other characteristics, a complex pattern of behavioral or cognitive abnormalities inconsistent with developmental level and unexplainable by genetic composition)

ARND (symptoms of central nervous system damage associated with FAS but without the facial anomalies typical of FAS)

ARBD (physical defects such as malformations of the heart, bone, kidney, and vision or hearing systems)

Severity

ARBD = alcohol-related birth defects; ARND = alcohol-related neurodevelopmental disorders; FAS = fetal alcohol syndrome; pFAS = partial fetal alcohol syndrome

Figure 2.1 Fetal alcohol spectrum disorder subtypes. ARBD = alcohol-related birth defects; ARND = alcohol-related neurodevelopmental disorder; FAS = fetal alcohol syndrome; pFAS = partial fetal alcohol syndrome.

There are no national statistics on the incidence or prevalence of FASD in Canada. A cross-sectional survey of FASD clinical activity in northwestern Canada (Alberta, British Columbia, Manitoba, Saskatchewan and the Yukon) conducted by Clarren and Lutke [6] reported that, during a 16-month period, about 23% of referrals to 27 clinical programs for FASD diagnosis were found to have FAS or pFAS, and that another 44% had other conditions classified as FASD. Clarren and Lutke [6] suggested that, if these clinic-based estimates were projected to the general population, it could be estimated that approximately 1% of the general population would have FASD, and that this would be likely an underestimate of the true prevalence.

FASD is associated with prenatal alcohol exposure [7]. The teratogenic effect of alcohol on the developing fetus has been described in numerous animal and clinical studies [8–11]. However, the mechanisms of prenatal alcohol damage are not yet fully understood, and it is not known whether there is a safe amount of alcohol or a "safe" time to drink during pregnancy.

The impairments experienced by individuals with FASD are thought to persist throughout their lives. Retrospective and prospective studies of the epigenetics, epidemiology, associated risk factors, history and prognosis of FASD have shown that individuals who were prenatally exposed to alcohol and subsequently developed FASD suffer long-lasting disturbances in their brain architecture [12, 13], psychological and cognitive functioning [14, 15], mental health, health risk behaviors, and social functioning [16]. The implications of these disturbances across the lifespan are not yet fully understood, due in part to the fact that the diagnosis of FASD is difficult and individuals with FASD may, therefore, struggle with an undetected disability throughout their lives. Some of the physical and psychosocial impairments in individuals with an established diagnosis of FASD are primary disabilities, such as a loss of intellectual potential, severe vision problems, dyslexia, learning disabilities, behavioral problems, and low levels of adaptive functioning [17, 18]. Secondary disabilities include mental health issues, such as attention-deficit disorders, hyperactivity, extreme impulsiveness, little or no capacity for moral judgment or interpersonal empathy, and sociopathic behavior [19]. Failure to identify and treat FASD increases the risk that the individual will experience disruptions in education, trouble with the law, unemployment, alcohol- and drug-related problems, loss of family, homelessness or dependent living, confinement in jail or treatment facilities, and premature death [3, 17]. The myriad negative effects associated with FASD that have been described in the scientific literature have led to a greater awareness of the need to prevent and diagnose FASD, as well as to treat individuals with FASD and provide support to them and their families.

The prevention, identification, and management of FASD are public health priorities. Success in these areas not only improves outcomes for affected individuals and their families, but also benefits the health system and society at large. It is impossible to work successfully in FASD prevention, diagnosis, and treatment without the support of a strong evidence base and knowledge with which to guide clinical practice and policy decisions. Clinicians and policy makers need to know what evidence is available, and which questions have not yet been addressed. The conducting of systematic reviews is considered to be the best method for identifying and evaluating the available evidence [20]. However, it is unknown whether systematic reviews in the areas of FASD prevention, diagnosis and treatment have been conducted according to a structured methodological approach that ensures the control of systematic errors in the review process. Evaluating systematic reviews allows for greater confidence in their results and conclusions. The primary aim of this overview is to provide a comprehensive collection and synthesis of the evidence summarized in systematic reviews on the best options for the prevention, diagnosis and treatment of FASD across the lifespan.

2.2
Objective and Scope

This overview of systematic reviews aims to provide an up-to-date synthesis of the evidence on the best practices for the prevention, diagnosis, and treatment of FASD.

2.3
Methodological Approach

2.3.1
Elements of Assessment

A prospectively designed protocol was developed for conducting an overview of systematic reviews that evaluate any approach to prevention, diagnosis, and treatment of FASD. An overview of reviews is defined as an integration of the evidence from multiple systematic reviews into one accessible and usable document [21]. This entails using explicit and reproducible methods for systematically identifying and selecting systematic reviews, assessing the validity of the reported results in the reviews, and analyzing the information in the reviews with regards to the diagnosis, prevention, and treatment of FASD. The analytic framework outlining this approach to the overview of reviews is shown in Figure 2.2.

A detailed description of the methodology of the overview is provided in Appendix 2.A. Briefly, comprehensive searches of biomedical electronic databases were

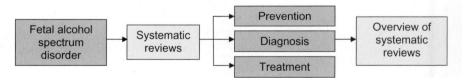

Figure 2.2 Analytic framework for an overview of reviews on prevention, diagnosis and treatment of FASD.

conducted for the period between 2004 and March 2010. The search strategy comprised both controlled vocabulary and keywords; in addition, Internet searches via Google and Google Scholar were supplemented with hand searches of the reference lists of articles retrieved in the search. Finally, the authors of reviews were contacted to identify other potentially relevant reviews. Gray literature searches were conducted to identify literature reviews from nontraditional sources, such as proceedings of relevant scientific meetings, government documents, theses and dissertations, and ongoing reviews. The search was limited to reviews published in English.

Two reviewers independently applied a set of inclusion and exclusion criteria to select the reviews, and assessed their methodological quality. Data were extracted by one reviewer and verified independently by a second reviewer. A narrative synthesis of review results was undertaken. Evidence tables were constructed to describe review characteristics, methodological quality, and results.

2.4
Results

2.4.1
Search Results

The systematic search (electronic, gray literature, and manual searches) resulted in the identification of 139 citations. After a screening of titles and abstracts, the full text of 29 potentially relevant articles was retrieved and evaluated for inclusion in the overview. The application of the selection criteria to the 29 articles resulted in nine articles being considered for inclusion, and 20 being excluded. Of the nine included articles, one article was identified as a multiple publication; this was not considered a unique study, and any additional information that it provided was included in the data reported in the main publication. One of the eight remaining articles addressed all three questions of the overview, and was regarded as three systematic reviews. Therefore, this overview included eight unique reports of 10 systematic reviews that evaluated approaches to the prevention, diagnosis, and treatment of FASD. The study retrieval and selection for the review are outlined in Figure 2.3.

The primary reasons for excluding studies from the overview were:

- The study was not a systematic review ($n = 11$).
- The full text of the study was not retrieved ($n = 3$).
- The study was primary research ($n = 2$).
- The study topic was not prevention, diagnosis, or treatment of FASD ($n = 2$).
- The study did not report measurable data for the analysis and synthesis of the results ($n = 2$).

The excluded studies, and the reasons for their exclusion from the overview, are listed in Table 2.B.1 of Appendix 2.B.

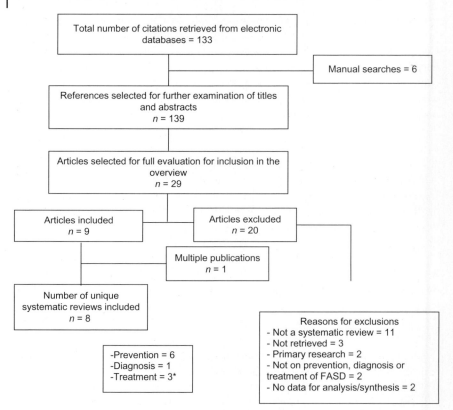

* One report included three systematic reviews evaluating prevention, diagnosis and treatment strategies for FASD

Figure 2.3 Flow-diagram for study retrieval and selection for the overview.

2.4.1.1 Characteristics of Systematic Reviews Included in the Overview

Eight reports of systematic reviews [22–29] met the selection criteria. One of the eight reports [22] was regarded as three unique systematic reviews because it included data for all three questions of the overview. Therefore, a total of 10 systematic reviews was included in this overview of prevention, diagnosis, and treatment strategies for FASD. Six systematic reviews [22–25, 28, 29] addressed questions related to the effectiveness of prevention approaches aimed at reducing prenatal alcohol use and preventing the occurrence of FASD. One systematic review [22] evaluated evidence pertaining to the accuracy of postnatal screening and diagnostic tools used to identify individuals who may have FASD. Three systematic reviews [22, 26, 27] assessed evidence on the effectiveness of therapeutic interventions for children and youth with FASD.

The systematic reviews were published between 1993 and 2010, the median year of publication being 2008 (interquartile range [IQR]: 2005, 2009). Three of the systematic reviews (two on FASD treatment [26, 27] and one on FASD prevention [23]) were published as peer-reviewed journal articles. Two systematic reviews [23, 29] on preventive approaches to reducing alcohol consumption during pregnancy were published as Cochrane reviews. Three systematic reviews (one on FASD prevention, diagnosis and treatment [22] and two on FASD prevention and reduction of alcohol use during pregnancy [24, 25]) have not been published in the mainstream scientific literature.

Four of the systematic reviews on FASD were produced in Canada: three systematic reviews [24, 25, 29] on the prevention of prenatal alcohol use and FASD, and one review [27] on treatment strategies for children and youth with FASD. Three reviews were produced in New Zealand (one report [22] of systematic reviews on FASD prevention, diagnosis, and treatment). Two reviews, one on FASD prevention [23] and the other on FASD treatment [26], were produced in Australia; and one systematic review [28] on prevention of prenatal alcohol use was produced in the USA.

All but one [28] of the systematic reviews included in the overview reported their sources of funding. Six reviews [22, 24–26] were funded by government agencies, two [23, 29] were funded internally, and another systematic review [27] received funding from a foundation.

The key characteristics of the systematic reviews are outlined in Tables 2.C.1–2.C.3 of Appendix 2.C. The characteristics and results of the systematic reviews are summarized by the research questions addressed (i.e., prevention, diagnosis and treatment) in the following subsections.

2.4.2
Systematic Reviews on Prevention of FASD and Prenatal Alcohol Use

2.4.2.1 General Characteristics

Six systematic reviews [22–25, 28, 29] addressed questions related to the effectiveness of approaches to reducing prenatal alcohol use, and thus preventing the occurrence of FASD. The systematic reviews were published between 1993 and 2010, the median year of publication being 2008 (IQR: 2002, 2009). Two systematic reviews [22, 24] directly addressed the topic of preventive approaches to FASD, whereas four [23, 25, 28, 29] evaluated evidence pertaining to preventive interventions to reduce alcohol use in pregnancy or during the childbearing years. The selection criteria and PICOD (population, intervention, comparator, outcomes and design) components that guided the selection of individual studies to be included in the systematic reviews of prevention approaches to FASD and alcohol use in pregnancy are summarized in Table 2.1.

All six systematic reviews evaluated the scientific evidence from primary studies that assessed FASD-prevention interventions targeting prenatal alcohol use by pregnant women. All of these reviews except two [23, 28] also included primary studies of interventions targeting women of childbearing age. Only two systematic reviews [22, 24] included primary studies that assessed FASD-prevention interventions targeting the general population. None of the systematic reviews

Table 2.1 Selection criteria applied in systematic reviews of prevention approaches to FASD and alcohol use in pregnancy.

Systematic review	Population	Interventions	Comparators	Outcomes	Study design of individual studies
Doggett *et al.* [23]	Pregnant or postpartum women with alcohol problems (i.e., self-report of alcohol abuse/binge)	Home visits commencing during pregnancy and/or after birth	No home visits or different type of home visiting intervention	Drug and alcohol use during pregnancy, pregnancy and puerperium outcomes, psychosocial outcomes	RCT, CCT
Elliott *et al.* [22]	General population, pregnant women, women at high risk of having a child with FASD	Any strategy aimed at reducing FASD incidence; any alcohol screening tool designed to evaluate a woman's risk of having a child with FASD	Any	Changes in FASD incidence, alcohol use during pregnancy; sensitivity and specificity of screening tools	Any
Ospina *et al.* [24]	General population, pregnant women and partners of reproductive age who have previously abused alcohol during pregnancy or who have had a child with FASD	Universal, selective, indicated prevention approaches to FASD	Any	Changes in FASD incidence, alcohol consumption during pregnancy, neonatal and infant outcomes, risk-reduction measures, maternal outcomes (drinking behavior, relapse), legal, family, economic and healthcare	RCT, CCT, case-control studies, analytical cohort studies, ITS, before-and-after studies

Parkes et al. [25]	Pregnant women and women in childbearing years	Identification, assessment and screening for alcohol use in pregnancy; brief interventions with pregnant women and women in their childbearing years; intensive interventions for pregnant women and mothers	NR	Self-reported alcohol use, reduction in alcohol-exposed pregnancies, contraceptive behavior	NR
Schorling [28]	Pregnant women	Prenatal education and counseling to reduce prenatal alcohol use	NR	Alcohol use	NR
Stade et al. [29]	Pregnant women or women planning for pregnancy who consume alcohol (i.e., self-report or urine/blood screening for alcohol)	Psychological and educational interventions for reducing consumption of alcohol	No intervention, routine care, other educational and/or psychological interventions	Abstinence from alcohol during pregnancy, reduction of alcohol consumption during pregnancy to less than seven standard drinks per week, maternal and neonatal outcomes	RCT

CCT = controlled clinical trials; FASD = fetal alcohol spectrum disorder; ITS = interrupted time series; NR = not reported; RCT = randomized controlled trials.

reported a subgroup analysis of special populations (e.g., Aboriginal groups, low-socioeconomic or underserved populations).

The prevention interventions for FASD and prenatal alcohol use that were evaluated in the systematic reviews varied widely in their characteristics and purpose. One systematic review [23] included studies that assessed home visits during pregnancy and/or after birth, a highly specific prevention strategy to reduce prenatal alcohol use. Two reviews [28, 29] included only studies that assessed psychological and educational interventions for reducing prenatal alcohol use, whereas three systematic reviews [22, 24, 25] included studies that evaluated any strategy aimed at reducing FASD incidence and prenatal alcohol use. Two systematic reviews [22, 25] assessed the effectiveness of screening for alcohol use during pregnancy.

In the selection of studies for inclusion in the systematic reviews, few restrictions were imposed on the comparison groups used in studies. Therefore, primary studies with comparison groups that received no intervention, routine care, or other active interventions were considered for inclusion in the majority of systematic reviews [22, 23, 24, 29]. Two systematic reviews did not report the types of comparison groups that were considered in the selection process [25, 28].

Outcomes that were assessed in the systematic reviews on FASD prevention included alcohol use during pregnancy [22–25, 28, 29], changes in the incidence of FASD [22, 24], psychosocial outcomes [23, 24], and other maternal and neonatal outcomes [23, 24, 29].

Three systematic reviews explicitly reported the methodological design criteria that primary studies had to meet in order to be considered for inclusion in the reviews. Three systematic reviews [23, 24, 29] included RCTs or CCTs. One of the reviews [24] also included case-control studies, analytical cohort studies, interrupted-time series (ITS), and before-and-after studies. One systematic review [22] stated that studies of any methodological design were considered for inclusion, whereas two systematic reviews [25, 28] did not explicitly report which study designs were acceptable for inclusion.

2.4.2.2 Methodological Characteristics of Systematic Reviews on Prevention of FASD and Prenatal Alcohol Use

All of the systematic reviews conducted searches in electronic bibliographic databases to identify primary studies that evaluated preventive approaches for FASD and prenatal alcohol use. The median number of databases searched was five (IQR: 1, 15). All of the systematic reviews conducted electronic searches in MEDLINE®. Other electronic databases frequently used were the Cochrane Library® and Embase® (four reviews each [22–24, 29]), CINAHL® (four reviews [23–25, 29]), and PsycINFO®/PsycLIT® (three reviews [24, 25, 29]). The time periods for which searches were conducted overlapped among the reviews within the time span from 1966 to 2010. All of the systematic reviews supplemented the electronic searches by tracking the references lists of included studies. Other commonly used search strategies and sources included hand searches of journals and conference proceedings (four reviews each [22–24, 29]), free searches of the Internet and key websites (three reviews [22, 24, 25]), and contact with experts or authors in the field of study (three reviews [23, 24, 29]). Two systematic reviews [23, 29] did not set language restrictions in their searches, whereas three systematic reviews explicitly [22, 24, 25] disclosed that searches were restricted to studies published in English. One review [28] did not report whether the language of publication was restricted. No restrictions by publication status were made in three of the systematic reviews [23, 24, 29], whereas one review [22] reported that only peer-reviewed literature was sought and that unpublished research was not considered. Two reviews [25, 28] did not explicitly report whether publication restrictions were applied.

There was some variation in methodology among the systematic reviews of the evidence on prevention approaches for FASD and prenatal alcohol use. Three reviews [23–25] reported that two reviewers independently applied a set of eligibility criteria to select primary studies for the reviews. One review [29] reported that five reviewers screened the studies, but it is unknown whether the study selection was made independently by at least two reviewers. One review [22] had only one reviewer scanning the titles and abstracts of primary studies and applying the selection criteria. One review [28] did not report the study-selection methods used.

Data extraction by at least two reviewers was reported in two reviews [23, 29]. Two other reviews [22, 24] disclosed that data from primary studies were extracted by one reviewer and verified by a second reviewer. Two reviews [25, 28] did not report explicitly how data were extracted from primary studies or the number of reviewers who participated at that stage of the review process.

All of the systematic reviews on FASD prevention assessed the methodological quality of the primary studies reviewed; that is, how well the studies controlled for systematic errors or bias. However, there was no uniformity among the reviews in the quality-assessment instruments used. These included: the Schultz criteria [30] for allocation concealment; the Public Health Research, Education and Development/Effective Public Health Practice Project (PHRED/EPHPP) quality tool [31]; the Cochrane "risk of bias" approach [32]; the National Institute for Health and Clinical Excellence (NICE) Public Health Guidance Methods critical appraisal checklists [33]; the National Health and Medical Research Council (NHMRC) quality checklist [34]; and eight methodological standards adapted from Goldstein et al. [35], Sackett et al. [36], and Windsor et al. [37] to assess threats to internal and external validity. Only two systematic reviews [24, 25] explicitly reported that at least two reviewers independently assessed the methodological quality of the studies included in the reviews.

One systematic review [23] conducted a meta-analysis of primary studies, which was to evaluate the effectiveness of a preventive intervention to reduce alcohol consumption during pregnancy. The other five reviews conducted a narrative synthesis of the results from primary studies on prevention of FASD and prenatal alcohol use.

Table 2.2 Overall quality of systematic reviews assessing the effectiveness of prevention approaches to FASD and prenatal alcohol use.

Systematic review	Interventions	Quality (AMSTAR score)
Doggett *et al.* [23]	Home visits commencing during pregnancy and after birth	High (10/11)
Elliott *et al.* [22]	Any strategy aimed at FASD incidence; any alcohol-screening tool designed to evaluate a woman's risk of having a child with FASD	Moderate (8/11)
Ospina *et al.* [24]	Universal, selective and indicated prevention approaches to FASD	High (10/11)
Parkes *et al.* [25]	Identification, assessment and screening for alcohol use in pregnancy; brief interventions with pregnant women and women in their childbearing years; intensive interventions for pregnant women and mothers	Moderate (6/11)
Schorling [28]	Prenatal education and counseling to reduce prenatal alcohol use	Low (4/11)
Stade *et al.* [29]	Psychological and educational interventions for reducing consumption of alcohol	High (9/11)

AMSTAR = Assessment of Multiple Systematic Reviews; FASD = fetal alcohol spectrum disorder.

2.4.3
Methodological Quality of Systematic Reviews on Prevention of FASD and Prenatal Alcohol Use

Overall, the methodological quality of systematic reviews on prevention of FASD and prenatal alcohol use was rated moderate to high (median AMSTAR score: 8.5/11; IQR: 5.5, 10). As shown in Table 2.2, three reviews [23, 24, 29] were considered of high quality (AMSTAR scores 9–11); two reviews [22, 25] were rated moderate in quality (AMSTAR scores 5–8); and one review [28] was considered of low quality (AMSTAR score ≤4). A description of the methodological components of each systematic review, as rated by the AMSTAR tool, is provided in Table 2.D.1 of Appendix 2.D.

An overview of how well the systematic reviews were able to control for biases in locating, selecting, appraising and synthesizing the evidence from individual studies, is provided in Table 2.3. Most of the systematic reviews reported the methods used to control for biases in the location and appraisal of individual studies. Overall, the most common methodological weaknesses were related to a lack of independent and duplicate study selection and data extraction (reported in

Table 2.3 Methodological quality of systematic reviews assessing the effectiveness of prevention approaches to FASD and prenatal alcohol use.

Domains of Methodological Quality from AMSTAR	Yes	No	Can't answer/NA
"A priori" design provided	6	–	–
Duplicate study selection and data extraction	2	2	2
Comprehensive literature search	5	1	–
Status of publication (i.e., gray literature) used as an inclusion criterion	4	2	–
List of studies (included and excluded) provided	4	2	–
Characteristics of the included studies provided	6	–	–
Scientific quality of the included studies assessed and documented	6	–	–
Scientific quality of the included studies used appropriately in formulating conclusions	5	1	–
Appropriate methods used to combine the findings of studies	2	–	4
Likelihood of publication bias assessed	2	4	–
Conflict of interest stated	5	1	–

AMSTAR = Assessment of Multiple Systematic Reviews; NA = not applicable.

two reviews only [23, 29]), and a lack of assessment of the likelihood of publication bias (reported in two reviews only [22, 24]). Only two reviews explicitly reported the criteria used to decide on the pooling of individual study results [22, 24]. Finally, all of the reviews except one [28] reported their source of funding and whether conflict of interest may have affected the review process.

2.4.3.1 Characteristics of the Evidence Presented in the Systematic Reviews on Prevention Approaches to FASD and Prenatal Alcohol Use

The six systematic reviews on prevention of FASD and prenatal alcohol use included a median of 22 studies per review (IQR: 5, 55). An analysis of the geographic distribution of the evidence in these systematic reviews (Figure 2.4) showed that the majority of the evidence was produced in high-income countries, predominantly in the USA. The generalizability of the evidence to Canada is limited. The maximum proportion of Canadian studies represented in the systematic reviews on FASD and prenatal alcohol use prevention was 4% in one systematic review [24]. Studies carried out in French-speaking Canada and published in French were not included in the reviews.

The studies included in the systematic reviews had a variety of study designs that ranged from RCTs to case-series studies. Figure 2.5 displays radar plots that

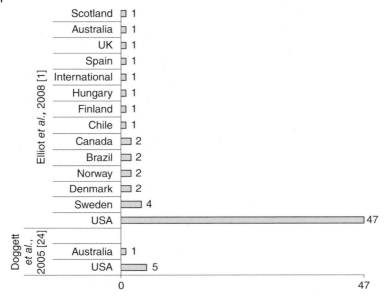

Figure 2.4 Distribution of the evidence on the effectiveness of prevention approaches to FASD and prenatal alcohol use by geographic location.

describe the distribution, by study design, of the evidence that was used to formulate conclusions in each systematic review.

Only two systematic reviews (one [23] on the effectiveness of home visits and the other [29] on the effectiveness of psycho-educational prevention interventions) based their conclusions on evidence provided by RCTs exclusively. All of the other systematic reviews expanded their evidence base to include studies with a variety of methodological designs (CCTs, observational analytical studies, and studies with no control groups). Two systematic reviews [22, 25] incorporated data from other systematic reviews and clinical practice guidelines into their summaries of the evidence on the effectiveness of prevention approaches for FASD and prenatal alcohol use.

2.4.3.2 Qualitative Synthesis of the Evidence on the Effectiveness of Prevention Approaches to FASD and Prenatal Alcohol Use

A qualitative synthesis was conducted of the evidence presented in systematic reviews that assessed the effectiveness of a variety of prevention approaches to FASD.

The review of Doggett *et al.* [23] was a Cochrane systematic review that evaluated the effects of home visits commencing during pregnancy or after birth for women with an alcohol-related and other drug-related problem. Six primary studies, all of which were RCTs conducted between 1994 and 2003, met the criteria of relevance for the review. The quality components of the RCTs were summarized individu-

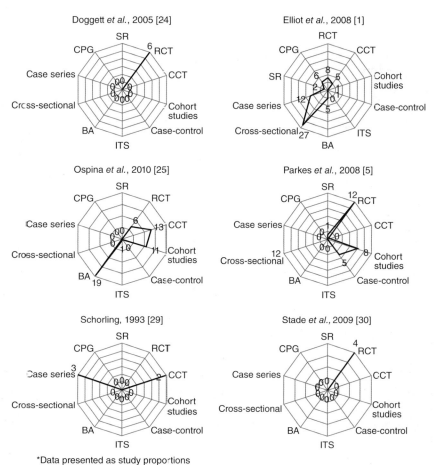

Figure 2.5 Distribution of the evidence on the effectiveness of prevention approaches to FASD and prenatal alcohol use by primary study design. BA = before-and-after study; CCT = controlled clinical trial; CPG = clinical practice guidelines; ITS = interrupted time series; RCT = randomized controlled trial; SR = systematic review.

ally The review authors considered that most of the trials had methodological weaknesses. All of the studies reported correct allocation sequence to treatment, and half of them reported adequate randomization procedures; however, none of the studies reported blinding of intervention, and the loss to follow-up was large in the majority of the studies. The main focus of the review was the effectiveness of home visits commencing during pregnancy or after birth by teams of doctors, nurses, social workers, or trained lay people. The effects on a variety of alcohol-related, pregnancy and puerperium, infant/child and psychosocial outcomes were evaluated in a meta-analysis of RCT data. The following are the main results of the review:

- There were no significant differences in continued alcohol use between the group that received home visits and the control groups (two studies; risk ratio [RR] 1.08; 95% confidence interval [CI] 0.83, 1.41).

- The risk of adverse outcomes in pregnancy and delivery was not reported in the studies.

- There were no significant differences between the home visit groups and control groups in the Bayley Mental Development Index (MDI) (three studies; weighted mean difference [WMD] 2.89; 95% CI: 1.17, 6.95).

- There were no significant differences between the home visit groups and control groups in the Bayley Psychomotor Development Index (PDI) (three studies; WMD 3.14; 95% CI: 0.03, 6.32).

- Results for other outcomes reported in individual RCTs, such as breastfeeding at six months, nonaccidental injury, nonvoluntary foster care, child behavioral problems, and involvement with child-protection services, did not favor the intervention group over the control groups.

Doggett *et al.* [23] concluded that there was insufficient evidence to recommend the routine use of home visits for women with a drug- or alcohol-related problem. The systematic review by Doggett *et al.* [23] was of high methodological quality.

The review by Elliott *et al.* [22] was a systematic review of the evidence pertaining to the relative effectiveness of various strategies to reduce the burden of FASD, including preventive approaches to FASD offered to populations with varied levels of exposure and risk for alcohol consumption during pregnancy. In total, 67 studies conducted between 1986 and 2007 met the criteria of relevance for the review: two systematic reviews; eight RCTs; six CCTs; one cohort study; five ITS; 27 cross-sectional studies; 12 case-series studies; and six clinical practice guidelines. Some 50% of the studies were considered to be of "fair" methodological quality, whereas 40% and 10% were rated "poor" and "good" in methodological quality, respectively. The main focus of the review findings was the effectiveness of prenatal screening (27 studies) and strategies to prevent prenatal alcohol drinking and FASD incidence (described as primary, secondary and tertiary interventions; 40 studies). No formal meta-analysis was conducted due to heterogeneity in the populations, interventions and outcomes of interest among the primary studies. The following were the main results of the review:

1) **Prenatal screening:** Evidence from five studies (study design not reported) indicated that biomarkers to detect prenatal alcohol consumption, such as serum gamma-glutamyl transferase, aspartate aminotransferases, and alanine aminotransferases, are ineffective. Evidence from seven (cross-sectional) studies indicated that the Tolerance, Annoyed, Cut down, Eye-opener (T-ACE) and the Tolerance, Worried, Eye-opener, Amnesia, and K/Cut down (TWEAK) tools were effective in detecting even low levels of alcohol consumption among pregnant women. The remaining 15 studies (study designs not indicated) were considered of very poor quality, and no conclusions were drawn from their results.

2) **Primary prevention strategies:** The review authors reported that a few papers have been published on the effect of primary prevention strategies on drinking behavior during pregnancy. Evidence from six studies (five ITS, one CCT) indicated that there is no strong evidence that any one primary prevention strategy (such as alcohol bans, warning labels on alcohol bottles, educational campaigns) is more effective than others at reducing alcohol use during pregnancy. The authors warned that this result should be considered in the context of the small number of published studies and the low quality of the available evidence.

3) **Secondary prevention strategies:** Evidence regarding the effectiveness of secondary prevention strategies was inconsistent across the 13 studies (three RCTs, four CCTs, six case-series studies) that evaluated these interventions. Only three studies – all of which assessed the effectiveness of educational interventions – reported a significant reduction in alcohol consumption in the intervention groups compared to control groups.

4) **Tertiary prevention strategies:** Thirteen studies (five RCTs, one CCT, one cohort study, six case-series studies) contributed data to this analysis. Only one of the 13 studies provided evidence that a tertiary prevention intervention significantly reduced prenatal alcohol consumption relative to the control group. The study was of poor methodological quality however, and therefore no conclusions were stated regarding the benefits of the intervention.

Elliott et al. [22] concluded that T-ACE and TWEAK are the most appropriate screening tools to use in clinical settings. With regards to primary, secondary, and tertiary preventive interventions, the review authors considered that, while a small number of prevention strategies appeared to reduce alcohol use among pregnant women, these results must be interpreted cautiously due to the potential that bias affected the quality of the evidence. The authors concluded that simple interventions (such as advising pregnant women about the effects of alcohol during pregnancy through a healthcare provider or educational strategy) may be effective, and that more intensive interventions do not necessary increase the effectiveness. The systematic review by Elliott et al. [22] was of high methodological quality. The main methodological weaknesses of the review were related to potential bias in the study selection process and the exclusion of gray literature from the review.

Ospina et al. [24] conducted a systematic review of scientific literature that evaluated the effectiveness of preventive approaches to FASD offered to populations with varied levels of exposure and risk for alcohol consumption during pregnancy. A total of 50 studies conducted between 1983 and 2010 met the criteria of relevance for the review; these included six RCTs, 13 CCTs, 19 before-and-after studies, 11 cohort studies, and one ITS study. The majority of the studies were considered of poor methodological quality (37 rated as weak, 12 as moderate, one as strong). The main focus of the review findings was the effectiveness of universal approaches (18 studies), selective approaches (23 studies) and indicated approaches (nine studies) to preventing FASD. No formal meta-analysis was conducted due to heterogeneity in the populations, interventions, and outcomes of interest among the primary studies. The following were the main results of the review:

1) **Universal preventive interventions:** Results from three CCTs, five cohort studies, nine before-and-after studies, and one ITS study indicated that the best evidence regarding the effectiveness of universal prevention approaches is available for a multimedia education program aimed at youth in school settings. The evidence to support the effectiveness of other universal prevention approaches, such as alcohol-related warning messages, alcohol bans, and other social marketing strategies, is limited, as the studies did not demonstrate that these interventions produced significant modifications in FASD knowledge, attitudes or changes in alcohol use during pregnancy.

2) **Selective preventive interventions:** Results from six CCTs, eight CCTs, four cohort studies, and five before-and-after studies indicated that the best evidence regarding the effectiveness of FASD selective prevention approaches is available for counseling activities and health education programs directed towards women of childbearing age who consume alcohol, pregnant women, and women at risk of an alcohol-exposed pregnancy (AEP).

3) **Indicated preventive interventions:** Results from two CCTs, five before-and-after studies and two cohort studies indicated that the evidence to support the effectiveness of indicated preventive approaches is weak.

Ospina *et al.* [24] concluded that the evidence to support decisions regarding the effectiveness of preventive interventions for FASD is weak, particularly for universal and indicated approaches. Moderate to strong evidence supporting counseling activities for pregnant women and women at risk of AEP were identified. The systematic review by Ospina *et al.* [24] was of high methodological quality. The main methodological limitation of the review was related to the lack of double data extraction from individual studies.

Parkes *et al.* [25] conducted a systematic review that evaluated evidence from the peer-reviewed literature on brief and intensive interventions to reduce alcohol use in pregnant women or women in their childbearing years. A total of 38 studies conducted between 1996 and 2007 met the criteria of relevance for the review: 12 RCTs, 12 cross-sectional studies, eight cohort studies, five case-control studies, and one systematic review. The formal methodological components of individual studies were not described; however, the studies were categorized by study type (types 1 to 4) and graded on the basis of methodological rigor indicators such as suitable control groups, appropriate measures, statistical analyses, attrition rates, and other sources of bias. Of these studies, 45% were rated as evidence type 2+, 24% were evidence type 1++, 21% were evidence type 2++, 7% were type 1+, and 3% were type 1–. The main focus of the review findings was the effectiveness of identification and screening tools for detecting perinatal alcohol use (evaluated in 11 cross-sectional studies, two case-control studies, three RCTs, and one cohort study), brief interventions (evaluated in nine RCTs, one cohort study, and one cross-sectional study), and intensive or in-depth interventions to reduce alcohol use among pregnant women or women of childbearing age (evaluated in six cohort studies, two case-control studies, and one meta-analysis). No formal meta-analysis was conducted due to the heterogeneity in populations, interventions, and outcomes of interest among the primary studies. The following were the main results of the review:

1) **Identification and screening tools for perinatal alcohol use:** Evidence from 11 cross-sectional studies, two case-control studies, three RCTs, and one cohort study indicated that, overall, using screening tools is more effective in identifying potential alcohol use during pregnancy than usual care, or than not using a screening tool. The most sensitive validated screening instruments were the T-ACE and the TWEAK. Self-administered tools were more accurate than staff-applied questionnaires.

2) **Brief interventions:** Evidence from nine RCTs, one cohort study and one cross-sectional study indicated that brief interventions can help to reduce alcohol consumption among pregnant women and women of childbearing age. However, the findings were mixed in the studies that evaluated the effectiveness of interventions for pregnant women. The review authors concluded that the interventions likely have differing impacts on different subgroups of women (such as heavy drinkers). Brief interventions were successful in reducing the risk of AEP among women of childbearing age.

3) **Intensive interventions:** Evidence from six cohort studies, two case-control studies, and one meta-analysis of RCTs indicated that intensive interventions may be very successful in reducing alcohol use during pregnancy and improving other maternal and fetal outcomes.

Parkes et al. [25] concluded that the use of screening tools is an efficient way to identify prenatal alcohol use. There is some evidence that brief, intensive interventions can help to reduce alcohol consumption among women who are pregnant or of childbearing age. However, there was a wide range of study designs in the research that evaluated these interventions, and the review authors acknowledged that some of them were limited in their ability to yield causal attributions. The systematic review by Parkes et al. [25] was of moderate methodological quality. The main methodological weaknesses of the review were potential bias in the selection of studies for the review, poor reporting of studies excluded from the review, and poor incorporation of aspects of methodological quality in individual studies when making recommendations and conclusions.

Schorling [28] conducted a systematic review to evaluate the effectiveness of prevention interventions for prenatal alcohol use. Five studies met the criteria of relevance for the review; these were conducted more than two decades ago (between 1983 and 1990). Of these five studies, two were CCTs, and three were case-series studies. No RCTs were identified. The quality of the included studies was summarized by individual components, and none of the studies met more than 50% of the methodological standards of quality. The main methodological deficiencies of individual studies were related to a lack of control groups (in case-series studies) and to substantial losses to follow-up and limited collection of baseline data in the treatment groups. The main focus of the review findings was the effectiveness of prenatal education offered to pregnant women (evaluated in two CCTs and one case-series study) and counseling interventions for heavy drinkers at a high risk of AEP (evaluated in two case-series studies). No formal meta-analysis was conducted due to the heterogeneity in populations, interventions, and outcomes of interest among the primary studies; however, the reviewers computed a 95% CI around the differences in effect between control and intervention groups reported in the individual studies. The following were the main results of the review:

1) **Prenatal education:** Two CCTs and one case-series study contributed data on the effectiveness of prenatal education interventions to prevent alcohol use during pregnancy. Prenatal education strategies included midwife and social worker visits, and written information with verbal reinforcement. Evidence from the individual studies showed that a majority of women reduced or eliminated their alcohol consumption by the end of their pregnancies; however, similar reductions were also noted among women in the control groups. The review authors found that the maximum difference between control and intervention groups in the two CCTs was 0.14, indicating that the intervention had a relatively small effect.

2) **Counseling:** Data from three case-series studies were used in the analysis of the effectiveness of counseling in the prevention or reduction of alcohol use during pregnancy among women who were heavy drinkers. The characteristics of the counseling interventions were not detailed. Evidence from case-series reports indicated that women reduced their alcohol use during pregnancy after receiving counseling; however, due to the lack of control groups in the studies, it is unknown whether the reductions in alcohol use were due to the intervention, or to some other factor.

Schorling [28] concluded that the primary studies failed to show that the interventions to prevent alcohol use during pregnancy had any clear benefit. The systematic review by Schorling [28] was of low methodological quality. The main methodological weaknesses of the review were potential bias in study selection, a lack of inclusion of gray literature, and poor incorporation of the methodological quality of individual studies in the analysis of the results.

The review by Stade *et al.* [29] was a Cochrane systematic review that evaluated the effectiveness of psychological and educational interventions aimed at reducing alcohol consumption in pregnant women and women planning pregnancy. Four RCTs conducted between 1995 and 2007 met the criteria of relevance for the review. The quality components of the RCTs were summarized individually, and an overall measure of risk of bias was provided for each trial. The method of allocation sequence was rated as adequate in only one RCT, and only two RCTs reported the blinding of outcome assessors. Levels of attrition were low in two studies. The risk of bias was mixed, with none of the studies providing full information about the methods used. The main focus of the review findings was the effectiveness of an educational counseling intervention (one study), a motivational interview (one study), a brief intervention to encourage alcohol reduction (one study), and a cognitive-behavioral self-help intervention (one study). The descriptions of the interventions and the methods of outcome assessment were not clear in the individual studies. No formal meta-analysis was conducted due to heterogeneity in the populations, interventions, and outcomes of interest among the primary studies. The following were the main results of the review:

1) **Educational counseling:** Data from one RCT showed that the rate of alcohol abstinence among the treatment groups was not statistically different from that of control groups. However, the intervention had a positive effect in maintaining the levels of alcohol abstinence among women who were abstinent at the beginning of the study. There were no statistically significant differences in the mean number of drinking episodes during pregnancy among the treatment groups.

2) **Motivational interview:** Data from one RCT showed a positive effect for the motivational interview group in post-intervention levels of alcohol abstinence. There were no statistically significant differences among the treatment groups in the mean number of alcohol drinks per month during pregnancy.

3) **Brief intervention:** Data from one RCT showed higher rates of alcohol abstinence in the intervention group. The brief intervention was also associated with a greater reduction in alcohol consumption during the third trimester.

4) **Cognitive-behavioral self-help intervention:** Data from one RCT showed that the alcohol abstinence rates among the treatment groups were not statistically different. There were no statistically significant differences among the treatment groups in the mean number of alcohol drinks consumed per month during pregnancy.

Stade *et al.* [29] concluded that the evidence from a limited number of studies suggests that some psychological interventions may result in abstinence from alcohol, or a reduction in alcohol consumption during pregnancy. The systematic review by Stade *et al.* [29] was of high methodological quality. The main methodological limitation of the review was related to a lack of evaluation of publication bias.

2.4.3.3 Highlights of the Overall Results

A summary of the results from systematic reviews assessing the effectiveness of prevention approaches to FASD and prenatal alcohol use is presented in Table 2.4. The following are highlights of the main results:

- One high-quality systematic review [23] identified evidence of moderate quality regarding the effectiveness of home visits during or after pregnancy to women with an alcohol-use problem. Results were inconsistent across the studies, and did not allow for the formulation of clear conclusions regarding the effectiveness of the intervention.

Table 2.4 Summary of results from systematic reviews assessing the effectiveness of prevention approaches to FASD and prenatal alcohol use.

Systematic review	Intervention	Population	Evidence type	Conclusions support the effectiveness of the intervention	Quality of the evidence reported in systematic reviews
Doggett et al. [23]	Home visits during or after pregnancy	Pregnant women with an alcohol-abuse problem	RCT = 6	Unclear	Moderate
Elliott et al. [22]	Prenatal screening (T-ACE and TWEAK)	Pregnant women	Cross-sectional = 7	Yes	Moderate
	Primary prevention	General public, women of childbearing age, pregnant women	CCT = 1 ITS = 5	Unclear	Low
	Secondary prevention	Pregnant women	RCT = 1 CCT = 4 Case-series = 6	Unclear	Low
	Tertiary prevention	Pregnant women	RCT = 5 CCT = 1 Cohort = 1 Case-series = 6	Unclear	Low
Ospina et al. [24]	Universal preventive approaches	General public, women of childbearing age, pregnant women	CCT = 3 Cohort = 5 BA = 9 ITS = 1	Unclear	Low
	Selective preventive approaches	Women of childbearing age, pregnant women	RCT = 6 CCT = 8 Cohort = 4 BA = 5	Yes	Moderate

	Indicated preventive approaches	Women of childbearing age, pregnant women at high risk of AEP	CCT = 2 Cohort = 2 BA = 5	Unclear	Low
Parkes *et al.* [25]	Identification and screening tools for perinatal alcohol use	Pregnant women	RCTs = 3 Cohort = 1 Case-control = 2 Cross-sectional = 11	Yes	Moderate
	Brief intervention (MI)	Pregnant women and women of childbearing age	RCTs = 9 Cohort = 1 Cross-sectional = 1	Yes	Low
	Intensive interventions	Pregnant women at high risk of AEP	MA = 1 Cohort = 6 Case-control = 2	Yes	Moderate
Schorling [28]	Prenatal education	Pregnant women	CCT = 2 Case-series = 1	No	Low
	Counseling	Pregnant women	Case-series = 2	Unclear	Low
Stade *et al.* [29]	Educational counseling intervention	Pregnant women	RCT = 1	Yes	Low
	MI	Pregnant women	RCT = 1	Yes	Low
	Brief intervention	Pregnant women	RCT = 1	Yes	Low
	Cognitive-behavioral self-help intervention	Pregnant women	RCT = 1	No	Low

AEP = alcohol-exposed pregnancy; BA = before-and-after study; CCT = controlled clinical trial; ITS = interrupted-time series; MA = meta-analysis; MI = motivational interview; RCT = randomized controlled trial; T-ACE = Tolerance, Annoyed, Cut down, Eye-opener; TWEAK = Tolerance, Worried, Eye-opener, Amnesia, and K/Cut down.

- Two moderate-quality systematic reviews [22, 25] identified evidence of moderate quality that the use of prenatal alcohol screening is an efficient strategy for identifying prenatal alcohol use.

- One moderate-quality systematic review [22] identified evidence of low quality on the effectiveness of primary, secondary, and tertiary prevention approaches. The results of individual studies did not allow for the formulation of clear conclusions regarding the benefits of these approaches.

- One high-quality systematic review [24] identified low-quality evidence on the effectiveness of universal and indicated prevention approaches. The results did not allow for the formulation of clear conclusions regarding the benefits of these approaches. There was evidence of moderate quality that selective prevention approaches might be effective in reducing alcohol use in pregnant women and women of childbearing age.

- Two systematic reviews, one of moderate quality [25] and one of high quality [29], identified evidence of low quality that brief interventions (including motivational interviews) can reduce the risk of AEP among women of childbearing age.

- One moderate-quality systematic review [25] found moderate-quality evidence that intensive interventions may be successful in reducing alcohol use during pregnancy.

- The evidence for the effectiveness of education and counseling reported in two systematic reviews, one of low quality [28] and one of high quality [29], was of low quality and did not allow for the formulation of clear conclusions regarding the benefits of these interventions.

- The evidence reported in one high-quality systematic review [29] on the effectiveness of cognitive-behavioral self-help intervention was limited, and did not show that the intervention led to any reduction in alcohol use during pregnancy.

2.4.4
Systematic Reviews on the Diagnosis of FASD

2.4.4.1 General Characteristics

One systematic review [22] addressed questions related to the effectiveness of postnatal screening tools in identifying individuals who should undergo a full diagnostic evaluation for FASD, and the accuracy of diagnostic tools used to identify cases of FASD. The selection criteria and PICOD components that guided the selection of studies to be included in the systematic review of postnatal screening and diagnosis of FASD are summarized in Table 2.5.

The systematic review by Elliot *et al.* [22] included reports of any strategy aimed at identifying individuals who may have FASD, as well as tools used to confirm the FASD diagnosis. Systematic reviews, diagnostic criteria, clinical guidelines,

Table 2.5 Selection criteria applied in a systematic review of postnatal screening and diagnosis of FASD.

Systematic review	Population	Interventions	Comparators	Outcomes	Study design of individual studies
Elliott *et al.* [22]	Individuals who may have FASD or mothers of individuals who may have FASD	Any strategy aimed at identifying an individual who may have FASD or diagnosing an individual with FASD	Any	Sensitivity and specificity of FASD diagnosis	Systematic reviews, diagnostic criteria or guidelines, primary research except case reports

FASD = fetal alcohol spectrum disorder.

and primary research (excluding case reports) were considered for inclusion in the review. The review also considered studies targeting mothers of individuals suspected of having FASD. No analysis of studies conducted on special populations (e g., Aboriginal groups, low-socioeconomic or underserved populations) was planned. No restrictions were imposed in regard to the type of comparison groups used in the primary studies. The outcomes of interest were measures of the efficiency of diagnostic tests, such as sensitivity and specificity.

2.4.4.2 Methodological Characteristics of the Systematic Review on Diagnosis of FASD

Elliot *et al.* [22] conducted searches in electronic bibliographic databases such as MEDLINE®, the Cochrane Library®, Embase®, and Scopus® for the period between 1966 and 2008. Nonelectronic search methods included reference tracking and hand searches of journals, conference proceedings, and health technology assessment websites. The systematic review explicitly disclosed that only English-language publications were considered for inclusion.

Only one reviewer scanned the titles and abstracts of primary studies and applied the selection criteria for inclusion in the review. Data from publications were extracted by one reviewer, and verified by a second reviewer. The systematic review did not report the approach used to assess the methodological quality of included publications. The review conducted a narrative synthesis of the reports on diagnostic approaches to FASD.

2.4.4.3 Methodological Quality of Systematic Reviews on Diagnosis of FASD

The methodological quality of the systematic review on postnatal screening and diagnosis of FASD was rated as moderate (AMSTAR score: 8). An overview of how well the review was able to control for biases in locating, selecting, appraising and synthesizing the evidence from individual studies is provided in Table 2.6. Methodological weaknesses were related to the lack of independent and duplicate study

Table 2.6 Methodological quality of systematic review of postnatal screening and diagnosis of FASD.

Domains of Methodological Quality from AMSTAR	Yes	No	Can't answer/NA
"A priori" design provided	1	–	–
Duplicate study selection and data extraction	–	1	–
Comprehensive literature search	1	–	–
Status of publication (i.e., gray literature) used as an inclusion criterion	–	1	–
List of studies (included and excluded) provided	1	–	–
Characteristics of the included studies provided	1	–	–
Scientific quality of the included studies assessed and documented	–	1	–
Scientific quality of the included studies used appropriately in formulating conclusions	–	1	–
Appropriate methods used to combine the findings of studies	–	–	1
Likelihood of publication bias assessed	1	–	–
Conflict of interest stated	1	–	–

AMSTAR = Assessment of Multiple Systematic Reviews; NA = not applicable.

selection and data extraction, a lack of assessment of the methodological quality of individual reports, and a lack of incorporation of methodological quality in formulating the conclusions of the review.

2.4.4.4 Characteristics of the Evidence Presented in the Systematic Review on the Effectiveness of Diagnostic Approaches to FASD

The systematic review by Elliott *et al.* [22] included six publications. An analysis of the geographic distribution of the evidence on the effectiveness of postnatal screening and diagnostic tools for FASD reported in the review (Figure 2.6) showed that the largest proportion of the evidence was produced in the USA. Only one Canadian report of guidelines for diagnosis was included in the summary of the evidence.

The systematic review by Elliot *et al.* [22] did not identify primary research or systematic reviews on the effectiveness of postnatal screening and diagnostic tools. Rather, the evidence collected consisted of data provided by clinical practice guidelines. Radar plots that describe the distribution, by study design, of the evidence that was used to formulate conclusions in the systematic review by Elliot *et al.* [22] Figure 2.7.

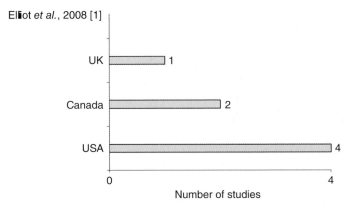

Figure 2.6 Distribution of the evidence on the effectiveness of diagnosis approaches to FASD by geographic location.

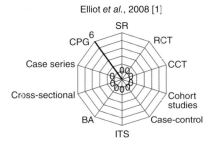

Figure 2.7 Distribution of the evidence on the effectiveness of diagnostic approaches to FASD by primary study design. BA = before-and-after study; CCT = controlled clinical trial; CPG = clinical practice guidelines; ITS = interrupted time series; RCT = randomized controlled trial; SR = systematic review.

2.4.4.5 Qualitative Synthesis of the Evidence on the Effectiveness of Diagnostic Approaches to FASD

The following is a synthesis of the main recommendations provided in the guidelines and diagnostic criteria identified in the review of Elliott *et al.* [22]:

1) **Diagnostic Criteria:**
   - **Institute of Medicine:** The first diagnostic criteria for FASD were published by the Institute of Medicine [3]. Five diagnostic categories are described: FAS with and without a confirmed history of alcohol exposure, partial FASD, ARBD, and ARND. The diagnostic criteria are facial abnormalities, growth retardation, central nervous system neurodevelopmental abnormalities, and known maternal alcohol use. These diagnostic criteria were based on recommendations by a panel of experts and no formal evaluation of the efficiency of the diagnostic approach was provided.

- **4-Digit Diagnostic Code [2]:** This was developed in response to concerns that the guidelines of the Institute of Medicine were not specific enough to ensure the accuracy or precision of the diagnostic criteria. The 4-Digit Diagnostic Code can be used to diagnose FASD as well as other FASD-related conditions. The four-digit system refers to the four key diagnostic features in FAS: growth deficiency; FAS facial phenotype; central nervous system damage; and gestational alcohol exposure. The magnitude of the expression of each feature is rated on a four-point Likert scale (1 = complete absence; 4 = extreme expression). No information was provided regarding the efficiency of the diagnostic criteria.

- **Hoyme Updated Institute of Medicine Criteria:** The Institute of Medicine criteria were updated in 2005 by Hoyme *et al.* [4] to provide more extensive definitions of the four FASD diagnostic criteria. No information was provided regarding the efficiency of the diagnostic criteria.

2) **Guidelines:**
- **Public Health Agency of Canada FASD-Referral Guidelines:** Referral guidelines [38] developed by the Public Health Agency of Canada's National Advisory Committee on FASD recommend screening for facial anomalies, known exposure to alcohol, or learning and behavioral difficulties. The guidelines further state that referral to specialty clinics and trained professionals is necessary. No information was provided regarding the evidence base that supports these recommendations.

- **The Centers for Disease Control (CDC) [39]:** The CDC developed guidelines for the referral of children with suspected FAS. The guidelines state that if the mother's alcohol consumption was high during pregnancy, but no other screening criteria are present, then the primary healthcare provider should document this exposure and closely monitor the child over time. The guidelines aim to assist in the referral decision, rather than to serve as a screening or diagnostic tool. No information was provided regarding the evidence base that supports these recommendations.

- **Canadian Guidelines for the Diagnosis of FASD [40]:** These were developed by a subcommittee of the Public Health Agency of Canada's National Advisory Committee on FASD. The guidelines combine the descriptive terminology of the Institute of Medicine criteria with the objective measures of the 4-Digit Diagnostic Code. The guidelines describe a diagnostic process of screening and referral, physical examination and differential diagnosis, and neurobehavioral assessment. No information was provided regarding the evidence base that supports these recommendations.

The guidelines and diagnostic criteria for FASD postnatal screening and diagnosis identified by Elliott *et al.* [22] are based on the opinions of panels of clinicians. Therefore, they represent the lowest level of evidence available for informing decisions on the most effective postnatal screening and diagnostic options for FASD.

Table 2.7 Summary of results from systematic review assessing the effectiveness of diagnostic approaches to FASD.

Systematic review	Diagnostic approach	Evidence type	Conclusions support the effectiveness of the diagnostic approach	Quality of the evidence reported
Elliott *et al.* [22]	Institute of Medicine diagnostic criteria	Expert opinion	NR	Low
	4-Digit Diagnostic Code	Expert opinion	NR	Low
	Hoyme updated Institute of Medicine criteria	Expert opinion	NR	Low
	Public Health Agency of Canada FASD referral guidelines	CPG based on expert opinion	NR	Low
	CDC guidelines	CPG based on expert opinion	NR	Low
	Canadian guidelines for the diagnosis of FASD	CPG based on expert opinion	NR	Low

CDC = Centers for Disease Control; CPG = clinical practice guidelines; FASD = fetal alcohol spectrum disorder; NR = not reported.

The systematic review by Elliott *et al.* [22] was of moderate methodological quality. The main methodological weaknesses of the review were related to potential bias in the selection of reports for the review and the lack of formal quality assessment of the evidence on diagnostic approaches for FASD.

2.4.4.6 Highlights of the Overall Results
A summary of the evidence presented in the systematic review on FASD diagnosis [22] is presented in Table 2.7. No primary studies have evaluated the efficiency of tools or classification systems used to diagnose FASD.

2.4.5
Systematic Reviews on the Treatment of FASD

2.4.5.1 General Characteristics
Three systematic reviews [22, 26, 27] addressed questions related to the effectiveness of treatment approaches for individuals with FASD. The systematic reviews were published between 2007 and 2009, the median year of publication being 2008 (IQR: 2007, 2009). The selection criteria and PICOD components that guided the inclusion of individual studies in the systematic reviews of treatment approaches to FASD are summarized in Table 2.8.

Two systematic reviews [26, 27] evaluated the scientific evidence from primary studies that assessed therapeutic interventions for FASD, and one review [22] included only systematic reviews and guidelines in the evidence synthesis.

Table 2.8 Selection criteria applied in systematic reviews of the effectiveness of therapeutic approaches to FASD.

Systematic review	Population	Interventions	Comparators	Outcomes	Study design of individual studies
Elliot *et al.* [22]	Individuals with FASD	Any strategy aimed at improving FASD clinical outcomes	Any	Reduction in severity of primary or secondary disabilities or deficits associated with FASD	SR, CPG, review articles
Peadon *et al.* [26]	Individuals under 18 years of age with a diagnosis of FASD	Pharmacological, behavioral, speech therapy, occupational therapy, physiotherapy, psychosocial and educational interventions and early intervention programs	No treatment, waiting list, usual therapy, placebo	Measures of physical and mental health, developmental status, cognitive status, quality of life, educational attainment, employment, contact with the law; substance-abuse measures during and immediately after the intervention and/or in adolescence and adulthood	RCT, CCT, before-and-after intervention studies
Premji *et al.* [27]	Individuals under 18 years of age with diagnosis or evidence of FAS, FASD or equivalent	Early interventions, strategies, education, medication. Intervention may target an individual with FASD, caregiver, or family of an affected individual	NR	Measures of cognitive status, impulsive behavior	RCT, CCT

CCT = controlled clinical trials; CPG = clinical practice guidelines; FASD = fetal alcohol spectrum disorder; NR = not reported; RCT = randomized controlled trials; SR = systematic reviews.

All of the reviews evaluated the scientific evidence from assessments of therapeutic interventions for individuals with FASD. Two systematic reviews [26, 27] were restricted to studies conducted in children and youth under 18 years of age. None of the systematic reviews evaluated the effectiveness of therapeutic approaches to FASD delivered to special populations (e.g., Aboriginal groups, low-socioeconomic and underserved populations).

None of the systematic reviews examined a single therapeutic intervention for FASD, but rather considered for inclusion a broad spectrum of interventions, such as pharmacological treatment, behavioral therapy, speech therapy, occupational therapy, physiotherapy and psychosocial, and educational interventions.

Few restrictions were imposed with regard to the type of comparison groups used in the primary studies. The two systematic reviews that included only primary studies [26, 27] considered no intervention, routine care, or other active interventions as valid comparison groups.

The outcomes that were assessed in the two systematic reviews of therapeutic interventions for FASD were measures of physical and mental health, developmental and cognitive status, behavior, quality of life, educational and employment attainment, substance abuse and primary, or secondary disabilities associated with FASD.

All of the systematic reviews explicitly reported the methodological design criteria that studies were required to meet in order to be considered for inclusion. One systematic review was restricted to systematic reviews and clinical practice guidelines. Two reviews [26, 27] included individual studies that used experimental methods, such as RCTs and CCTs. One of these [26] expanded the inclusion criteria to before-and-after intervention studies.

2.4.5.2 Methodological Characteristics of Systematic Reviews on Therapeutic Approaches to FASD

All of the systematic reviews conducted searches in electronic bibliographic databases to identify relevant studies. Two systematic reviews conducted electronic searches in four [22] and six [26] databases, respectively, whereas one systematic review [27] reported that 40 peer-reviewed databases and 23 gray literature databases were searched (although the names of the databases were not provided). Electronic databases that were used included MEDLINE®, Embase®, Cochrane Library® (all three systematic reviews), CINAHL®, PsycINFO®/PsycLIT®, Eric ® (one review [26]), and Scopus® (one review [22]).

The time periods for which searches were conducted overlapped among the reviews, and ranged from 1950 to 2009. All of the systematic reviews supplemented the electronic searches by tracking the lists of references of included studies. Other commonly used search strategies and sources included hand searches of journals [22, 27] and conference proceedings [22, 26], free searches in the Internet and key websites [22], and contact with experts in the field of study [26, 27]. Two systematic reviews [26, 27] did not set language restrictions in their searches, whereas one review explicitly [22] disclosed that searches were restricted to literature published in English. No restrictions by publication status were made in two of the systematic reviews [26, 27], whereas one review [22] reported that only peer-reviewed literature was sought and that unpublished research was not considered for inclusion.

There was some variation in the methodology adopted in the systematic reviews of therapeutic approaches for FASD. Two systematic reviews [26, 27] reported that two reviewers independently applied a set of selection criteria to decide the eligibility of studies for the reviews. One review [22] had only one reviewer scanning the titles and abstracts of potentially relevant studies, applying the selection criteria for inclusion in the review and conducting quality assessment and data extraction. Two systematic reviews [26, 27] reported that study quality assessment and data extraction were undertaken independently by two reviewers.

Two of the systematic reviews [26, 27] on the treatment of FASD appraised the internal validity of the primary studies reviewed; that is, how well their design and execution controlled for systematic errors or bias. One of the reviews [26] appraised individual dimensions of quality, such as the method of randomization, allocation concealment, blinding of outcome assessment, use of standardized measures, and intention-to-treat analysis. The other review [27] applied the Schultz criteria [30] for allocation concealment, and the Jadad scale [41] to evaluate the quality of individual studies. The systematic review that included secondary material [22] (i.e., systematic reviews, clinical guidelines, and review articles) did not use any methodological quality tool, but reported the levels of the evidence for the selected reviews.

None of the systematic reviews conducted a meta-analysis of primary studies to evaluate the effectiveness of therapeutic intervention to reduce FASD-associated problems. All of them conducted a narrative synthesis of findings from primary or secondary sources of evidence.

2.4.5.3 Methodological Quality of Systematic Reviews on Therapeutic Approaches to FASD

The methodological quality of systematic reviews on therapeutic approaches to FASD was rated as moderate overall (median AMSTAR score: 8; IQR: 6, 8) (Table 2.9). The individual methodological components of each systematic review, as rated by the AMSTAR tool, are described in Table 2.D.2 of Appendix 2.D.

An overview of how well the systematic reviews were able to control for biases in locating, selecting, appraising, and synthesizing the evidence from studies is provided in Table 2.10. Most of the systematic reviews reported the methods used to control for bias in the search for individual studies. The methodological weaknesses were related to a lack of assessment of the likelihood of publication bias (reported in one review only [22]). Finally, all of the reviews reported their sources of funding and whether conflict of interest may have affected the review process.

2.4.5.4 Characteristics of the Evidence Presented in the Systematic Reviews on Therapeutic Approaches to FASD

The systematic reviews on treatment of FASD included a median of six studies per review (IQR: 3, 12). An analysis of the geographic distribution of the evidence

Table 2.9 Overall quality of systematic reviews assessing the effectiveness of therapeutic approaches to FASD.

Systematic review	Interventions	Quality (AMSTAR score)
Elliott *et al.* [22]	Any strategy aimed at improving FASD clinical outcomes	Low (6/11)
Peadon *et al.* [26]	Pharmacological, behavioral, speech therapy, occupational therapy, physiotherapy, psychosocial and educational interventions and early intervention programs	Moderate (8/11)
Premji *et al.* [27]	Early interventions, strategies, education, medication. Intervention may target an individual with FASD, caregiver, or family of an affected individual	Moderate (8/11)

AMSTAR = Assessment of Multiple Systematic Reviews; FASD = fetal alcohol spectrum disorder.

Table 2.10 Methodological quality of systematic reviews assessing the effectiveness of therapeutic approaches to FASD.

Domains of Methodological Quality from AMSTAR	Yes	No	Can't answer/NA
1. "A priori" design provided	3	–	–
2. Duplicate study selection and data extraction	2	1	–
3. Comprehensive literature search	3	–	–
4. Status of publication (i.e., gray literature) used as an inclusion criterion	2	1	–
5. List of studies (included and excluded) provided	1	2	–
6. Characteristics of the included studies provided	3	–	–
7. Scientific quality of the included studies assessed and documented	2	1	–
8. Scientific quality of the included studies used appropriately in formulating conclusions	2	1	–
9. Appropriate methods used to combine the findings of studies	–	–	3
10. Likelihood of publication bias assessed	1	2	–
11. Conflict of interest stated	3	–	–

AMSTAR = Assessment of Multiple Systematic Reviews; NA = not applicable.

on the effectiveness of therapeutic approaches for FASD that was summarized in the three systematic reviews (Figure 2.8) shows that the evidence was produced predominantly in high-income countries; however, studies conducted in developing countries such as South Africa have also contributed to the evidence base regarding the effectiveness of FASD therapeutics. The evidence is generalizable

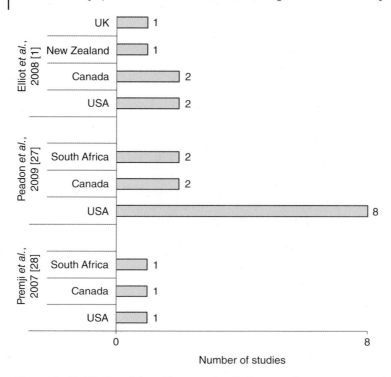

Figure 2.8 Distribution of the evidence on the effectiveness of treatment approaches to FASD by geographic location.

to Canada. Canadian studies were represented in the three systematic reviews on FASD treatment. Studies carried out in French-speaking Canada and published in French were not included in the reviews.

Radar plots that describe, by study design, the distribution of the evidence that was used to formulate conclusions in each systematic review, are displayed in Figure 2.9. One systematic review [22] incorporated data from other systematic reviews and clinical practice guidelines into an evidence summary on the effectiveness of treatment approaches for FASD. The two other reviews based their conclusions on the evidence provided by experimental research; that is, RCTs [26, 27], CCTs [26, 27], and before-and-after studies [26].

2.4.5.5 Qualitative Synthesis of the Evidence on the Effectiveness of Therapeutic Approaches to FASD

A qualitative synthesis was conducted of the evidence presented in systematic reviews that assessed the effectiveness of a variety of therapeutic approaches to FASD.

Elliott *et al.* [22] conducted a systematic review to evaluate the evidence on interventions to support the clinical management of individuals diagnosed with FASD, and to minimize the effect of primary disabilities and prevent secondary disabili-

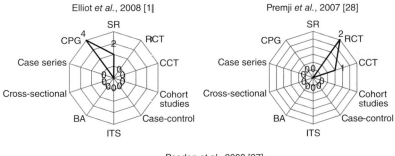

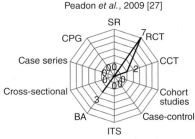

Figure 2.9 Distribution of the evidence on the effectiveness of treatment approaches to FASD by primary study design. BA = before-and-after study; CCT = controlled clinical trial; CPG = clinical practice guidelines; ITT = interrupted time series; RCT = randomized controlled trial; SR = systematic review.

ties. Only systematic reviews (two) and published guidelines (four) met the criteria of relevance for the review; all of these were published between 2004 and 2007. The methodological quality of the systematic reviews and guidelines was not summarized, but a narrative synthesis of their main results was provided.

The systematic reviews identified by Elliott *et al.* [22] focused on the effectiveness of nursing interventions to prevent secondary disabilities associated with FASD (one systematic review), and any research-based intervention for children and youth with FASD (one systematic review). Unfortunately, the review on nursing interventions to prevent secondary disabilities did not identify any relevant publications and, therefore, was not further discussed. The following are the main findings of the Elliott *et al.* [22] review:

1) **Cognitive control therapy:** One systematic review provided evidence on the effectiveness of cognitive control therapy for children with FASD. The review was severely limited by a lack of scientific rigor in the individual studies included in it. The authors did not make any final conclusions regarding the effectiveness of cognitive control therapy in improving attention deficits, impulsiveness and hyperactivity in children and youth diagnosed with FASD.

2) **Psychostimulant medications:** One systematic review provided evidence on the effectiveness of psychostimulant medications for children diagnosed with FASD and ADHD. The reviewers found that psychostimulant medications

reduced hyperactivity; however, no changes in attention or impulsivity were identified. Elliott *et al.* [22] concluded that psychostimulant medications are potentially effective in children with FASD and ADHD.

The four published guidelines identified by Elliott *et al.* [22] based their discussions of FASD management strategies on the opinions of panels of clinicians. Therefore, these represent the lowest level of evidence available for informing decisions on the most effective treatment options for FASD. The following is a synthesis of the main recommendations in the four published guidelines:

- A guideline developed by Alcohol Healthwatch [42] in New Zealand describes New Zealand policy and action on FASD. FASD is not considered a disability in New Zealand; however, individuals diagnosed with FASD qualify for disability support if they meet a threshold of intellectual disability (IQ of 70 or less). The report did not recommend specific treatment strategies.

- Canadian guidelines on the management of FASD [40] were developed by a subcommittee of the Public Health Agency of Canada's National Advisory Committee on FASD. The guidelines recommend that individuals diagnosed with FASD and their families be educated about the disorder and its potential psychosocial impact, and that they be linked to resources and services that may improve outcome. The guidelines do not state which specific resources and services are needed.

- The CDC [39] developed guidelines in the USA that recommend general services that may benefit individuals with FAS. The CDC guidelines emphasize the importance of educating parents and caregivers about therapeutic options; recommend early interventions (between birth and three years of age) as being vital to prevent disabilities secondary to FASD; and recommend that FASD diagnostic centers or trained clinicians be available, as well as appropriate services (physical, occupational, speech, behavioral, mental health and other related services) and vocational training focusing on the skills of daily living.

- Guidelines developed by the British Medical Association (BMA) in the UK state that there has been very little research into the therapeutic options available for FASD, and that there is no framework for the clinical management of FASD in the UK. Services recommended by the BMA include education, social support, and vocational training.

Elliott *et al.* [22] concluded that there was insufficient evidence in the literature to recommend specific management strategies. The systematic review by Elliott *et al.* [22] was of moderate methodological quality. The main methodological deficiencies of the review were related to potential bias in the selection of studies for the review and a lack of formal quality-assessment of the evidence on therapeutic interventions for FASD.

Peadon *et al.* [26] conducted a systematic review to identify and evaluate the evidence for pharmacological and nonpharmacological interventions for children and youth (under 18 years of age) with FASD. Twelve studies met the criteria of relevance for the review; these were conducted during the last decade (between 1997 and 2008) and included seven RCTs, two CCTs, and three before-and-after-studies. The methodological quality of individual studies was not described using a rating score but, rather, some quality components of the individual studies were summarized individually. The reviewers found that most (six out of seven) of the RCTs did not provide clear information regarding the methods of randomization, and none of them described the method for concealment of allocation. None of the studies described whether an intention-to-treat analysis was conducted, or the number of study withdrawals and losses to follow-up. No formal meta-analysis was conducted due to the heterogeneity in populations, interventions, and out-comes of interest among the primary studies; rather, a narrative synthesis of the results was provided. The main focus of the review findings was the effectiveness of educational and learning strategies (reported in four RCTs, one CCT, and two before-and-after studies), psychostimulant medications (reported in one RCT and one CCT), social skills and social communication interventions (one CCT and one before-and-after study), and behavioral strategies (one RCT) as treatment options for individuals with FASD. The following were the main findings of the Peadon *et al.* [26] review:

1) **Educational and learning strategies:** A variety of educational and learning strategies were evaluated in the individual studies that were reviewed: cognitive control therapy and a language intervention focused on basic literacy skills (one RCT each), mathematics interventions (one RCT and one CCT), virtual-reality game interventions for increasing knowledge of fire, home and street safety (one RCT and one before-and-after study), and teacher modeling strategies (one before-and-after study).

   - Evidence from one RCT on the effectiveness of cognitive control therapy indicated improvement in children's behavior in the intervention group compared with a control group.

   - Evidence from one RCT indicated that a language intervention focused on basic literacy skills led to improvements in reading, spelling, and some pre-literacy domains in the intervention group compared to a control group.

   - Evidence from one RCT and one CCT indicated that mathematics interventions produced significant improvements in mathematics knowledge and digit span memory.

   - Evidence from one RCT and one before-and-after study indicated that a virtual reality game increased children's knowledge of fire, home and street safety.

   - Evidence from one before-and-after study indicated that modeling as a teaching strategy did not produce improvements in perceptual skills.

2) **Psychostimulant medications:** One RCT and one CCT contributed data on the effectiveness of psychostimulant medications in improving attention skills or reducing hyperactivity scores in children diagnosed with FAS or pFAS and attention-deficit and hyperactivity disorder (ADHD). The evidence from the two studies did not agree.

3) **Social skills and social communication interventions:** Social skills and social communication interventions were evaluated by two studies in the review by Peadon *et al.* [26] Evidence from one CCT on parent-assisted child friendship training indicated improvements in knowledge of appropriate social behavior. Evidence from one before-and-after study indicated improvements in child's social communication skills.

4) **Behavioral interventions:** A behavioral intervention consisting of attention process training was evaluated in one RCT. Importantly, this intervention was evaluated in a small sample ($n = 20$) of Inuit children in Canada. Evidence from the RCT indicated significant improvements on measures of sustained attention and nonverbal reasoning ability, but no improvement on measures of executive function.

Peadon *et al.* [26] concluded that there is limited good quality scientific evidence for specific interventions for managing FASD. The systematic review by Peadon *et al.* [26] was of moderate methodological quality. The main methodological weakness was a lack of reporting of the studies that were excluded from the review.

Premji *et al.* [27] conducted a systematic review to identify efficacious interventions for children and youth (under 18 years of age) affected with FASD. The objective of this review was to identify the best FASD treatment practices in order to inform policy decisions and to identify priority areas for future research. Two RCTs and one CCT conducted between 1997 and 2003 met the criteria of relevance for the review. The quality components of the included studies were summarized individually. Briefly, the reviewers considered that the randomization sequence and exclusions after randomization were not clearly described in the individual studies. Similarly, the reviewers considered that individual studies were not blinded with regards to the concealment of treatment allocation. No formal meta-analysis was conducted due to heterogeneity in study populations, interventions, and outcomes of interest; rather, a narrative synthesis of the results was provided. The main focus of the review findings was the effectiveness of cognitive control therapy (reported in one RCT) and psychostimulant medications (reported in one RCT and one CCT) as treatment options for individuals with FASD. The following were the main results of the review:

1) **Cognitive control therapy:** One RCT contributed data on the effectiveness of cognitive control therapy administered in an educational setting to children with FASD. The characteristics of the intervention were not clearly described in the RCT. The evidence did not indicate a statistically significant difference in neuropsychological or intelligence tests between the intervention group and

a control group; however, behavioral improvements following the intervention were reported anecdotally.

2) **Psychostimulant medications:** One RCT and one CCT contributed data on the effectiveness of psychostimulant medications in the short-term reduction of hyperactivity and improvement of attention in children diagnosed with FAS or pFAS, and ADHD. The evidence from the two studies did not agree.

Premji et al. [27] concluded that there is limited scientific evidence upon which to draw recommendations regarding efficacious interventions for children and youth with FASD. The systematic review by Premji et al. [27] was of moderate methodological quality. The main methodological limitation was a lack of reporting of the studies that were excluded from the review.

2.4.5.6 Highlights of the Overall Results

A summary of the results from systematic reviews assessing the effectiveness of therapeutic approaches to FASD is presented in Table 2.11. The highlights of these results were as follows:

- Three moderate-quality systematic reviews [22, 26, 27] summarized moderate-quality evidence from studies on the effectiveness of cognitive control therapy for individuals with FASD. Results were inconsistent across the studies, and did not allow for the formulation of clear conclusions regarding the benefits of this intervention.

- Three moderate-quality systematic reviews [22, 26, 27] on the effectiveness of psychostimulant medications for individuals with FASD and ADHD showed inconsistent results across the studies. No clear conclusions could be made regarding the benefits of this intervention.

- There was moderate-quality evidence reported in one moderate-quality systematic review [26] that interventions aimed at increasing basic literacy skills, math skills, social skills and communication, and children's safety could be effective in treating certain cognitive and social disabilities secondary to FASD.

- Moderate-quality evidence reported in one moderate-quality systematic review [26] regarding the effectiveness of behavioral interventions for FASD was unclear, and did not allow for the formulation of clear conclusions.

- Moderate-quality evidence from one moderate-quality systematic review [26] failed to show any clear benefit from teacher modeling strategies as a treatment option for FASD.

2.5
Discussion

This overview has summarized the evidence presented in systematic reviews of scientific literature published during the past 25 years on the prevention, diagnostic,

Table 2.11 Summary of results from systematic reviews assessing the effectiveness of treatment approaches to FASD.

Systematic review	Intervention	Population	Evidence type	Conclusions support the effectiveness of the intervention	Quality of the evidence reported in systematic reviews
Elliott *et al.* [22]	Cognitive control therapy	FASD	SR = 1	Unclear	Moderate
	Psychostimulant medications	FASD plus ADHD	SR = 1	Yes	Moderate
Peadon *et al.* [26]	Cognitive control therapy	FASD	RCT = 1	Yes	Moderate
	Language intervention focused on basic literacy skills	FASD	RCT = 1	Yes	Moderate
	Math intervention	FASD	RCT = 1; CCT = 1	Yes	Moderate
	Virtual reality game intervention on safety	FAS, pFAS	RCT = 1	Yes	Moderate
	Teacher modeling strategy	FASD	BA = 1	No	Moderate
	Psychostimulant medications	FAS or pFAS plus ADHD	RCT = 1 CCT = 1	Unclear	Moderate
	Social skills and social communication interventions	FASD	CCT = 1; BA = 1	Yes	Moderate
	Behavioral interventions	FASD	RCT = 1	Unclear	Moderate
Premji *et al.* [27]	Cognitive control therapy	FASD	RCT = 1	No	Moderate
	Psychostimulant medications	FAS or pFAS plus ADHD	RCT = 1 CCT = 1	Unclear	Moderate

ADHD = attention deficit and hyperactivity disorder; BA = before-and-after study; FAS = fetal alcohol syndrome; FASD = fetal alcohol spectrum disorder; pFAS = partial fetal alcohol syndrome.

and treatment approaches to FASD. Four of the systematic reviews were produced in Canada (three systematic reviews on the prevention of prenatal alcohol use and FASD occurrence, and one review on treatment strategies for children and youth with FASD); however, most of the evidence analyzed in the reviews is derived from primary studies conducted in the USA.

2.5.1
FASD Prevention

The majority of systematic reviews on the prevention of FASD have evaluated the evidence on the effectiveness of prevention interventions to reduce prenatal alcohol use and FASD occurrence. The main focus of these reviews has been the effect of these interventions in women of childbearing age, in pregnant adult women, and in adult women at risk of an alcohol-exposed pregnancy. Therefore, evidence related to the effect of prevention strategies directed to youth (females under the age of 18), women's partners or other family members is scarce compared to that which has been collected for adult women.

The evidence analyzed in this overview indicates that prenatal screening tools such as ACE-T and TWEAK are likely to be effective in identifying prenatal alcohol use. The identification of women who consume alcohol during pregnancy is a crucial step toward implementing interventions aimed at reducing the rate of AEP and, eventually, the incidence of FASD [43, 44]. However, the lack of evidence on how culturally sensitive instruments can be implemented indicates a gap in the research.

There is some evidence that brief interventions can help to reduce the risk of AEP among women of childbearing age. It has been suggested that, in addition to brief interventions which provide clinical advice and counseling regarding the risk posed by prenatal alcohol exposure, a follow-up should be conducted which would include referral to intensive interventions or to community-group interventions that support women seeking to reduce hazardous alcohol use [43]. The importance of establishing formal alcohol screening and brief intervention programs that are culturally and linguistically appropriate for pregnant women and women of childbearing age is emphasized.

The evidence regarding the implementation of other prevention approaches, such as home visits, education, and counseling interventions, is unclear. It is important to continue expanding the evidence base with regards to the effectiveness of these interventions, and also to promote the evaluation of culturally sensitive intervention methods in multiple settings in which women are seen.

Because of the complexity of the problem of FASD, preventive initiatives should originate from many levels (community, regional, provincial, and federal), in order to make significant gains to reduce this serious public health problem. Intersectoral approaches involving the social services, the education system, and the healthcare system are necessary to address the multiple needs of those women who are at risk of using alcohol prenatally.

It is also important to ensure that the prevention of prenatal alcohol use and the occurrence of FASD is addressed in the context of the broader determinants of health. An understanding of the broader social and systemic root causes of alcohol use during pregnancy, and the social and cultural dynamics of this practice in society, are fundamental to the development of effective prevention and screening initiatives.

Clearly, there is a great need to promote the research and implementation of empirically validated prevention interventions targeting the general population. This overview of systematic reviews did not identify any evidence supporting the use of universal massive community campaigns to reduce prenatal alcohol use or FASD. In theory, such social strategies may play an important role in educating the general public and raising awareness about FASD, and they should therefore be part of a comprehensive and multilevel FASD-prevention approach. However, current evidence to support their wide implementation is weak, and further research is required to determine the magnitude of the effect of these interventions on alcohol use patterns and reproductive health outcomes, including the incidence of FASD among the population.

Both, population-based strategies and more targeted individual-level interventions to reduce prenatal alcohol exposure should be evaluated. Partnerships across government agencies, academia, medical, education and social service delivery systems, as well as with the general public, are essential to strengthen evidence-based services aimed at reducing the risk of AEP in pregnant women and women of childbearing age [43].

2.5.2
FASD Diagnosis

The systematic reviews included in the overview did not identify primary studies that evaluated the efficiency of tools or classification systems to diagnose FASD. The evidence presented in the systematic review on diagnostic approaches consists of guidelines and diagnostic criteria for FASD derived from the opinions of panels of clinicians. This represents the lowest level of evidence available for informing decisions on the postnatal and diagnostic options for FASD. Therefore, conclusions regarding the best way to identify and diagnose individuals with FASD remain elusive. The lack of reliable and validated methods has also precluded an accurate description of the epidemiology of FASD in the general population.

The diagnosis of FASD is a highly debated issue [45] and a difficult task, particularly in those cases in which a physical marker of *in-utero* alcohol exposure is not readily observed. Efforts to identify FASD are further complicated by the fact that the definition of the condition identifies the mother's use of alcohol during pregnancy as the root of the problem. This circumstance increases a fear of stigmatization that may discourage families from seeking diagnosis or treatment [44].

There remain important gaps in our knowledge of what is the best approach towards identifying cases of FASD. Diagnostic tools that are culturally sensitive and that capture information regarding the considerable variability in the manifestation of FASD in different individuals and over the lifespan should be evaluated and implemented. In particular, it has been considered that early identification allows for a more effective intervention for children who have been affected by prenatal alcohol exposure.

2.5.3
FASD Treatment

This overview found that the evidence from systematic reviews on cognitive control therapy and psychostimulant medications for FASD does not indicate agreement about their effectiveness; therefore, no conclusions can be drawn regarding the benefits of these interventions. The best evidence is available for interventions that target cognitive and communication deficiencies which appear as disabilities secondary to FASD.

This overview emphasizes the importance of developing evidence-based treatments for individuals with FASD and their families across the entire lifespan. Since the first identification of FASD during the 1970s, the implications of treating FASD in adulthood are now coming to the fore. There is, at the present time, very little knowledge and virtually no evidence-based evaluation of services for individuals with FASD in their middle and old age.

A wide variety of barriers have precluded access to services directed to individuals with FASD. One of these is related to the fact that the term FASD is not intended for use as a clinical diagnosis, and many individuals who experience the detrimental consequences of prenatal alcohol exposure have to struggle with an often-misdiagnosed disability, encountering at every developmental phase an overwhelming set of barriers to finding appropriate resources [44]. Researchers and clinicians alike have underscored the importance of intervening with the entire spectrum of alcohol-exposed individuals [46]. There is a need to expand the evidence base that supports the effectiveness of interventions aimed at reducing the secondary disabilities commonly associated with FASD.

2.5.4
Methodological Quality of the Overview of Systematic Reviews

2.5.4.1 Strengths and Limitations
The strengths of this overview of systematic reviews pertain to the rigor of its literature searches, the criterion-based selection of relevant evidence, the rigorous appraisal of validity, and the evidence-based inferences. The search strategy is likely to have identified the majority of systematic reviews that evaluate preventive, diagnostic, or therapeutic interventions for FASD. The identification of multiple publications is also an important strength of this overview, as it prevented the inclusion of duplicate data that may have skewed the evidence in the analysis of the results.

In order to assess the methodological quality of the systematic reviews included in the overview, we adopted a comprehensive strategy that focused mainly on the control of bias that can affect the systematic review process. The AMSTAR tool is currently used in overviews published in the peer-reviewed literature [47–50], and this has been recommended as a first-line tool to evaluate the methodological quality of systematic reviews [51–53].

One potential limitation of this overview is its restriction to English-language publications. There is no evidence on the impact of the language of publication on the results of overviews of systematic reviews. It is, therefore, difficult to predict how the exclusion of non-English reviews may have biased the results of this overview. It should also be noted that, although only systematic reviews published in English language were included in this overview, some of the included reviews did not set language restrictions in their searches for primary studies.

2.6
Conclusions

The development, evaluation, and dissemination of preventive, diagnostic tools, and therapeutic evidence-based interventions for FASD and prenatal alcohol use have lagged significantly since the disorder was first identified during the 1970s. Encouragingly, some evidence has accumulated regarding the effectiveness of prenatal alcohol screening tools; certain preventive approaches to FASD and pre-natal alcohol use, such as brief and intensive interventions; and therapeutic options aimed at reducing cognitive and social disabilities experienced by individuals with FASD. It is important to increase efforts to expand the evidence base that is needed to inform policy and healthcare decisions regarding prevention, diagnosis, and treatment options for individuals with FASD and their families.

Appendix 2.A: Methodology

Search Strategy

Comprehensive searches of biomedical electronic databases listed in Table 2.A.1 were conducted for the period from 2004 to March 2010 to identify systematic reviews of the prevention, diagnosis, and treatment of FASD. The search strategy was designed by an Information Specialist at the Institute of Health Economics (IHE) and comprised both controlled vocabulary and keywords. The publication type was limited to systematic reviews/meta-analysis. In addition, reference lists of reviews and retrieved articles were browsed for relevant studies. Gray literature searches were conducted to identify literature from nontraditional sources, includ-ing proceedings from relevant scientific meetings, government documents, theses and dissertations, unpublished studies, and ongoing studies. The search was limited to English-language articles.

Study Selection Process

Two reviewers (M.O., C.M.) independently examined the titles and abstracts generated from the searches to identify potentially relevant systematic reviews

Table 2.A.1   Databases searched for relevant studies.

Database	Edition or date searched	Search Terms
Core Databases		
Cochrane Database of Systematic Review http://www. thecochranelibrary.com	2004 – Issue 1, 2010 (March 9, 2010)	f?etal alcohol in Title, Abstract or Keywords or (alcohol* or ethanol) AND (pregnan* OR fetus OR fetal OR prenatal OR in utero OR intrauterine) in Title, Abstract or Keywords
MEDLINE (OVID Interface) includes in process	2004 – March 9, 2010	1) Fetal Alcohol Syndrome/ 2) f?etal alcohol.tw. 3) ((alcohol* or ethanol) adj3 (birth defects or congenital malformations or neurodevelopmental)).mp 4) fasd.tw. 5) fae.tw. 6) arnd.tw. 7) arbd.tw. 8) or/1–7 9) Alcoholism/ 10) Alcoholic Intoxication/ 11) Alcohol-Induced Disorders/ 12) Alcohol-Related Disorders/ 13) Substance-Related Disorders/ and (alcohol* or ethanol).tw. 14) exp Alcoholic Beverages/ 15) Alcohol Drinking/ 16) Ethanol/ 17) or/9-16 18) exp Fetus/ 19) pregnancy/ or pregnancy, high-risk/ or exp pregnancy outcome/ 20) prenatal injuries/ or prenatal exposure delayed effects/ 21) Pregnancy Complications/ 22) Maternal Exposure/ 23) or/18–22 24) 17 and 23 25) ((alcohol* or ethanol or (drinking not drinking water)) and (pregnan* or fetus or fetal or prenatal or in utero or intrauterine)).tw. 26) limit 25 to ("in data review" or in process or "pubmed not medline") 27) 8 or 24 or 26 28) meta-analy*.mp,pt. 29) ([systematic* adj2 review*] or Medline or pubmed or psychinfo or psycinfo or search*).tw. 30) 28 or 29 31) 27 and 30 32) limit 31 to yr="2004–2010"

(Continued)

Table 2.A.1 *(Continued)*

Database	Edition or date searched	Search Terms
Embase (OVID Interface)	2004–March 9, 2010	1) fetal alcohol syndrome/ 2) f?etal alcohol.tw. 3) ([alcohol* or ethanol] adj3 [birth defects or congenital malformations or neurodevelopmental]).tw. 4) (fasd or fae or arnd or arbd).tw. 5) or/1–4 6) alcohol abuse/ 7) alcoholism/ 8) alcohol/ 9) exp alcoholic beverage/ 10) alcohol consumption/ 11) alcohol intoxication/ 12) or/6–11 13) pregnancy/ 14) fetus/ 15) prenatal*.mp. 16) or/13–15 17) 12 and 16 18) 5 or 17 19) meta-analy*.mp,pt. 20) systematic review/ 21) ((systematic* adj2 review*) or (MEDLINE or pubmed or psychinfo or psycinfo)).tw. 22) 19 or 20 or 21 23) 18 and 22 24) limit 23 to yr="2004 –Current"
CRD Databases (DARE, HTA & NHS EED)	2004–March 9, 2010	#1 "fetal alcohol" OR "fetal alcohol" #2 (alcohol* OR ethanol) AND (pregnancy OR fetus OR prenatal OR "birth defects") #1 OR #2
Google	March 17, 2010	Fetal alcohol systematic-review OR meta-analysis -pubmed -wiley -bmj

on prevention, diagnosis, or treatment of FASD. The full text of all studies deemed relevant was retrieved for a closer inspection. Two reviewers independently appraised the full manuscripts of potentially relevant studies to determine their eligibility for inclusion in the overview. Disagreements about eligibility were resolved through discussions among reviewers until consensus was reached.

Table 2.A.2 summarizes the eligibility criteria for the overview of reviews. Briefly, systematic reviews written or published in English were eligible for

Table 2.A.2 Study eligibility criteria.

Criterion	Description
Study topic	Prevention, diagnosis and treatment of FASD
Study design	Systematic reviews defined as scientific investigations with pre-planned methods that synthesize the results of multiple primary investigations by using strategies that limit bias and random [20]. They must: (1) have a clearly formulated research question; (2) define the search strategy used to identify studies for inclusion; (3) use explicit, reproducible and uniformly applied criteria for article selection; (4) critically appraise the included studies using a quality-assessment tool or checklist; and (5) attempt to analyze the data from primary studies.
Population	The reviews must focus on participants with a variety of risk-exposure levels for FASD across the lifespan.
Intervention	Reviews must assess the evidence from primary studies on an approach for prevention, diagnosis or treatment of FASD.
Language of publication	English only

FASD = fetal alcohol spectrum disorder.

inclusion in this overview of reviews. In order to be considered systematic, a review was required to: (1) have a clearly formulated research question; (2) define a search strategy for identifying studies for inclusion; (3) use explicit, reproducible, and uniformly applied criteria for article selection; (4) incorporate a critical appraisal of the included studies, using a quality-assessment tool or checklist; and (5) attempt to analyze the data from primary studies [20]. Reviews that statistically pooled results in a meta-analysis and those that conducted qualitative or semi-qualitative analysis were both eligible for inclusion. No restrictions were made on the study design of the primary research included in the systematic reviews. Excluded were editorials, correspondence, narrative reviews, abstracts, position papers and clinical practice guidelines.

Data Extraction

Data were extracted by one reviewer (M.O.) and cross-checked for accuracy and completeness by a second reviewer (C.M.). Information was collected on the topic of the review (i.e., prevention, diagnosis, treatment), the characteristics of the review (e.g., country, year, publication status, update status, funding sources), the PICOD components of the review, methodological characteristics (search strategy, language and publication restrictions, study selection process, methods for quality assessment of primary studies, and type of analysis), results (number of primary studies included, effect size, direction of the results, adverse events), and conclusions and recommendations for practice. Study selection, methodological quality assessment, and data extraction were managed with Microsoft Excel™ (Microsoft Corporation, Redmond, WA, USA).

Methodological Quality Assessment

The methodological quality of systematic reviews was assessed independently by two reviewers (M.O., C.M.) using the Assessment of Multiple Systematic Reviews tool (AMSTAR) [54] (Table 2.A.3). AMSTAR is an 11-item instrument that assesses the key attributes of a well-conducted systematic review (i.e., search strategy, study selection, quality assessment, data synthesis, publication bias, and declaration of potential conflict of interests). Each question has four responses: "yes", "no", "can't answer", and "not applicable." A "yes" gives a score of 1; any other response results in a score of 0. The overall score is out of 11. AMSTAR scores between 0 and 4 indicate that the review has low quality; scores between 5 and 8 indicate moderate quality; and scores of 9 to 11 indicate that the review is of high quality [54]. The AMSTAR tool has been shown to have high content validity and reliability [55, 56]. It is currently used in overviews published in the peer-reviewed literature [47–50], and has been recommended as a first-line tool for evaluating the methodological quality of systematic reviews [51–53]. Disagreements about methodological quality were resolved through discussions among reviewers until consensus was reached.

Table 2.A.3 Assessment of Multiple Systematic Reviews tool (AMSTAR).

Item	Rating
1. Was an "a priori" design provided? The research question and inclusion criteria should be established before the conduct of the review.	☐ Yes (1) ☐ No ☐ Can't answer ☐ Not applicable
2. Was there duplicate study selection and data extraction? There should be at least two independent data extractors and a consensus procedure for disagreements should be in place.	☐ Yes (1) ☐ No ☐ Can't answer ☐ Not applicable
3. Was a comprehensive literature search performed? At least two electronic sources should be searched. The report must include years and databases used (e.g., Central, Embase and MEDLINE). Key words and/or MESH terms must be stated and, where feasible, the search strategy should be provided. All searches should be supplemented by consulting reviews, textbooks, specialized registers, or experts in the particular field of study, and by reviewing the references in the studies found.	☐ Yes (1) ☐ No ☐ Can't answer ☐ Not applicable
4. Was the status of publication (i.e., gray literature) used as an inclusion criterion? The authors should state that they searched for reports, regardless of their publication type. The authors should state whether or not they excluded any reports (from the systematic review), based on their publication status, language, etc.	☐ Yes (1) ☐ No ☐ Can't answer ☐ Not applicable
5. Was a list of studies (included and excluded) provided? A list of included and excluded studies should be provided.	☐ Yes (1) ☐ No ☐ Can't answer ☐ Not applicable

(Continued)

Table 2.A.3 *(Continued)*

Item	Rating
6. Were the characteristics of the included studies provided? In an aggregated form such as a table, data from the original studies should be provided on the participants, interventions and outcomes. The ranges of characteristics in all the studies analyzed (e.g., age, race, gender, relevant socioeconomic data, disease status, duration, severity, or other diseases) should be reported.	☐ Yes (1) ☐ No ☐ Can't answer ☐ Not applicable
7. Was the scientific quality of the included studies assessed and documented? "A priori" methods of assessment should be provided (e.g., for effectiveness studies if the author(s) chose to include only randomized, double-blind, placebo-controlled studies, or allocation concealment as inclusion criteria; for other types of studies, alternative items will be relevant).	☐ Yes (1) ☐ No ☐ Can't answer ☐ Not applicable
8. Was the scientific quality of the included studies used appropriately in formulating conclusions? The results of the methodological rigor and scientific quality should be considered in the analysis and the conclusions of the review, and explicitly stated in formulating recommendations.	☐ Yes (1) ☐ No ☐ Can't answer ☐ Not applicable
9. Were the methods used to combine the findings of studies appropriate? For the pooled results, a test should be done to ensure the studies were combinable, to assess their homogeneity (i.e., chi-squared test for homogeneity, I^2). If heterogeneity exists, a random effects model should be used and/or the clinical appropriateness of combining should be taken into consideration (i.e., is it sensible to combine?).	☐ Yes (1) ☐ No ☐ Can't answer ☐ Not applicable
10. Was the likelihood of publication bias assessed? An assessment of publication bias should include a combination of graphical aids (e.g., funnel plot, other available tests) and/or statistical tests (e.g., Egger regression test).	☐ Yes (1) ☐ No ☐ Can't answer ☐ Not applicable
11. Was the conflict of interest stated? Potential sources of support should be clearly acknowledged in both the systematic review and the included studies.	☐ Yes (1) ☐ No ☐ Can't answer ☐ Not applicable

FINAL SCORE
Add up all "Yes" (scored as 1):

Data Analysis and Synthesis of the Results

Systematic reviews were classified and analyzed under the following major topics of interest: prevention, diagnosis, and treatment. Characteristics of the systematic reviews were summarized descriptively. Details were provided on the population studied, the research designs used, and the number of studies and participants on which the reviews were based. Evidence tables were prepared to synthesize the review characteristics and conclusions of selected systematic reviews. For each of the categories of prevention, diagnosis and treatment, evidence profiles were incorporated in the tables to evaluate the quality and type of evidence evaluated in the systematic reviews. For each systematic review, a radar plot was created to describe the distribution of the evidence, by study design, that was used to formulate the review conclusions.

Appendix 2.B: Excluded Studies and Multiple Publications

Excluded Research Studies

The application of the selection criteria resulted in 20 excluded studies. The main reasons for exclusion of studies from the overview were as follows: (1) the study was not a systematic review ($n = 11$); (2) the full text of the study was not retrieved ($n = 3$); (3) the study was primary research ($n = 2$); (4) the study topic was not prevention, diagnosis, or treatment of FASD ($n = 2$); and (5) the study did not report measurable data for the analysis/synthesis of the results ($n = 2$). The excluded studies, and the reasons for their exclusion from the overview, are listed in Table 2.B.1.

Table 2.B.1 Excluded research studies.

Main reason for exclusion:
The study was not a systematic review ($n = 11$)

Basford, D.L., Thorpe, K., and William, R. *State of the evidence: fetal alcohol spectrum disorder (FASD) prevention.* Edmonton, AB: Alberta Centre for Child, Family & Community Research/ University of Lethbridge, 2004.

Burd, L. and Hofer, R. Biomarkers for detection of prenatal alcohol exposure: a critical review of fatty acid ethyl esters in meconium. *Birth Defects Res.* 2008;82(7):487–493.

Caley, L.M., Shipkey, N., Winkelman, T., Dunlap, C., and Rivera, S. Evidence-based review of nursing interventions to prevent secondary disabilities in fetal alcohol spectrum disorder. *Pediatr. Nurs.* 2006;32(2):155–162.

Clarren, S.K. and Smith, D.W. The fetal alcohol syndrome: experience with 65 patients and a review of the world literature. *N. Engl. J. Med.* 1978;298:1063–1067.

(Continued)

Table 2.B.1 *(Continued)*

Main reason for exclusion:
The study was not a systematic review (*n* = 11**)**

D'Angiulli, A., Grunau, P., Maggi, S., and Herdman, A. Electroencephalographic correlates of prenatal exposure to alcohol in infants and children: a review of findings and implications for neurocognitive development. *Alcohol* 2006;40(2):127–133.

Finkelstein, N. Treatment Programming for Alcohol and Drug-Dependent Pregnant Women. *Int. J. Addict.* 1993;28(13):1275–1308.

Institute of Medicine (eds K. Stratton, C. Howe, and F. Battaglia), *Fetal Alcohol Syndrome: Diagnosis, Epidemiology, Prevention, and Treatment.* Washington, DC: National Academy Press; 1996.

May, P.A. Prevention of alcohol misuse: A review of health promotion efforts among American Indians. *Am. J. Health Promot.* 1995;9(4):288–299.

Murphy-Brennan, M.G. and Oei, T.P. Is there evidence to show that fetal alcohol syndrome can be prevented? *J. Drug Educ.* 1999;29(1):5–24.

Nayak, R.B. and Murthy, P. Fetal alcohol spectrum disorder. *Indian Pediatr.* 2008;45(12): 977–983.

Sokol, R.J., Delaney-Black, V., and Nordstrom, B. Fetal alcohol spectrum disorder. *JAMA* 2003;290:2996–2999.

Main reason for exclusion:
The full text of the study was not retrieved (*n* = 3**)**

Gronimus, R. Maternal alcohol consumption. *London J. Primary Care* 2009;(1):28–35.

Kodituwakku, P.W. Neurocognitive profile in children with fetal alcohol spectrum disorders. *Dev. Disabil. Res. Rev.* 2009;15(3):218–224.

Norman, A.L., Crocker, N., Mattson, S.N., and Riley, E.P. Neuroimaging and fetal alcohol spectrum disorders. *Dev. Disabil. Res. Rev.* 2009;15(3):209–217.

Main reason for exclusion:
The study was primary research (*n* = 2**)**

Astley, S.J. and Clarren, S.K. Diagnosing the full spectrum of fetal alcohol-exposed individuals: introducing the 4-digit diagnostic code. *Alcohol Alcohol.* 2000;35:400–410.

Leslie, M. and Roberts, G. *Enhancing fetal alcohol syndrome (FAS)-related interventions at the prenatal and early childhood stages in Canada.* Ottawa, ON: Canadian Center on Substance Abuse; 2001.

Main reason for exclusion:
The study topic was not prevention, diagnosis or treatment of FASD (*n* = 2**)**

Ashley, O.S. Effectiveness of substance abuse treatment programming for women: a review. *Am. J. Drug Alcohol Abuse* 2003;29(1):19–53.

Table 2.B.1 *(Continued)*

Main reason for exclusion:
The study topic was not prevention, diagnosis or treatment of FASD (*n* = 2)

Rayburn, W.F. and Bogenschutz, M.P. Pharmacotherapy for pregnant women with addictions. *Am. J. Obstet. Gynecol.* 2004;191(6):1885–1897.

Main reason for exclusion:
The study did not report measurable data for the analysis/synthesis of the results (*n* = 2)

Lui, S., Terplan, M., and Smith, E.J. Psychosocial interventions for women enrolled in alcohol treatment during pregnancy. *Cochrane Database of Systematic Reviews* 2008;(3):CD006753.

Smith, E.J., Lui, S., and Terplan, M. Pharmacologic interventions for pregnant women enrolled in alcohol treatment. *Cochrane Database of Systematic Reviews* 2009;(3):CD007361.

Multiple Publications of Studies Included in the Review

Of eight included articles, one was identified as a multiple publication; that is, a case in which the same study was published more than once. The multiple publication was not considered to be a unique review, and any information that was provided in it was incorporated into the data reported in the main publication of the review.

Table 2.B.2 Multiple publications.

Multiple publications of studies included in the review (*n* = 1)

Peadon, R. Health professionals making a difference: fetal alcohol spectrum disorder, alcohol and substance use in pregnancy, and breastfeeding. Perth, Western Australia; 2007. Available at: http://www.childhealthresearch.com.au/files/user22/E_Peadon_0.pdf. Associated publication of Peadon *et al.* (2009) [26]

Appendix 2.C: Summary Tables of Overall Characteristics of Systematic Reviews on Prevention, Diagnosis, and Treatment of FASD

Table 2.C.1   Characteristics of systematic reviews on prevention of FASD.

General information	Objective	Type and source of the evidence	Selection criteria	Review procedures	Review findings supporting effectiveness of the intervention; AMSTAR score
Doggett et al. [23]; Funding: Internal	*Objective* To determine the effects of home visits during pregnancy and/or after birth for pregnant women with a drug or alcohol problem. To examine the evidence for the timing, duration, intensity/frequency of the intervention, content of visits and effect of modifying factors	*Databases searched (n):* (5) Cochrane Pregnancy and Childbirth Trials Register, CENTRAL, MEDLINE, Embase, CINAHL. *Search periods:* 1966 to 2004 *Other sources:* Reference tracking, hand searches of journals, conference proceedings, contact with experts *Language restrictions:* No *Publication restrictions:* No	*Population* Pregnant or postpartum women with alcohol problems (i.e., self-report of alcohol abuse/binge) *Interventions* Home visits commencing during pregnancy and/or after birth *Comparisons* No home visits or a different type of home visiting intervention *Outcomes* Drug- and alcohol-related outcomes, pregnancy and puerperium outcomes, psychosocial outcomes *Study designs* RCT, CCT	*Procedures* Assessment of trials for inclusion performed independently and unblinded by all review authors. Data extraction performed independently by all authors using prepared DE forms *Quality assessment:* Allocation concealment criteria (Schultz)[30] *Type of analysis:* Quantitative (meta-analysis)	Unclear AMSTAR quality score: 10/11

Elliott *et al.* [22] Funding: Government	*Databases searched (n):* (4) Cochrane Library, MEDLINE, Embase, Scopus	*Population* General population, pregnant women, women at high risk of having a child with FASD	*Procedures* One reviewer scanned titles and abstracts and applied selection criteria for inclusion and appraisal in the review. DE by one reviewer and verified by another. Unclear how many assessed QA
Objective To evaluate the evidence pertaining to the relative effectiveness of various strategies to reduce the burden of FASD.	*Search periods:* 1966 to 2008	*Interventions* Any strategy aimed at FASD incidence; any alcohol screening tool designed to evaluate a woman's risk of having a child with FASD	*Quality assessment.* NHMRC quality checklist[34]
	Other sources: Reference tracking, hand searches of journals, conference proceedings, HTA websites	*Comparisons* Any	*Type of analysis:* Narrative synthesis
	Language restrictions: Yes	*Outcomes* – Prevention and prenatal screening: reduction in the incidence of FASD, reduction in alcohol use during pregnancy; sensitivity and specificity of screening tool; – Diagnosis and treatment: reduction in severity of primary/secondary disabilities or deficits associated with FASD; information on cost or cost-effectiveness of strategies to reduce the incidence and financial burden of FASD	– Prenatal screening (T-ACE and TWEAK) = Yes – Primary prevention = Unclear – Secondary prevention = Unclear – Tertiary prevention = Unclear AMSTAR quality score: 8/11
	Publication restrictions: Yes	*Study designs* Any	

(*Continued*)

Table 2.C.1 (*Continued*)

General information	Objective	Type and source of the evidence	Selection criteria	Review procedures	Review findings supporting effectiveness of the intervention; AMSTAR score
Ospina *et al.* [24]: Funding: Government	*Objective* To identify and evaluate the evidence on the effectiveness of universal, selective and indicated approaches to prevent the occurrence of FASD	*Databases searched (n):* (16) Cochrane Library, MEDLINE, Embase, CRD, CINAHL, Web of Science, PsycINFO, Sociological Abstracts, SocIndex, Social Services Abstracts, CBCA, CPI.Q, Canadian Research Index, AMA Clinical Practice Guidelines, CMA Infobase, National Guideline Clearinghouse *Search periods:* 1970 to 2010 *Other sources:* Reference tracking, hand searches of journals, conference proceedings, HTA websites, government reports, theses and dissertations, ongoing studies, contact with experts/ authors *Language restrictions:* Yes *Publication restrictions:* No	*Population* General population, pregnant women and partners at reproductive age, who have previously abused alcohol during pregnancy or who have had a child with FASD *Interventions* Universal, selective, indicated prevention approaches to FASD *Comparisons* Any *Outcomes* FASD incidence, alcohol consumption during pregnancy, neonatal and infant outcomes, risk-reduction measures, maternal outcomes (drinking behavior, relapse), legal, family, economic and health care utilization outcomes *Study designs* RCT, CCT, case-control studies, analytical cohort studies, ITS, before-and-after studies	*Procedures* Two reviewers independently assessed eligibility and quality; one reviewer extracted data and verified by a second reviewer *Quality assessment:* PHRED/ EPHPP quality tool [31] *Type of analysis:* Narrative synthesis	–Universal preventive approaches = Unclear – Selective preventive approaches = Yes Indicated preventive approaches = Unclear AMSTAR quality score: 10/11

Parkes et al. [25]
Funding: Government

Objective
To review the evidence from peer-reviewed literature on FASD-identification tools and brief and intensive interventions aimed at supporting women to reduce their use of alcohol in pregnancy or in the childbearing years

Databases searched (n):
(15) ASSIA, Australian Medical Index, CDSR, CINAHL, DARE, Drugscope, EBSCO Host, Eric, Ingenta, MD Consult, MEDLINE, PsycINFO, PubMed, Sociofile

Search periods:
1995 to 2007

Other sources:
Reference tracking, key websites

Language restrictions: Yes

Publication restrictions: NR

Population
Pregnant women and women in childbearing years

Interventions
Identification, assessment and screening for alcohol use in pregnancy; brief interventions with pregnant women and women in their childbearing years; intensive interventions for pregnant women and mothers

Comparisons
NR

Outcomes
Self-reported alcohol use, reduction in alcohol-exposed pregnancies, contraceptive behavior

Study designs
NR

Procedures
Titles were scanned; two independent reviewers assessed abstracts to select those that met the inclusion criteria; two reviewers independently rated the strength of the evidence, a better practices approach was used. Unclear how many did DE

Quality assessment: NICE Public Health Guidance Methods critical appraisal checklists [33]

Type of analysis: Narrative synthesis

– Identification and screening tools for perinatal alcohol use = Yes
– Brief intervention (MI) = Yes
– Intensive interventions = Yes

AMSTAR quality score: 6/11

Schorling [28]
Funding: NR

Objective
To critically review intervention studies on the prevention of prenatal alcohol use

Databases searched (n):
(2) MEDLINE, ETOH (Alcohol and Alcohol Problems Science) database

Search periods:
1973 to 1991

Other sources:
Reference tracking

Language restrictions: NR

Publication restrictions: NR

Population
Pregnant women

Interventions
Prenatal education and counseling to reduce prenatal alcohol use

Comparisons
NR

Outcomes
Alcohol use

Study designs
NR

Procedures
NR

Quality assessment: Eight methodological standards to assess threats to internal (n = 6) and external (n = 2) validity. Standards adapted from Goldstein et al. [35]; Sackett et al. [36] and Windsor et al. [37]

Type of analysis: Narrative synthesis

– Prenatal education = Yes
– Counseling = Yes

AMSTAR quality score: 4/11

(Continued)

Table 2.C.1 (Continued)

General information	Objective	Type and source of the evidence	Selection criteria	Review procedures	Review findings supporting effectiveness of the intervention; AMSTAR score
Stade et al. [29] Funding: Internal	*Objective* To determine the effectiveness of psychological and educational interventions to reduce alcohol consumption during pregnancy in pregnant women or women planning pregnancy. To describe any adverse effects on the mother or the fetus when psychological and/or educational interventions are used to reduce prenatal alcohol consumption	*Databases searched (n):* (6) Cochrane Library, CENTRAL, MEDLINE, Embase, CINAHL, PsycLIT *Search periods:* 1966 to 2008 *Other sources:* Reference tracking, hand searches of journals, conference proceedings, contact with experts *Language restrictions:* No *Publication restrictions:* No	*Population* Pregnant women or women planning for pregnancy who consume alcohol (i.e., self-report or urine/blood screening for alcohol) *Interventions* Psychological and educational interventions for reducing consumption of alcohol *Comparisons* No intervention, routine care, other educational and/or psychological interventions *Outcomes* Abstinence from alcohol during pregnancy, reduction of alcohol consumption during pregnancy to less than seven standard drinks a week, maternal and neonatal outcomes *Study designs* RCT	*Procedures* Five reviewers screened the studies; two reviewers independently abstracted information from studies. Unclear how many assessed QA *Quality assessment:* Risk of bias approach *Type of analysis:* Narrative synthesis	– Educational counseling intervention = Yes – MI = Yes – Brief intervention = Yes – Cognitive behavioral self-help intervention = Yes AMSTAR quality score: 9/11

AMSTAR = Assessment of Multiple Systematic Reviews; BA = before-and-after study; CCT = controlled clinical trial; DE = data extraction; EPHPP = Effective Public Health Practice Project; HTA = health technology assessment; ITS = interrupted time series; MA = meta-analysis; MI = motivational interview; NHMRC = National Health and Medical Research Council; NICE = National Institute for Health and Clinical Excellence; NR = not reported; PHRED = Public Health Research, Education and Development; QA = quality assessment; RCT = randomized controlled trial; T-ACE = Tolerance, Annoyed, Cut down, Eye-opener; TWEAK = Tolerance, Worried, Eye-opener, Amnesia, and K/Cut down.

Table 2.C.2 Characteristics of systematic reviews on diagnosis of FASD.

General information	Objective	Type and source of the evidence	Selection criteria	Review procedures	Review findings supporting effectiveness of the diagnostic approach; AMSTAR score
Elliott *et al.* [22] Funding: Government	*Objective* To evaluate the evidence pertaining to the relative effectiveness of various strategies to reduce the burden of FASD.	*Databases searched (n):* (4) Cochrane Library, MEDLINE, Embase, Scopus *Search periods:* 1966 to 2008 *Other sources:* Reference tracking, hand searches of journals, conference proceedings, HTA websites *Language restrictions:* Yes *Publication restrictions:* Yes	*Population* Individuals who may have FASD or mothers of individuals who may have FASD *Interventions* Any strategy aimed at identifying an individual who may have FASD or to diagnose an individual with FASD *Comparisons* Any *Outcomes* Sensitivity and specificity of FASD diagnosis *Study designs* Systematic reviews, diagnostic criteria or guidelines, primary research except case reports	*Procedures* One reviewer scanned titles and abstracts and applied selection criteria for inclusion and appraisal in the review *Quality assessment:* NR *Type of analysis:* Narrative synthesis	– Institute of Medicine diagnostic criteria = NR – 4-Digit Diagnostic Code = NR – Hoyme Updated Institute of Medicine Criteria = NR – Public Health Agency of Canada FASD referral guidelines = NR – CDC guidelines = NR – Canadian guidelines for the diagnosis of FASD = NR AMSTAR quality score: 6/11

AMSTAR = Assessment of Multiple Systematic Reviews; CDC = Center for Disease Control; FASD = fetal alcohol spectrum disorder; HTA = health technology assessment; NR = not reported.

Table 2.C.3 Characteristics of systematic reviews on treatment of FASD.

General information	Objective	Type and source of the evidence	Selection criteria	Review procedures	Review findings supporting effectiveness of the therapeutic approach; AMSTAR score
Elliott *et al.* [22] Funding: Government	*Objective* To evaluate the evidence pertaining to the relative effectiveness of various strategies to reduce the burden of FASD. To review the economics of FASD, i.e., the cost and cost-effectiveness of strategies targeting FASD, as well as the financial burden of FASD	*Databases searched (n):* (4) Cochrane Library, MEDLINE, Embase, Scopus *Search periods:* 1966 to 2008 *Other sources:* Reference tracking, hand searches of journals, conference proceedings, HTA websites *Language restrictions:* Yes *Publication restrictions:* Yes	*Population* Individuals with FASD *Interventions* Any strategy aimed at improving clinical outcomes *Comparisons* Any *Outcomes* Reduction in severity of primary/ secondary disabilities or deficits associated with FASD *Study designs* SR, CPG, review articles	*Procedures* One reviewer scanned titles and abstracts and applied selection criteria for inclusion and appraisal in the review *Quality assessment:* NR *Type of analysis:* Narrative synthesis	– Cognitive control therapy = Unclear – Psychostimulant medications = Yes AMSTAR quality score: 6/11

Peadon *et al.* [26] Funding: Government	*Objective* To identify and evaluate the evidence for pharmacological and non-pharmacological interventions for children with FASD	*Databases searched (n):* (6) Cochrane Library, MEDLINE, Embase, PsychINFO, CINAHL, Eric *Search periods:* 1950 to 2009 *Other sources:* Reference tracking, conference proceedings, contact with experts *Language restrictions:* No *Publication restrictions:* No	*Population* Individuals under 18 years of age with a diagnosis of FASD *Interventions* Pharmacological, behavioral, speech therapy, occupational therapy, physiotherapy, psychosocial and educational interventions and early intervention programs *Comparisons* No treatment, waiting list, usual therapy, placebo *Outcomes* Measures of physical and mental health, developmental status, cognitive status, quality of life, educational attainment, employment, contact with the law and substance abuse measures during and immediately after the intervention and/or in adolescence and adulthood *Study designs* RCT, CCT, before-and-after intervention studies	*Procedures* Selection of studies for inclusion, assessment of study quality and data extraction was undertaken independently by two reviewers *Quality assessment:* Individual components approach, blinding of outcome assessment, use of standardized measures. For RCTs: method of randomization, allocation concealment and ITT analysis *Type of analysis:* Narrative synthesis	– Cognitive control therapy = Yes – Language intervention focused on basic literacy skills = Yes – Math intervention = Yes – Virtual reality game interventions for child's safety = Yes – Teacher modeling strategy = Yes – Psychostimulant medications = Unclear – Social skills and social communication interventions = Yes – Behavioral interventions = Unclear AMSTAR quality score:8/11

(Continued)

Table 2.C.3 *(Continued)*

General information	Objective	Type and source of the evidence	Selection criteria	Review procedures	Review findings supporting effectiveness of the therapeutic approach; AMSTAR score
Premji *et al.* [27] Funding: Foundation	*Objective* To identify research-based interventions for children and youth with FASD	*Databases searched (n):* (63) Peer-reviewed and gray literature databases (MEDLINE, Embase, others no further specified) *Search periods:* 1973 to 2004 *Other sources:* Reference tracking, hand searches of journals, contact with experts *Language restrictions:* No *Publication restrictions:* No	*Population* Individuals under 18 years of age with a diagnosis of FASD *Interventions* Early interventions, strategies, education, medication. Intervention may target an individual with FASD, caregiver, or family of an affected individual *Comparisons* NR *Outcomes* Measures of cognitive status, impulsive behavior *Study designs* RCT, CCT	*Procedures* Two reviewers independently assessed eligibility and quality, and extracted data *Quality assessment:* Jadad scale [41], Allocation concealment criteria (Schultz) [30] *Type of analysis:* Narrative synthesis	– Cognitive control therapy = No – Psychostimulant medications = Unclear AMSTAR quality score:8/11

AMSTAR = Assessment of Multiple Systematic Reviews; CCT = controlled clinical trials; CPG = clinical practice guidelines; FASD = fetal alcohol spectrum disorder; ITT = intention to treat; NR = not reported; RCT = randomized controlled trials; SR = systematic reviews.

Appendix 2.D: Methodological Quality of Systematic Reviews Included in the Overview

Table 2.D.1 Methodological quality assessment of systematic reviews on prevention of FASD.

Systematic review	AM1	AM 2	AM3	AM4	AM5	AM6	AM7	AM8	AM9	AM10	AM11	Total AMSTAR score
Doggett, C. et al. [23]	Yes	Yes	Yes	Yes	Yes	Yes	Yes	Yes	Yes	No	Yes	10
Elliott, L. et al. [22]	Yes	No	Yes	No	Yes	Yes	Yes	Yes	Not applicable	Yes	Yes	8
Ospina, M. et al. [24]	Yes	Can't answer	Yes	Yes	Yes	Yes	Yes	Yes	Yes	Yes	Yes	10
Parkes, T. et al. [25]	Yes	No	Yes	Yes	No	Yes	Yes	No	Not applicable	No	Yes	6
Schorling, J.B. [28]	Yes	Can't answer	No	No	No	Yes	Yes	Yes	Not applicable	No	No	4
Stade, B.C. et al. [29]	Yes	Yes	Yes	Yes	Yes	Yes	Yes	Yes	Not applicable	No	Yes	9

AMSTAR = Assessment of Multiple Systematic Reviews; AM1 = Was an "a priori" design provided?; AM2 = Was there duplicate study selection and data extraction?; AM3 = Was a comprehensive literature search performed?; AM4 = Was the status of publication (i.e., gray literature) used as an inclusion criterion?; AM5 = Was a list of studies (included and excluded) provided?; AM6 = Were the characteristics of the included studies provided?; AM7 = Was the scientific quality of the included studies assessed and documented?; AM8 = Was the scientific quality of the included studies used appropriately in formulating conclusions?; AM9 = Were the methods used to combine the findings of studies appropriate?; AM10 = Was potential conflict of interest stated?

Table 2.D.2 Methodological quality assessment of systematic reviews on diagnosis of FASD.

Systematic review	AM1	AM2	AM3	AM4	AM5	AM6	AM7	AM8	AM9	AM10	AM11	Total AMSTAR score
Elliott, L. *et al.* [22]	Yes	No	Yes	No	Yes	Yes	No	No	Not applicable	Yes	Yes	6

AMSTAR = Assessment of Multiple Systematic Reviews: AM1 = Was an "a priori" design provided?; AM2 = Was there duplicate study selection and data extraction?; AM3 = Was a comprehensive literature search performed?; AM4 = Was the status of publication (i.e., gray literature) used as an inclusion criterion?; AM5 = Was a list of studies (included and excluded) provided?; AM6 = Were the characteristics of the included studies provided?; AM7 = Was the scientific quality of the included studies assessed and documented?; AM8 = Was the scientific quality of the included studies used appropriately in formulating conclusions?; AM9 = Were the methods used to combine the findings of studies appropriate?; AM10 = Was potential conflict of interest stated?

Table 2.D.3 Methodological quality assessment of systematic reviews on treatment of FASD.

Systematic review	AM1	AM2	AM3	AM4	AM5	AM6	AM7	AM8	AM9	AM10	AM11	Total AMSTAR score
Elliott, L. *et al.* [22]	Yes	No	Yes	No	Yes	Yes	Yes	Yes	Not applicable	Yes	Yes	8
Peadon, E. *et al.* [26]	Yes	Yes	Yes	Yes	No	Yes	Yes	Yes	Not applicable	No	Yes	8
Premji, S. *et al.* [27]	Yes	Yes	Yes	Yes	No	Yes	Yes	Yes	Not applicable	No	Yes	8

AMSTAR = Assessment of Multiple Systematic Reviews; AM1 = Was an "a priori" design provided?; AM2 = Was there duplicate study selection and data extraction?; AM3 = Was a comprehensive literature search performed?; AM4 = Was the status of publication (i.e., gray literature) used as an inclusion criterion?; AM5 = Was a list of studies (included and excluded) provided?; AM6 = Were the characteristics of the included studies provided?; AM7 = Was the scientific quality of the included studies assessed and documented?; AM8 = Was the scientific quality of the included studies used appropriately in formulating conclusions?; AM9 = Were the methods used to combine the findings of studies appropriate?; AM10 = Was potential conflict of interest stated?

References

1 Sokol, R.J., Delaney-Black, V., and Nordstrom, B. (2003) Fetal alcohol spectrum disorder. *JAMA*, **290**, 2996–2999.

2 Astley, S.J. and Clarren, S.K. (2000) Diagnosing the full spectrum of fetal alcohol-exposed individuals: introducing the 4-digit diagnostic code. *Alcohol Alcohol.*, **35**, 400–410.

3 Institute of Medicine (1996) *Fetal Alcohol Syndrome: Diagnosis, Epidemiology, Prevention, and Treatment*, National Academy Press, Washington, DC.

4 Hoyme, H.E., May, P.A., Kalberg, W.O., Kodituwakkn, P., Gossage, J.P., Trujillo, P.M., *et al.* (2005) A practical clinical approach to diagnosis of fetal alcohol spectrum disorders: clarification of the 1996 Institute of Medicine criteria. *Pediatrics*, **115** (1), 39–47.

5 May, P.A., Gossage, J.P., Kalberg, W.O., Robinson, L.K., Buckley, D., Manning, M., *et al.* (2009) Prevalence and epidemiologic characteristics of FASD from various research methods with an emphasis on recent in-school studies. *Dev. Disabil. Res. Rev.*, **15**, 176–192.

6 Clarren, S.K. and Lutke, J. (2008) Building clinical capacity for fetal alcohol spectrum disorder diagnoses in western and northern Canada. *Can. J. Clin . Pharmacol.*, **15** (2), 223–237.

7 Abel, E.L. and Hannigan, J.H. (1995) Maternal risk factors in fetal alcohol syndrome: provocative and permissive influences. *Neurotoxicol. Teratol.*, **17**, 445–462.

8 Kelly, S.J., Goodlett, C.R., and Hannigan, J.H. (2009) Animal models of fetal alcohol spectrum disorders: impact of the social environment. *Dev. Disabil. Res. Rev.*, **15** (3), 200–208.

9 Majewski, F. (1993) Alcohol embryopathy: experience in 200 patients. *Dev. Brain Dysfunc.*, **6**, 248–265.

10 Clarren, S.K. and Smith, D.W. (1978) The fetal alcohol syndrome: experience with 65 patients and a review of the world literature. *N. Engl. J. Med.*, **298**, 1063–1067.

11 Guerri, C., Bazinet, A., and Riley, E.P. (2009) Foetal alcohol spectrum disorders and alterations in brain and behaviour. *Alcohol Alcohol.*, **44** (2), 108–114.

12 Norman, A.L., Crocker, N., Mattson, S.N., and Riley, E.P. (2009) Neuroimaging and fetal alcohol spectrum disorders. *Dev. Disabil. Res. Rev.*, **15** (3), 209–217.

13 Fukui, Y. and Sakata-Haga, H. (2009) Intrauterine environment-genome interaction and children's development (1): ethanol: a teratogen in developing brain. *J. Toxicol. Sci.*, **34** (Suppl. 2), SP273–SP278.

14 Manji, S., Pei, J., Loomes, C., and Rasmussen, C.A. (2009) review of the verbal and visual memory impairments in children with foetal alcohol spectrum disorders. *Dev. Neurorehabil.*, **12** (4), 239–247.

15 Kodituwakku, P.W. (2009) Neurocognitive profile in children with fetal alcohol spectrum disorders. *Dev. Disabil. Res. Rev.*, **15** (3), 218–224.

16 Spohr, H.L. and Steinhausen, H.C. (2008) Fetal alcohol spectrum disorders and their persisting sequelae in adult life. *Dtsch. Arztebl. Int.*, **105** (41), 693–698.

17 Streissguth, A.P., Barr, H.M., Kogan, J., and Bookstein, F. (1996) *Understanding the Occurrence of Secondary Disabilities in Clients with Fetal Alcohol Syndrome (FAS) and Fetal Alcohol Effects (FAE). Final Report to the Centers for Disease Control and Prevention (CDC)*, University of Washington, Fetal Alcohol and Drug Unit, Seattle.

18 Steinhausen, H.C., Willms, J., and Spohr, H.L. (1993) The long-term psychopathological and cognitive outcome of children with fetal alcohol syndrome. *J. Am. Acad. Child Adolesc. Psychiatry*, **32**, 990–994.

19 Streissguth, A. and Kanter, J. (1997) *The Challenge of Fetal Alcohol Syndrome: Overcoming Secondary Disabilities*, University of Washington Press, Seattle.

20 Cook, D.J. and Mulrow, C.D. (1997) Systematic reviews: synthesis of best evidence for clinical decisions. *Ann. Intern. Med.*, **126**, 376–380.

21 Becker, L.A. and Oxman, A. (2008) Overview of reviews, in *Cochrane*

Handbook for Systematic Reviews of Interventions (eds J.P.T. Higgins and S. Green), John Wiley & Sons, Chichester, UK.

22 Elliott, L., Coleman, K., Suebwongpat, A., and Norris, S. (2008) Fetal Alcohol Spectrum Disorders (FASD): systematic reviews of prevention, diagnosis and management. Health Services Assessment Collaboration Report, 1 (9), i–535.

23 Doggett, C., Burrett, S., and Osborn, D.A. (2005) Home visits during pregnancy and after birth for women with an alcohol or drug problem. *Cochrane Database Syst. Rev.* 4 (Art. No.: 004456).

24 Ospina, M.B., Moga, C., Dennett, L., and Harstall, C. (2011) *A systematic review of the effectiveness of prevention approaches for fetal alcohol spectrum disorder, in Prevention of Fetal Alcohol Spectrum Disorder FASD: Who is Responsible?* (eds S.K. Clarren, A. Salmon and E. Jonsson), Wiley-Blackwell.

25 Parkes, T., Poole, N., Salmon, A., Greaves, L., and Urquhart, C. (2008) *Double Exposure: A Better Practices Review on Alcohol Interventions during Pregnancy*, Centre of Excellence for Women's Health, Vancouver, BC.

26 Peadon, E., Rhys-Jones, B., Bower, C., and Elliott, E.J. (2009) Systematic review of interventions for children with Fetal Alcohol Spectrum Disorders. *BMC Pediatr.*, 9, 35.

27 Premji, S., Benzies, K., Serrett, K., and Hayden, K.A. (2007) Research-based interventions for children and youth with a Fetal Alcohol Spectrum Disorder: revealing the gap. *Child Care Health Dev.*, 33 (4), 389–397.

28 Schorling, J.B. (1993) The prevention of prenatal alcohol use: a critical analysis of intervention studies. *J. Stud. Alcohol*, 54 (3), 261–267.

29 Stade, B.C., Bailey, C., Dzendoletas, D., Sgro, M., Dowswell, T., and Bennett, D. (2009) Psychological and/or educational interventions for reducing alcohol consumption in pregnant women and women planning pregnancy. *Cochrane Database Syst. Rev.* 2 (Art. No.: 004228).

30 Schulz, K.F., Chalmers, I., Hayes, R.J., and Altman, D.G. (1995) Empirical evidence of bias: dimensions of methodological quality associated with estimates of treatment effects in controlled trials. *JAMA*, 273, 408–412.

31 Thomas, H., Ciliska, D., Dobbins, M., and Micucci, S. (2004) A process for systematically reviewing the literature: providing the research evidence for public health nursing interventions26. *Worldviews Evid. Based Nurs.*, 2, 91–99.

32 Higgins, J.P.T. and Green, S. (eds) (2008) *Cochrane Handbook for Systematic Reviews of Interventions*, John Wiley & Sons, Ltd, Chichester, UK.

33 National Institute for Health and Clinical Excellence (2007) *The Guidelines Manual*, NICE, London, UK.

34 National Health and Medical Research Council (2000) *How to Review the Evidence: Systematic Identification and Review of the Scientific Literature*, NHMRC, Canberra.

35 Goldstein, M.S., Surber, M., and Wilner, D.M. (1984) Outcome evaluations in substance abuse: a comparison of alcoholism, drug abuse, and other mental health interventions. *Int. J. Addict.*, 19, 479–502.

36 Sackett, D.L., Haynes, P.B., and Tugwell, P. (1991) *Clinical Epidemiology: A Basic Science for Clinical Medicine*, 2nd edn, Little, Brown & Co, Boston.

37 Windsor, R.A., Baranowski, T., Clark, N., and Cutter, G. (1984) *Evaluation of Health Promotion and Education Programs*, Mayfield Publishing Co, Palo Alto, CA.

38 Public Health Agency of Canada (2005) *Fetal Alcohol Spectrum Disorder (FASD): A Framework for Action*, Public Health Agency of Canada, Ottawa.

39 National Center on Birth Defects and Developmental Disabilities (2004) *Fetal Alcohol Syndrome: Guidelines for Referral and Diagnosis*, Centers for Disease Control and Prevention, Atlanta, GA.

40 Chudley, A.E., Conry, J., Cook, J.L., Loock, C., Rosales, T., and LeBlanc, N. (2005) Fetal alcohol spectrum disorder: Canadian guidelines for diagnosis. *Can. Med. Assoc. J.*, 172 (5 Suppl.), S1–S21.

41 Jadad, A.R., Moore, R.A., Carroll, D., Jenkinson, C., Reynolds, D.J., Gavaghan, D.J., *et al.* (1996) Assessing the quality of reports of randomized clinical trials: is

blinding necessary? *Controlled Clin. Trials*, **17** (1), 1–12.

42 Alcohol Healthwatch (2007) *Fetal Alcohol Spectrum Disorder in New Zealand: Activating the Awareness and Intervention Continuum*, Alcohol Healthwatch, Auckland.

43 Floyd, R.L., Weber, M.K., Denny, C., and O'Connor, M.J. (2009) Prevention of fetal alcohol spectrum disorders. *Dev. Disabil. Res. Rev.*, **15**, 193–199.

44 Paley, B. (2009) Introduction: fetal alcohol spectrum disorders: shedding light on an unseen disability. *Dev. Disabil. Res. Rev.*, **15**, 167–169.

45 Mancinelli, R., Ceccanti, M., and Laviola, G. (2007) Fetal alcohol spectrum disorders (FASD): from experimental biology to the search for treatment. *Neurosci. Biobehav. Rev.*, **31** (2), 165–167.

46 Paley, B. and O'Connor, M.J. (2009) Intervention for individuals with fetal alcohol spectrum disorders: treatment approaches and case management. *Dev. Disabil. Res. Rev.*, **15**, 258–267.

47 Mikton, C. and Butchart, A. (2009) Child maltreatment prevention: a systematic review of reviews. *Bull. World Health Org.*, **87** (5), 353–361.

48 Prior, M., Guerin, M., and Grimmer-Somers, K. (2008) The effectiveness of clinical guideline implementation strategies: a synthesis of systematic review findings. *J. Eval. Clin. Pract.*, **14** (5), 888–897.

49 Kamioka, H., Tsutani, K., Okuizumi, H., Mutoh, Y., Ohta, M., Handa, S., *et al.* (2010) Effectiveness of aquatic exercise and balneotherapy: a summary of systematic reviews based on randomized controlled trials of water immersion therapies. *J. Epidemiol.*, **20** (1), 2–12.

50 Sakzewski, L., Ziviani, J., and Boyd, R. (2009) Systematic review and meta-analysis of therapeutic management of upper-limb dysfunction in children with congenital hemiplegia. *Pediatrics*, **123** (6), e1111–e1122.

51 Oxman, A.D., Schunemann, H.J., and Fretheim, A. (2006) Improving the use of research evidence in guideline development: synthesis and presentation of evidence. *Health Res. Policy Syst.*, **5**, 4–20.

52 Canadian Coordinating Office for Health Technology Assessment (2005) *Evaluation Tools for COMPUS*, Canadian Coordinating Office for Health Technology Assessment, Ottawa.

53 The Cochrane Collaboration (2009) *The Cochrane Collaboration Methods Groups Newsletter, 13*, The UK Cochrane Centre.

54 Shea, B., Grimshaw, J.M., Wells, G.A., Boers, M., Andresson, N., *et al.* (2007) Development of AMSTAR: a measurement tool to assess systematic reviews. *BMC Med. Res. Methodol.*, **7** (10); doi:10.1186/1471-2288-7-10.

55 West, S., King, V., Carey, T.S., Lohr, K.N., McKoy, N., Sutton, S.F., *et al.* (2002) Systems to rate the strength of scientific evidence. Evidence Report/ Technology Assessment No. 28. Rockville, MD: Agency for Healthcare Research and Quality.

56 Shea, B.J., Hamel, C., Wells, G.A., Bouter, L.M., Kristjansson, E., Grimshaw, J., *et al.* (2010) AMSTAR is a reliable and valid measurement tool to assess the methodological quality of systematic reviews. *J. Clin. Epidemiol.*, **62** (10), 1013–1020.

3

A Systematic Review of the Effectiveness of Prevention Approaches for Fetal Alcohol Spectrum Disorder

Maria Ospina, Carmen Moga, Liz Dennett, and Christa Harstall

Summary

Fetal alcohol spectrum disorder (FASD) is an umbrella term that refers to a group of disorders that are associated with prenatal alcohol exposure. FASD is characterized by prenatal and postnatal impairments, such as growth retardation, a unique cluster of facial anomalies, and a variety of neurological, cognitive, and behavioral disorders. Many preventive approaches have been proposed to reduce the risk of FASD by influencing women to reduce their alcohol consumption during pregnancy. Preventive approaches to FASD can be classified into three main categories—universal, selective, and indicated approaches—according to the breadth of the target group, the risk of having children with the disorder, and the cost–benefit ratio of committing resources to the prevention strategy:

- *Universal preventive approaches* are broad strategies targeting the general public or whole population groups that have not been identified on the basis of risk. These approaches aim to educate the public about the risks of drinking during pregnancy.

- *Selective preventive approaches* are more specifically targeted and intense than universal approaches. The targets of selective prevention strategies are subgroups of women and their partners from the general population who are at risk of having children with FASD (e.g., women of reproductive age and their partners who drink alcohol, women who drink while pregnant, and women who belong to vulnerable subgroups).

- *Indicated prevention strategies* target women who are at the highest risk of having a child with FASD (e.g., women who previously abused alcohol while pregnant, pregnant women who are experiencing early signs of alcohol abuse, women who already have a child with FASD, women with FASD, and women with alcohol problems who do not use effective contraception). This

(Continued)

Prevention of Fetal Alcohol Spectrum Disorder FASD: Who is Responsible?, First Edition. Edited by Sterling Clarren, Amy Salmon, Egon Jonsson.
© 2011 Wiley-VCH Verlag GmbH & Co. KGaA. Published 2011 by Wiley-VCH Verlag GmbH & Co. KGaA.

level of prevention includes treatment of alcoholism in women who are pregnant or likely to become pregnant.

The prevention of FASD is a public health priority, and a variety of programs have been developed to prevent drinking during pregnancy and thus reduce the incidence of FASD. However, some have argued that the paucity of evaluative research on FASD-prevention programs makes it difficult to draw convincing inferences about the effectiveness of FASD-prevention strategies. A scientifically rigorous evaluation of prevention strategies that have been implemented in clinical and community settings is needed to inform the selection and implementation of these programs.

Objectives

This is a systematic review of the scientific literature on preventive approaches to FASD. The objective of the review was to identify and evaluate evidence on the effectiveness of universal, selective, and indicated approaches to preventing the occurrence of FASD.

Results

General Characteristics

A total of 50 studies on the effectiveness of preventive approaches to FASD was included in this systematic review. Half of the studies were published at least a decade ago, and most were conducted in the United States. Two Canadian studies met the selection criteria of the review. The review includes 19 clinical trials (six randomized control trials [RCTs] and 13 controlled clinical trials [CCTs]), 19 before-and-after studies with no comparison group, 11 observational analytical cohort studies, and one interrupted time series study.

Populations and Settings

Most of the studies were conducted in urban health facilities with study populations consisting mainly of pregnant women and women at risk of an alcohol-exposed pregnancy (AEP). The studies did not include partners or support persons in the evaluation of the intervention. Five studies evaluated interventions directed only to Native American populations. None of the studies conducted in Canadian Aboriginal populations met the selection criteria for the review.

Types of Preventive Approaches to FASD

The most frequently studied FASD-prevention approaches were selective approaches (23 studies), followed by universal approaches (18 studies), and indicated approaches (9 studies). RCTs were conducted to evaluate selective prevention approaches only. Universal and indicated approaches were mainly evaluated by means of before-and-after studies with no comparison groups. Counseling activities were the most frequently implemented interventions in the

studies (25 studies), followed by health teaching (18 studies), and social market-
ng interventions (11 studies).

Outcomes

The effectiveness of FASD-prevention approaches was evaluated through the
assessment of a variety of outcomes. Of these, the majority ($n = 69$) were intermediate outcomes related to changes in drinking behavior, while 47 were ultimate outcomes that represented changes in the status of a condition in the
mother or the child. Immediate outcomes ($n = 32$) were less frequently addressed
in studies on FASD prevention.

The most frequently studied outcome was self-reported alcohol intake (i.e.,
abstinence, use, abuse; $n = 63$), followed by neonatal and infant outcomes
($n = 31$) and knowledge about alcohol use during pregnancy ($n = 17$).

Methodological Quality

The majority of the studies were of poor methodological quality. Of the 50
studies reviewed, 37 were rated as "weak," 12 as "moderate", and one was rated
"strong" in methodology. Overall, the studies that evaluated selective approaches
were of a higher quality than the studies assessing universal and indicated
approaches.

Evidence on the Effectiveness of FASD Universal Prevention Approaches

Evidence on the effectiveness of universal prevention approaches to FASD was
provided by 18 studies, including two of Canadian origin. The studies were
conducted mainly in health facilities or in the community, and targeted pregnant
women and the broad general public in urban settings. The majority of the
studies were conducted in non-Caucasian populations. Three of the studies
evaluated the impact of a universal preventive intervention in Native American
populations, while the remainder combined the results for participants of other
ethnicities. Social marketing activities were the most frequently implemented
universal interventions, followed by health teaching interventions. Individual
components of the interventions included education (e.g., audiovisual materials, mass media strategies, motivational messages, computer-based education)
and legal/system activities (e.g., warning messages on alcohol beverage labels,
alcohol bans in the community).

The effectiveness of universal prevention approaches was evaluated mainly
through assessing immediate outcomes. The most frequently studied outcome
was acquisition of knowledge regarding FASD and alcohol use during pregnancy
(15 outcomes), followed by changes in alcohol intake and attitudes toward
alcohol use during pregnancy.

A qualitative synthesis of individual study results showed that universal programs were generally of poor quality and mixed effect. When effective, the
improvements seemed to be in the area of knowledge acquisition. The best

(Continued)

evidence for the effectiveness of universal prevention approaches to FASD is from a nonrandomized clinical trial of moderate quality which showed that an educational multimedia program could significantly increase youths' knowledge of FASD after two weeks. No information was available as to whether this knowledge gain was sustained over time, however. Evidence on the effectiveness of other universal interventions, such as alcohol-related warning messages, health education activities, and alcohol bans, is based on studies of poor methodological quality. Overall, these studies did not show that universal interventions produced significant modifications over time in knowledge of FASD, attitudes toward drinking during pregnancy and the perception of risks associated with this behavior. In the few studies that evaluated changes in alcohol intake, none of the interventions significantly modified self-reported measures of alcohol intake. Only a few studies have been conducted during the past five years, and it is unknown whether universal interventions that were implemented 15–20 years ago are still relevant and sensitive to current societal and technological changes.

Evidence on the Effectiveness of FASD Selective Prevention Approaches

Evidence on the effectiveness of selective prevention approaches for FASD was provided in 23 studies, among which were six RCTs and eight CCTs. No Canadian studies of selective prevention approaches were identified. The studies were conducted mainly in urban health facilities among pregnant women and women at risk of an AEP. Only two studies focused exclusively on non-Caucasian populations (i.e., Native Americans and Hispanics). Counseling activities were the most frequent interventions, followed by health teaching, referrals and follow-up, and screening and case-finding activities. Individual components of the interventions included brief interventions (counseling) and education activities.

The most frequently studied outcomes were intermediate outcomes, such as self-reported alcohol intake, followed by neonatal and infant outcomes. A qualitative synthesis showed that the methodology of studies of selective prevention approaches was slightly better than that of studies of universal prevention approaches. Some studies provided evidence for making inferences regarding the effectiveness of selective prevention approaches. The best evidence was obtained from studies on counseling activities directed to pregnant women, women of childbearing age who consume alcohol, and women who were at risk of an AEP. One study that was rated strong in methodological quality and three studies of moderate quality concluded that counseling was effective at reducing the risk of an AEP and the frequency of alcohol consumption. Studies of moderate quality also reported that counseling had a positive effect on neonatal outcomes, such as birth weight and mortality rates. Selective programs that involved health education demonstrated at least short-term benefits. Two studies of moderate quality provided evidence that health education directed to pregnant women increased their knowledge of the effects of alcohol use during pregnancy, and reduced their alcohol consumption in the short term (less than three months of follow-up following intervention). There was no evidence that these effects were sustained over time, however. One study of moderate quality provided evidence that health education was effective in increasing the number of normal spontaneous vaginal deliveries. No other maternal outcomes related to alcohol exposure were evaluated.

The positive results associated with counseling and health education programs as selective FASD-prevention interventions should be interpreted with caution. A small number of studies of moderate quality did not find that these interventions had any significant effect on alcohol use during pregnancy. Compared to studies conducted many years ago on the effects of other preventive approaches, the results of recent studies of selective interventions may be more applicable to the current times.

Evidence on the Effectiveness of FASD Indicated Prevention Approaches

Evidence on the effectiveness of indicated approaches to FASD prevention was provided by nine studies, half of which were published before 1999. No Canadian studies on indicated prevention approaches to FASD were identified. More than half of the studies were before-and-after studies with no comparison group. The studies were conducted mainly in urban health facilities among women at a high risk of an AEP because of their level of alcohol consumption. Two studies focused exclusively on Native American populations. Counseling was the most frequent intervention, followed by case management, referrals, and follow-up activities. The most frequently studied outcomes were ultimate outcomes, such as neonatal and child-related outcomes, followed by intermediate outcomes such as self-reported measures of alcohol intake and abstinence.

A qualitative synthesis of the results of individual studies showed that, overall, there was limited evidence of the effectiveness of indicated programs. The methodological quality of the studies was poor, precluding the application of their results to inform practice. One study which assessed a multifaceted intervention (i.e., the Four-State FAS Consortium initiative) was considered to be of moderate quality, but it is unknown whether the intervention effectively modified such outcomes as alcohol use, perceptions of alcohol use, well-being, family functioning, and mental health status during pregnancy. The evidence base to support the effectiveness of indicated preventive approaches is weak.

Conclusions

There is a substantial gap in our knowledge of the effectiveness of preventive approaches to FASD. Most research on the potential benefits of prevention strategies has examined the effects of interventions in a range of clinical and community settings in the United States. Study participants have consisted mainly of pregnant adult women and adult women at risk of an AEP because

(Continued)

their use of alcohol was either suspected or confirmed. Only two Canadian studies – one conducted in Saskatchewan and another in Manitoba – met the inclusion criteria for the review. Both of these studies evaluated the effects of a universal FASD-prevention approach targeting the general public. Canadian studies evaluating the effects of selective and indicated FASD-prevention approaches are scarce in the scientific literature, and therefore no conclusions can be made regarding the applicability of the review findings to the Canadian population.

The evidence base to support decisions regarding preventive interventions for FASD is weak, particularly for universal and indicated approaches. Moderate to strong evidence supporting the counseling of pregnant women and women at risk of an AEP was identified. However, these results should be interpreted with caution. Many studies of prevention programs have significant methodological problems that make conclusions regarding the effectiveness of the programs tenuous.

Considering the importance of, and demand for, interventions to prevent FASD, and the current increase in new programs, a rigorous synthesis of high-quality evidence on the effectiveness of the spectrum of preventive interventions for FASD was undertaken to provide much-needed information for the clinical community, policy makers, researchers, and families. In spite of the published studies on the subject, there remains deep controversy and no definitive answer regarding the "best" approach to preventing the occurrence of FASD.

Management decisions should be guided by the needs of the community and the availability of resources for intervention. Research on new prevention strategies is recommended, as the majority of the studies summarized in this review were conducted before 2000, and the conditions under which the interventions were evaluated may have changed. Future studies on the effectiveness of preventive interventions need to be more rigorous. Only two Canadian studies were identified; hence, more effort should be made to publish and disseminate the results of research on prevention programs that have been implemented and evaluated in Canada. Yet, this body of evidence remains mostly unpublished and unknown to the broad public.

Methodology

Comprehensive searches of psychological, sociological, and biomedical electronic databases were conducted for articles published between 1970 (or database inception) and March 2010. In addition, the reference lists of retrieved articles were browsed for relevant studies. Other searches were conducted to identify literature from nontraditional sources, including proceedings from scientific meetings, government documents, theses and dissertations, unpublished studies, and ongoing studies. Two reviewers independently applied a set of inclusion and exclusion criteria to select the studies for the review, and also assessed the methodological quality of the included studies. Each study that met the selection criteria was classified into one of three categories of FASD-prevention approaches: universal, selective, or indicated. Due to the heterogeneity in study designs, populations, interventions, and outcomes, a meta-analysis of study data was not possible; therefore, a narrative synthesis of study results was undertaken. Evidence tables were constructed to describe study characteristics, methodological quality, and individual study results. Study outcomes were analyzed based on the report of statistically significant differences in the analysis of the individual studies.

3.1
Introduction

Fetal alcohol spectrum disorder (FASD) is an umbrella term that refers to a spectrum or range of clinical conditions associated with prenatal exposure to alcohol [1]. Four types of FASD have been described (Table 3.1) that are characterized by one or more of the following conditions: prenatal and postnatal growth retardation; a unique cluster of facial anomalies; central nervous system impairments (neurological, cognitive and behavioral) [2]; and physical defects.

The prevalence of fetal alcohol syndrome (FAS) in the United States has been estimated at one to three per 1000 live births [3] in most populations. In some communities, the rate of FASD surpasses these estimates, being as high as five to 10 cases per 1000 live births [4]. For example, FAS rates of about 10 per 1000 live births have been reported among Southwestern Plains Indians living on

Table 3.1 Fetal alcohol spectrum disorder subtypes.

Subtypes	Description
Fetal alcohol syndrome (FAS)	Diagnostic classification for individuals who were prenatally exposed to alcohol and who present with growth deficiency, height or weight below the 10th percentile, facial anomalies (e.g., small eyes, smooth philtrum and thin upper lip) and central nervous system damage (structural, neurological and/or functional impairment)
Partial Fetal Alcohol Syndrome (pFAS)	Diagnostic classification for individuals who were prenatally exposed to alcohol and who present with some, but not all, of the physiological symptoms of full FAS
Alcohol-related Neurodevelopmental Disorder (ARND)	Diagnostic classification for individuals who were prenatally exposed to alcohol and who have symptoms of central nervous system damage associated with FAS, but do not present the facial features typical of FAS
Alcohol-related Birth Defects (ARBD)	Diagnostic classification for individuals who were prenatally exposed to alcohol and who have physical defects, such as malformations of the heart, bones, kidney, and vision or hearing systems

reserves in the United States [3]. There are no national statistics on the rates of FASD in Canada, although some studies have estimated its prevalence in high-risk populations. An FASD prevalence of 190 per 1000 live births was estimated among individuals from an isolated Aboriginal community in British Columbia [5]. In northeastern Manitoba, an incidence of about 7.2 per 1000 live births was found [6]. In another study conducted in a First Nations community in Manitoba, the prevalence of FAS and partial fetal alcohol syndrome (pFAS) was estimated to be between 55 and 101 per 1000 live births [7]. The rate of FAS and related effects has been estimated at 46 per 1000 among Native Canadian children in the Yukon, and 25 per 1000 in northern British Columbia [8]. Variations in prevalence rates result from differences in the populations being studied, in the case definitions and the methods used to identify the cases.

FASD, which is caused by maternal alcohol use during pregnancy [7], is one of the leading causes of birth defects and developmental disabilities in Canadian children, along with spina bifida and Down syndrome [9]. However, it is the only one of the three conditions that is considered largely preventable [10, 11].

Children who are exposed to alcohol prenatally and develop FASD may experience longlasting effects on their physical and psychosocial development. Mild effects include the loss of some intellectual functioning, hearing and visual problems, and a higher than normal pain tolerance. Severe effects include the loss of intellectual potential, severe vision problems, dyslexia, serious maxillo-facial deformities, dental abnormalities, heart defects, immune system malfunc-tioning, behavioral problems, attention-deficit disorder, hyperactivity, extreme impulsiveness, poor judgment, difficulty with memory retention and retrieval, hearing disorders, little capacity for moral judgment or interpersonal empathy, sociopathic behavior, epilepsy, tremors, cerebral palsy, renal failure, heart failure, and death [4].

There is currently no consensus within the scientific community regarding the adverse and irreversible effects of low to moderate prenatal alcohol exposure, or whether a safe level of alcohol consumption during pregnancy exists [4, 12, 13]. The early identification of women at risk for an AEP and intervention before con-ception are critical to preventing FASD. Since FASD was first described in the medical literature almost 40 years ago, a number of efforts have been made to prevent its occurrence among women of childbearing age, and among high-risk subgroups in particular. Some efforts have been also directed towards including male partners in FASD-prevention activities. Although data relating to the possible role of paternal factors in the genesis of FASD is still sparse, the social, psychologi-cal, and supportive roles that male partners play during pregnancy is well estab-lished [4, 14]. Since women who drink heavily tend to associate with men who are also heavy drinkers [15], the importance of including men as a target of FASD-preventive activities has been increasingly recognized [4].

According to a conceptual framework proposed by the Institute of Medicine in the United States [4, 14], prevention approaches to FASD can be grouped into three main categories: universal, selective, and indicated approaches. These categories are organized along a targeted-audience continuum that takes into account the breadth of the target group, the risk of having a child with the disorder, and the

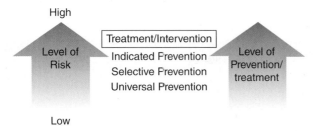

Figure 3.1 Frameworks to classify prevention strategies.

cost–benefit ratio of committing resources to the prevention strategy (Figure 3.1) [4]. The universal–selective–indicated model of prevention has been used widely in Alberta [16] in the health policy planning of FASD-prevention activities.

Universal approaches: These are broad, population-wide strategies targeted to the general public or a whole population group that has not been identified on the basis of individual risk [4]. These approaches aim to educate the broad public about the risks of drinking during pregnancy, and are regarded as being desirable for everyone. Activities often associated with universal prevention include awareness campaigns (through public-service announcements, billboards, pamphlets in physicians' offices, media advertisements), school drug-education programs, parenting programs, multicomponent community initiatives, and various measures to control the availability and price of alcoholic beverages [4].

Selective preventive interventions: These are targeted at people who are at greater risk of a particular outcome because they are members of a group known to be at a higher risk than the general population [4]. Targets of selective prevention strategies include subgroups of women and their partners from the general population who are determined to be at risk of having children with FASD (e.g., women of reproductive age and their partners who drink alcohol, women who drink while pregnant, and women who belong to vulnerable subgroups). Examples of selective preventive interventions are alcohol screening, counseling, and brief interventions to enhance coping skills and reduce alcohol consumption.

Indicated prevention strategies: These are targeted at women who are at the highest risk of having a child with FASD (e.g., women who have previously abused alcohol while pregnant, pregnant women who are experiencing early signs of alcohol abuse, women who already have a child with FASD, women with FASD, and women with alcohol problems who do not use effective contraception). This level of prevention includes treatment of alcoholism in women who are pregnant or likely to become pregnant [17].

One of the main challenges in FASD-prevention research is the gap that exists between what is known about the risk factors for FASD, and the use of that information in developing and evaluating prevention strategies and policies [17, 18]. Preventing FASD has been identified as a public health priority, and consequently the variety of programs to prevent drinking during pregnancy – and, thus, reduce the incidence of FASD–has expanded greatly. However, some have argued that limited evaluative research on FASD-prevention programs makes it difficult to draw convincing inferences about the effectiveness of FASD-prevention strategies [18].

Researchers who have reviewed and summarized the FASD-prevention literature [3, 4, 12, 18–20] have emphasized the need for scientifically rigorous evaluations of prevention strategies that have been implemented in clinical and community settings. Therefore, it is important to examine the evidence on the effectiveness of the spectrum of FASD-prevention efforts and to summarize recent research on FASD-prevention activities to inform the selection and implementation of these programs.

3.2
Objective and Scope

This document describes the objectives, methodology, analytical approach, and the results of a systematic review of published and unpublished studies that evaluated the effectiveness of preventive approaches to FASD. The objective of this systematic review is to identify and evaluate the evidence on the effectiveness of universal, selective, and indicated approaches to prevent the occurrence of FASD.

3.3
Methodological Approach

3.3.1
Elements of Assessment

A prospectively designed protocol was developed for this review. It included explicit and reproducible methods for systematically identifying and selecting studies, assessing the validity of reported results in the studies, and analyzing information on the effectiveness of strategies used to prevent FASD. Figure 3.2 presents the analytic framework outlining our approach to the review.

A detailed description of the methods for the systematic review is available in Appendix 3.A. Briefly, comprehensive searches of psychological, sociological, and biomedical electronic databases were conducted to identify English-language articles published from 1970 (or database inception) to March 2010. In addition, reference lists of retrieved articles were browsed for relevant studies. Other searches were conducted to identify literature from non-traditional sources, including proceedings from relevant scientific meetings, government documents, theses and dissertations, unpublished studies, and ongoing studies. Two reviewers independently applied a set of inclusion and exclusion criteria to select the studies for the review and assessed the methodological quality of the included studies. Each study that met the selection criteria was classified into one of three main categories of

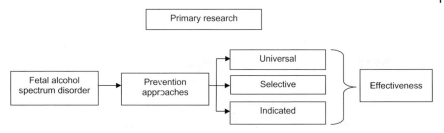

Figure 3.2 Analytic framework to evaluate the topic of the effectiveness of prevention approaches for FASD.

FASD-prevention approaches: universal, selective, or indicated. A narrative synthesis of study results was undertaken. Evidence tables were constructed to describe study characteristics, methodological quality, and individual study results. Data were extracted by one reviewer and verified independently by a second reviewer. Outcomes were analyzed based on the report of statistically significant differences in the analysis of the individual studies.

3.4
Studies on the Effectiveness of FASD Preventive Approaches

3.4.1
Search Results

The systematic search (electronic, gray literature, and manual searches) resulted in the identification of 2753 citations. After screening of titles and abstracts, the full text of 198 potentially relevant articles was retrieved and evaluated for inclusion in the review. The application of the selection criteria to the 198 articles resulted in 70 articles being included, and 128 being excluded. The study retrieval and selection for the review are outlined in Figure 3.3.

The primary reasons for the exclusion of studies from the systematic review were as follows:

- The study did not assess the effectiveness of a prevention approach to FASD ($n = 60$).
- The study was not original research (e.g., narrative review, commentary, editorial) ($n = 37$).
- The study did not report measurable data for the outcomes of interest ($n = 14$).
- The study did not use any of the study designs considered in the review ($n = 8$).
- The study did not target the populations of interest ($n = 5$).
- The full text of the study was not retrieved ($n = 4$).

The excluded studies, and the reasons for their exclusion from the systematic review, are listed on Table 3.B.1 in Appendix 3.B.

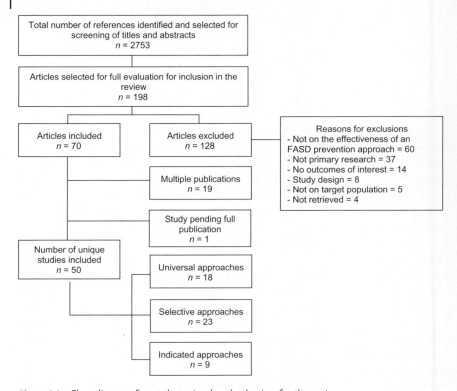

Figure 3.3 Flow diagram for study retrieval and selection for the review.

Of the 70 included articles, 19 were identified as multiple publications; that is, the same study was published more than once, or part of the data from an original report was republished [21–24]. The publication that included the largest sample size was regarded as the main publication. Multiple publications were not considered to be unique studies, and any information they provided was included with the data reported in the main study [25]. One study that was identified through gray literature searches and that met the selection criteria for the review is referenced but not included at this stage. After communication with the study authors, it was determined that study results are being prepared for final publication. The multiple publications of studies included in the review are listed in Table 3.B.2 in Appendix 3.B. Therefore, this review included 50 unique studies on the effectiveness of preventive approaches to FASD.

3.4.2
Characteristics of Included Studies

3.4.2.1 General Characteristics
Fifty studies [26–75] met the selection criteria of the systematic review and provided evidence regarding the effectiveness of prevention approaches for FASD.

The key characteristics of the studies included in the review are summarized in Tables 3.C.1 to 3.C.21 of Appendix 3.C.

The studies were published between 1983 and 2010, the median year of publication being 1999 (interquartile range [IQR]: 1993, 2005). Most of the studies ($n = 46$) were published as journal articles, two were dissertations, and two were presented at scientific conferences (see Table 3.C.2). Authors of primary studies were mainly from the USA (41 studies); only two Canadian studies met the selection criteria of the review (see Table 3.C.1). Other countries of origin of studies were Sweden (two studies) and Denmark, Finland, Norway, and the United Kingdom (one study each). Four Latin American countries (Argentina, Brazil, Cuba, and Mexico) participated in one study. Of the 50 studies, 19 were clinical trials (six RCTs and 13 CCTs), 19 were before-and-after studies with no comparison group, 11 were observational analytical cohort studies (five prospective and six retrospective analytical cohort studies), and one study was an interrupted time series study (Table 3.C.3).

Thirty-seven studies reported their sources of funding (Table 3.C.4). Of these studies, 26 were funded by government agencies [26–28, 33, 34, 37, 39, 40, 43, 44, 46, 48, 51, 52, 54–58, 61, 63, 64, 66, 69, 74, 75], three received funding from foundations or societies [32, 50, 60], one study was funded internally [70], and another study received funding from a private party [41]. A few studies received more than one type of funding. Four studies were funded by a government agency and a society [62, 65, 68, 73] and two studies [42, 47] used internal as well as government and society funds.

The studies were conducted in health facilities ($n = 35$), the community ($n = 8$), and schools ($n = 3$). Some studies were conducted in combined settings, such as community and health facilities ($n = 1$); community, health facilities and an urban jail ($n = 1$); and community, health facilities and schools ($n = 2$) (Table 3.C.5).

3.4.2.2 Characteristics of the Populations

The population most frequently targeted in the studies was pregnant women at risk of an AEP ($n = 19$), either because their use of alcohol was suspected or because it was confirmed (see Table 3.C.6). Other target populations included pregnant women ($n = 15$), the broad general public ($n = 7$), women of childbearing age ($n = 5$), and women of childbearing age who consume alcohol ($n = 3$). One study combined a population of pregnant women and women of childbearing age. Only two studies [28, 34] involved partners or support persons in the study sample. The residential settings of the target populations were mainly urban ($n = 20$). Other residential settings were suburban areas or inner cities ($n = 7$), rural settings ($n = 5$), and a mix of urban and rural areas ($n = 9$). Nine studies did not report the residential setting of their samples (Table 3.C.7). Forty-two studies [26, 28–30, 32, 33, 35–49, 51–53, 56, 57, 60–75] included only women participants whereas eight included samples of both male and females [27, 31, 34, 50, 54, 55, 58, 59] (Table 3 C.8).

Overall, the studies had moderate sample sizes, the median being 249 participants per study (IQR: 95, 799; data from 39 studies that reported the number of enrolled participants). The median age of study participants was 25 years

(IQR: 23.1, 28; data from 28 studies). Half of the studies ($n = 25$) included adult populations only (aged 18 years and older), whereas six studies included youth populations only (aged less than 18 years). Eleven studies included both adult and youth populations, and eight studies did not report the age range of the participants (Table 3.C.9).

Twenty-six studies included individuals of miscellaneous races. Eleven studies focused exclusively on non-Caucasian populations, whereas 13 studies did not report the race of participants (Table 3.C.10). Among studies conducted in non-Caucasian populations ($n = 11$), five [29, 54, 56–58] focused exclusively on Aboriginal groups (i.e., Native American populations). One study [61] included both Native American and Hispanic populations; two studies [46, 62] were conducted exclusively in African Americans, whereas one study [41] combined African Americans and Hispanics. Finally, two studies [28, 55] included Hispanic participants only. Six studies analyzed the data on the effectiveness of prevention approaches to FASD by race. Four of these studies [30, 39, 67, 68] included participants from miscellaneous races, and reported separate results by race. Two studies included non-Caucasian populations only and conducted subgroup analyzes by race: one of these [41] compared African Americans and Hispanics, and the other [58] compared Plains, Navajo, Alaska and Pueblo tribes, and acculturated Native American populations.

None of the studies in this review reported whether the study participants had past or concurrent exposure to other FASD-prevention interventions.

3.4.2.3 Characteristics of the Interventions

Three broad categories of prevention approaches were considered in this review: universal prevention approaches (evaluated in 18 studies), selective prevention approaches (evaluated in 23 studies), and indicated prevention approaches (evaluated in nine studies) (see Table 3.C.11; see also Appendix 3.D for an operational description of these categories). The types of prevention approach to FASD examined in clinical trials, observational analytical studies, before-and-after studies, and interrupted time series studies are reported in Table 3.2.

The preventive approaches were classified into categories that correspond to the three levels of public health practice: [76] directed to the community; directed to

Table 3.2 Prevention approaches to FASD examined in clinical trials and observational analytical studies.

Intervention	Clinical trials (n)		Observational analytical studies (n)		Before-and-after studies (n)	Interrupted time series studies (n)	Total (n)
	RCT	CCT	Prospective	Retrospective			
Universal	–	3	1	4	9	1	18
Selective	6	8	3	1	5	–	23
Indicated	–	2	1	1	5	–	9
Total	6	13	5	6	19	1	50

CCT = controlled clinical trial; RCT = randomized controlled trial.

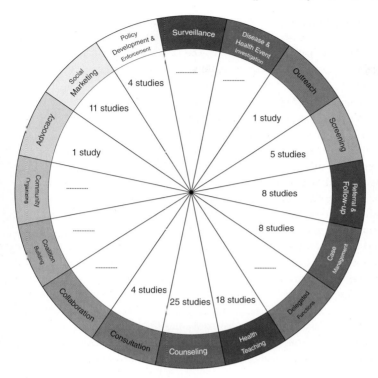

Figure 3.4 Types of public health preventive intervention implemented for FASD. Adapted from the Minnesota Department of Health Division of Community Health Services [76].

individuals; or directed system-wide (see Appendix 3.D for a description of these terms). The majority of studies evaluated preventive interventions that were directed toward individuals ($n = 36$), ten studies evaluated preventive interventions directed toward entire populations or target groups in the community, and one study evaluated an intervention implemented at a system-wide level (see Table 3.C.12). Three studies evaluated preventive approaches that operated at both the community and system-wide levels. The types of public health preventive interventions for FASD [76] that were implemented are described in Figure 3.4 (see Appendix 3.D for a description of terms). Some studies examined the implementation of more than one intervention; therefore, the number of interventions does not match the number of studies included in the review.

Counseling was the most frequently implemented preventive approach ($n = 25$), followed by health teaching ($n = 18$), social marketing interventions ($n = 11$), case management ($n = 8$), referrals and follow-up ($n = 8$), screening and case-finding activities ($n = 8$), consultation ($n = 4$), policy development or law enforcement activities ($n = 4$), outreach ($n = 1$), and advocacy ($n = 1$) (Table 3.C.13).

3.4 2.4 Components of the Interventions
The FASD prevention interventions varied widely in their theoretical underpinnings and components. Seventeen studies reported the theoretical framework

underlying their approach to prevention. These included social marketing theory ($n = 4$), social cognitive theory ($n = 3$), the cognitive-behavioral approach ($n = 4$), the activated health education model, the ecological model of social support, the health belief model, the health communication process model, the home visitation model, Miller's self-in-relation theory, the reasoned action and social learning theory, and a theoretical model that was not further specified (one study each). Thirty studies did not specify the theoretical model that supported the interventions (Table 3.C.14).

The preventive interventions were implemented in a variety of settings. The majority were implemented in health facilities ($n = 27$) and the community ($n = 14$). A small number of studies set the interventions at home ($n = 3$) or at schools ($n = 3$). Three studies implemented the preventive intervention both at health facilities and study participants' homes (Table 3.C.15).

The individual components of the FASD preventive interventions were further classified into three main categories according to the type of activities that were undertaken: education; legal activities; and counseling activities (Table 3.C.16). Educational components included the distribution of printed educational materials such as fact sheets and posters ($n = 11$), the use of audiovisual materials ($n = 8$) and motivational messages ($n = 7$), educational sessions and workshops ($n = 6$), mass media strategies ($n = 6$), computer-based education ($n = 2$), and school curriculum changes ($n = 2$). Some components of the interventions involved legal and policy decisions, such as the use of warning labels on alcohol beverages or an alcohol ban ($n = 5$). Counseling activities and brief interventions included individual counseling ($n = 23$), case management ($n = 9$), referral to available services ($n = 9$), skills training ($n = 6$), support groups ($n = 5$), and alcohol testing and counseling ($n = 1$).

Forty studies described the type of providers or resources that were used to deliver the preventive interventions (see Table 3.C.17). Eleven studies used self-applied materials that did not require the participation of other personnel. Multidisciplinary teams involving two or more providers were used in 12 studies. A variety of providers delivered the interventions. These included physicians ($n = 3$), health educators ($n = 3$), public health nurses, peers ($n = 2$), midwives ($n = 2$), counselors, clinical nurses, nutritionists, social workers, and substance abuse counselors (one study each). The composition of multidisciplinary teams was quite heterogeneous. The 12 studies that involved two or more providers included teams of nurses and certified alcoholism therapists [52]; prevention and case managers [57]; psychiatrists and counselors [68]; public health nurses, substance-abuse counselors, and a liaison team not further identified [35]; social workers and health educators [66]; social workers and obstetric nurses [28]; midwives and social workers [51]; nurses and medical students [75]; obstetric nurses and research staff [39]; social workers, nurse practitioners, case managers, consultants in medicine, addictions, psychology, and law/ethics [74]; social worker and substance-abuse treatment providers [26]; and an interdisciplinary team that was not further specified [53]. Only 14 studies [28, 34, 36, 39, 40, 42, 47, 53, 57, 61, 64, 66, 67, 75] reported that the providers received training prior to the intervention. Likewise, only seven studies [28, 33, 36, 39, 47, 64, 67] reported the use of a manual to guarantee the fidelity of the intervention.

3.4.2.5 Characteristics of the Outcomes

A total of 143 outcomes was reported in the 50 studies reviewed. The time to outcome assessment varied considerably among the studies, ranging from less than three months to more than one year. The types of outcome measures that were examined in studies on the effectiveness of prevention approaches for FASD are displayed in Table 3.3 (see also Table 3.C.18).

The effectiveness of FASD-prevention approaches was evaluated by measuring a variety of outcomes. The majority ($n = 65$) were intermediate outcomes related to changes in drinking behavior, while 47 were ultimate outcomes that represented changes of the status of a condition in the mother, the child, the family or the society. Immediate outcomes ($n = 31$) were less frequently addressed in the studies.

The most frequently reported outcomes were of self-reported alcohol intake (50 outcomes), followed by neonatal and infant outcomes (29 outcomes), knowledge about alcohol use during pregnancy and FASD (17 outcomes), and alcohol abstinence (nine outcomes). The majority of outcomes were assessed after follow-up periods of nine months to less than one year (61 outcomes), or at less than three months (30 outcomes). The most frequently reported assessments at less than three months and between three and six months of follow-up were measures of alcohol intake and acquisition of knowledge about alcohol use during pregnancy. Measures of alcohol intake were the predominant outcome assessments conducted at between six and nine months of follow-up. Between nine and 12 months of follow-up, neonatal outcomes were the most frequently evaluated, a trend that was maintained after one year of follow-up.

3.4.2.6 Types of Result Reported in the Individual Studies

The types of result reported in the 50 studies reviewed are listed in Table 3.4 (see also Table 3.C.19). They are described in terms of the report of statistically significant differences in the outcomes of interest and the support of the intervention under the study conclusions.

Among the 50 studies included in the review, 18 reported statistically significant results, whereas 16 failed to show any statistically significant differences in the outcome data. Sixteen studies did not report the results of tests to analyze whether statistically significant differences existed among the groups or study periods for the outcomes of interest.

In interpreting the results of their studies, the majority of primary authors ($n = 20$) claimed that the intervention under study was effective. Fifteen studies did not state definite conclusions regarding the effectiveness of the intervention, and ten studies did not support the effectiveness of the intervention under study. Five studies gave a partial endorsement to the preventive intervention under study, based on the interpretation of secondary outcome data.

Nine studies which were rated as weak in methodology yielded conclusions regarding the effectiveness of the FASD-prevention approach that were not

Table 3.3 Types of outcome measure examined in studies on prevention approaches to FASD.

Type of outcome		Number of outcomes assessed at different follow-up periods					
		≤3 months	>3 months and ≤6 months	>6 months and ≤9 months	>9 months and ≤1 year	>1 year	Total number of outcomes
Immediate	Knowledge about alcohol use during pregnancy/FASD	8	2	3	2	2	17
	Attitudes toward alcohol use during pregnancy	5	1	–	2	–	8
	Awareness of risk of alcohol use during pregnancy	–	1	–	1	1	3
	Perceptions about alcohol use during pregnancy	1	1	–	1	–	3
Intermediate	Alcohol intake	12	12	4	20	2	50
	Alcohol abstinence	2	–	2	2	3	9
	Binge drinking	1	–	1	1	1	4
	Alcohol-exposed pregnancy	1	–	1	–	–	2
Ultimate	Neonatal and infant outcomes	–	–	1	21	7	29
	Maternal outcomes	–	–	2	4	3	9
	FASD outcomes	–	–	–	4	1[a]	5
	Economic and health care utilization outcomes	–	–	–	2	–	2
	Family outcomes	–	–	–	–	1	1
	Legal outcomes	–	–	–	1	–	1
Total		30	17	14	61	21	143

a) The study did not report the maximum follow-up period for FASD outcome assessment.
FASD = fetal alcohol spectrum disorder.

Table 3.4 Types of result reported in the individual studies assessing the effectiveness of prevention approaches to FASD.

Report of statistically significant differences in the results	Study conclusion				Total number of studies
	No support of the effectiveness of the intervention (number of studies)	No conclusions regarding the effectiveness of the intervention (number of studies)	Partial support of the effectiveness of the Intervention (number of studies)	Support of the effectiveness of the intervention (number of studies)	
Study did not provide data on statistical testing of differences	2 ☺	11 ☺	–	3 ☹	16
Study found no statistically significant differences	8 ☺	3 ☺	2 ☹	3 ☹	16
Study reported statistically significant differences	–	1 ☹	3 ☺	14 ☺	18
Total number of studies	10	15	5	20	50

☺ = an appropriate conclusion based on study results; ☹ = an inappropriate conclusion based on study results; ☺ = an appropriate partial conclusion based on study results.

supported by the statistical analysis of the outcome data. Among the 16 studies that found no statistically significant differences in the data analysis, three concluded nevertheless that the preventive intervention was effective, and two granted partial support to the preventive intervention under study. Likewise, three studies supported the effectiveness of the intervention when, in fact, no statistical analysis was conducted to evaluate it. Finally, one study that reported statistically significant differences in the analysis of the outcomes did not offer firm conclusions regarding the effectiveness of the intervention.

3.4.3
Methodological Quality of the Studies

The majority of the studies were considered of poor methodological quality. Of the 50 studies, 37 were rated as weak, 12 as moderate, and only one study was rated as strong.

An overview of how well the studies were able to control for methodological weaknesses related to selection bias, allocation bias, confounding, blinding of outcome assessors, validity and reliability of data collection methods, and management of withdrawals and dropouts, is provided in Table 3.5 (see also Table 3.C.20).

Most of the studies were consistently rated as weak in all domains of methodological quality. The most common methodological weaknesses were related to a lack of blinding and an inadequate description of data collection methods, followed by a lack of control for confounders and bias in the selection of study populations. Overall, the studies rated highest in the domain of controlling for allocation bias. All of the studies received a rating of either moderate ($n = 26$) or strong ($n = 16$)

Table 3.5 Methodological quality of studies assessing the effectiveness of prevention approaches to FASD.

Domains of Methodological Quality	Number of studies rated as Weak	Number of studies rated as Moderate	Number of studies rated as Strong
Methods to control for selection bias	28	18	4
Methods to control for allocation bias	–	32	18
Methods to control for confounders	29	2	19
Methods of blinding	32	17	1
Data collection methods	30	4	16
Methods to handle withdrawals and dropouts	25	10	15
Global methodological quality	37	12	1

in this quality domain. This was due to the setting of a minimum standard of quality at the study selection phase, whereby only clinical trials, observational analytical studies and before-and-after studies were accepted for inclusion in the review.

Methodological aspects that go beyond the internal validity of the studies were also evaluated. More than half of the studies fully or partially reported the dates for starting and stopping accession of participants ($n = 32$). The majority of the studies ($n = 34$) provided information on how well the sample represented the criteria for selecting participants. Only five studies, however, fully reported the set of inclusion and exclusion criteria used in enrolling participants in their studies. A small proportion of studies ($n = 15$) stated the number of patients deemed ineligible before intervention took place.

The quality of reporting of the characteristics and conditions under which the interventions operated was variable. Only five studies [30, 34, 36, 64, 67] described the use of a method to monitor the fidelity with which the intervention was implemented. Likewise, the majority of studies did not state whether the participants received an unintended intervention that may have influenced the results. Only two studies [30, 72] provided some description of the method used to control for cointerventions that may have affected the outcomes. Half of the studies ($n = 25$) described the frequency of the intervention delivered, and a smaller proportion ($n = 16$) reported the duration of the intervention.

Some issues related to data analysis in the individual studies were also evaluated. Only five studies [30, 34, 39, 60, 61] reported that an intention-to-treat (ITT) approach was used in the analysis of the results. Ten studies [26, 27, 41, 48, 52, 55, 58, 59, 62, 64] did not take account of the unit of allocation in the data analysis; rather, they used individuals as the unit of analysis, whereas the unit of allocation to the interventions was an entire group of people (i.e., clusters).

3.4.4
Highlights of the Overall Results

- Fifty studies published between 1983 and 2010 were included in the review.

- Half of the studies were published at least a decade ago (the median year of publication was 1998).

- Most of the studies ($n = 41$) were conducted in the United States.

- Only two Canadian studies met the selection criteria of the review.

- The 50 studies included 19 clinical trials (six RCTs and 13 CCTs), 19 before-and-after studies with no comparison group, 11 observational analytical cohort studies (five prospective and six retrospective), and one interrupted time series study.

- The source of funding was declared in the majority of the studies. Funding was provided mainly by government agencies.

- The studies were conducted mainly in urban health facilities.

3.4.4.1 **Populations**

- The population that was most frequently targeted in the studies consisted of women at risk of an AEP and pregnant women. The median age of participants in the studies was 25 years.

- Only two studies involved partners or support persons in the evaluation of the intervention.

- Half of the studies evaluated the interventions in individuals of miscellaneous races. Fewer than one-quarter of the studies were conducted exclusively in non-Caucasian populations. Interventions directed only to Native American populations were evaluated in five studies.

- No studies conducted in Canadian Aboriginal populations met the selection criteria for the review.

3.4.4.2 **Interventions**

- The most frequently studied FASD-prevention approaches were selective approaches (23 studies) followed by universal approaches (18 studies) and indicated approaches (nine studies).

- RCTs were conducted only in the evaluation of selective prevention approaches. No RCTs on universal or indicated approaches were identified. Universal and indicated approaches were evaluated mainly by means of before-and-after studies with no comparison groups.

- Counseling was the most frequently implemented intervention in the studies (25 studies), followed by health teaching (18 studies), social marketing activities (11 studies), case management (eight studies), referrals and follow-up (eight studies), and screening and case-finding activities (eight studies).

3.4.4.3 **Outcomes**

- The majority of outcomes evaluated in the studies were intermediate outcomes related to changes in drinking behavior (65 outcomes); 47 were ultimate outcomes that represented changes of status of a condition in the mother, the child, the family, or the society; and 31 were immediate outcomes related to changes in knowledge and attitudes.

- The most frequently studied outcomes were those of self-reported alcohol intake (50 outcomes), followed by neonatal and infant outcomes (29 outcomes), knowledge about alcohol use during pregnancy and FASD (17 outcomes), and measures of alcohol abstinence (nine outcomes).

- Among the 50 studies in the review, 18 reported statistically significant results that favored the preventive intervention, whereas 16 studies reported that no statistically significant differences were found in the analysis of outcome data. Sixteen studies did not report on the results of statistical tests to determine the significance of differences among the groups or study periods for the outcomes of interest.

3.4.4.4 Methodological Quality

- The majority of the studies were considered to be of poor methodological quality. Of the 50 studies reviewed, 37 were rated as weak, 12 as moderate, and one study was rated as strong.

- The most common methodological weaknesses were related to a lack of blinding and an inadequate description of data collection methods, followed by a lack of control for confounders and bias in the selection of study populations.

3.5
Evidence on the Effectiveness of Universal Prevention Approaches for FASD

3.5.1
Characteristics of Included Studies

3.5.1.1 General Characteristics

Eighteen studies [27, 29–32, 41, 46, 48–50, 54, 55, 58, 59, 62, 65, 72, 73] provided evidence on the effectiveness of universal prevention approaches for FASD. The characteristics of the studies that were used to evaluate universal prevention approaches are summarized in Table 3.E.1 of Appendix 3.E.

The studies were published between 1989 and 2008, with the median year of publication being 1997 (IQR: 1992, 2005). The 18 studies were published as journal articles. The authors of the primary studies were mainly from the USA (14 studies [27, 29, 30, 41, 46, 48–50, 54, 55, 58, 59, 62, 72]); other countries of origin were Canada [31, 32], Denmark [65], and the United Kingdom [73]. The 18 studies included nine before-and-after studies with no comparison group [27, 31, 41, 48, 49, 54, 55, 58, 72], three CCTs [30, 50, 73], five observational analytical cohort studies (four retrospective analytical cohort studies [29, 32, 59, 65], one prospective analytical cohort study [62],) and one interrupted time series study [46]. No RCTs that evaluated a universal prevention approach for FASD were identified.

Twelve studies [27, 32, 41, 46, 48, 50, 54, 55, 58, 62, 65, 73] disclosed their sources of funding. Six studies [27, 46, 48, 54, 55, 58] were funded by government agencies, two [32, 50] received funding from foundations or societies, one study [41] was funded by a private party, and three studies [62, 65, 73] used both government and society funds.

Studies assessing universal prevention approaches for FASD were conducted mainly in the community (eight studies [27, 29, 31, 41, 48, 55, 59, 62]) or in health facilities (seven studies [30, 32, 46, 49, 65, 72, 73]). Two studies [50, 54] were undertaken in school settings, and one study [58] was conducted in both community and high school settings.

3.5.1.2 Characteristics of the Populations

The most frequently targeted populations in the studies on universal FASD-prevention approaches were the general public (seven studies [27, 31, 50, 54, 55, 58, 59]), pregnant women (six studies [29, 30, 46, 49, 65, 73]), and women of childbearing age (four studies [32, 41, 62, 72]). One study combined a population of pregnant women and women of childbearing age [48]. None of the studies involved partners or support persons as the target of the intervention. The residential settings of target populations were mainly urban (six studies [27, 41, 55, 62, 65, 73]). A smaller proportion of the studies were conducted in rural settings (three studies [29, 49, 58]) and suburban settings (two studies [46, 50]). Three studies [30–32] sampled populations from both urban and rural areas, while four studies [48, 54, 59, 72] did not report the residential setting of the samples.

Overall, the studies had large sample sizes, the median number of participants being 799 (IQR: 90, 2324; data from 11 studies that reported the number of enrolled participants). Eleven studies [29, 30, 32, 41, 46, 48, 49, 62, 65, 72, 73] involved only women, whereas seven [27, 31, 50, 54, 55, 58, 59] included samples of both men and women. The median age of participants in the studies was 23.7 years (IQR: 19.3, 30.4; data from five studies). Five studies [31, 55, 59, 62, 72] included adult populations, and three studies [41, 50, 54] were conducted in youth populations only. Five studies combined both adult and youth populations [27, 30, 32, 46, 58] , and five [29, 48, 49, 65, 73] did not report the participants' ages.

The majority of studies on universal preventive approaches to FASD were conducted in non-Caucasian populations (seven studies [29, 41, 46, 54, 55, 58, 62]). Four studies [27, 30, 50, 59] were conducted with participants of miscellaneous races, and the race composition of the samples was unknown in seven studies [31, 32, 48, 49, 65, 72, 73]. Among studies conducted in non-Caucasian populations (n = 8), three [29, 54, 58] included Aboriginal groups (i.e., Native American populations) exclusively. Two studies [46, 62] were conducted exclusively in African Americans, whereas one study [41] combined samples of both African Americans and Hispanics. Finally, one study [55] included Hispanic participants only. Only three studies [30, 41, 58] analyzed the data on the effectiveness of universal approaches by race. Among the four studies that included miscellaneous races, only one study [30] reported a subgroup analysis by race. Among the seven studies of non-Caucasian populations, two conducted a subgroup analysis by race: one study [41] compared African Americans and Hispanics, while the other [58] compared Plains, Navajo, Alaska and Pueblo tribes, and acculturated Native American populations.

It is unknown whether the populations included in the studies that evaluated universal preventive interventions for FASD had past or current exposure to similar or other prevention approaches.

3.5.1.3 Characteristics of the Interventions

The majority of universal preventive approaches targeted entire populations within the community (nine studies [27, 31, 32, 41, 46, 54, 58, 62, 65]). One study [29]

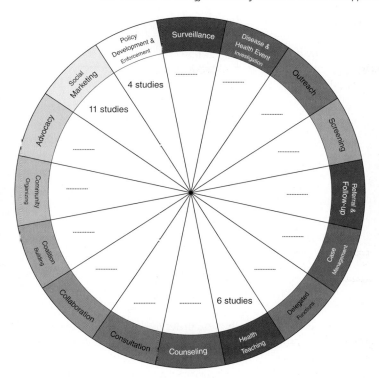

Figure 3.5 Types of public health preventive intervention implemented in the universal preventive approaches. Adapted from the Minnesota Department of Health Division of Community Health Services [76].

implemented the intervention at a policy and system-wide level. Five studies [30, 49, 50, 72, 73] evaluated universal interventions that were directed to individuals, and three studies [48, 55, 59] evaluated an approach that was both community and system-level focused.

The types of public health intervention that were implemented in the universal preventive approaches are described in Figure 3.5. Some studies implemented more than one intervention; therefore, the number of interventions does not match the number of studies.

Social marketing activities were the most frequently implemented interventions in the universal prevention approaches to FASD (11 studies [27, 31, 32, 41, 46, 48, 55, 59, 62, 65, 72]), followed by health teaching interventions evaluated in six studies [30, 49, 50, 54, 58, 73]. Four studies evaluated the implementation of interventions at a policy or law enforcement level [29, 48, 55, 59].

The FASD universal prevention approaches that were examined in individual studies and the populations targeted are detailed in Table 3.6. The studies are arranged by study design, from clinical trials to observational studies.

Table 3.6 FASD universal prevention approaches examined in individual studies.

Study	Study design	Intervention	Population
LaChausse [50]	CCT	Multimedia education program	Broad public
Calabro et al. [30]	CCT	Written health education materials	Pregnant women
Waterson [73]	CCT	Written health education materials	Pregnant women
Mengel et al. [62]	Prospective analytical cohort study	Public education campaign	Women of childbearing age
Mazis et al. [59]	Retrospective analytical cohort study	Alcohol beverage warning label	Broad public
Casiro et al. [32]	Retrospective analytical cohort study	Television public awareness campaign	Women of childbearing age
Bowerman [29]	Retrospective analytical cohort study	Alcohol ban	Pregnant women
Olsen et al. [65]	Retrospective analytical cohort study	Health campaign	Pregnant women
Hankin et al. [46]	Interrupted time series study	Alcohol beverage warning label	Pregnant women
Awopetu et al. [27]	Before-and-after study	Multimedia public education campaign	Broad public
Carr and Brand [31]	Before-and-after study	Multimedia public education campaign	Broad public
Ma [54]	Before-and-after study	Educational FAS-prevention program	Broad public
Marin [55]	Before-and-after study	Alcohol-related warning messages	Broad public
May and Hymbaugh [58]	Before-and-after study	Macro level FAS-education program	Broad public
Glik et al. [41]	Before-and-after study	Public education campaign	Women of childbearing age
Walker et al. [72]	Before-and-after study	Education brochure	Women of childbearing age
Kaskutas et al. [48]	Before-and-after study	Alcohol beverage warning label	Pregnant women and women of childbearing age
Kinzie et al. [49]	Before-and-after study	Interactive multimedia education program	Pregnant women

CCT = controlled clinical trial; FAS = fetal alcohol syndrome.

3 5.1.4 Components of the Interventions

Six studies described the theoretical framework underlying the universal approach under study. These frameworks included social marketing theory [32, 41, 62], a health communication process model [54], reasoned action and social learning theory [49], and a mix of health promotion, social marketing, communications, and instructional design theories [31].

The individual components of the universal preventive interventions fell within two main categories: education and legal-system activities. Educational components included the distribution of printed educational materials in nine studies [27, 30, 41, 54, 58, 62, 65, 72, 73], the distribution of audiovisual materials in six studies [49, 50, 54, 58, 62, 73], mass media strategies in five studies [27, 31, 32, 48, 62], and motivational messages [49, 73] and computer-based education [49, 50] in two studies each. Some individual components involved legal and policy decisions, such as banning alcohol in the community [29] or placing labels on alcohol beverages with messages warning of the effects of drinking alcohol during pregnancy [46, 48, 55, 59].

Interventions using media or printed materials alone did not require providers; however, other universal preventive interventions involved the participation of peers [50, 58] or doctors [73]. Six studies [29, 46, 54, 55, 59, 72] did not clearly describe whether providers were required in implementing the interventions. None of the studies reported whether providers received training prior to implementing the intervention. Likewise, the use of a manual to guarantee treatment fidelity was not described in any of the studies. A detailed description of the characteristics of the universal preventive approaches that were evaluated in the individual studies is provided in Table 3.F.1 in Appendix 3.F.

3.5.1.5 Characteristics of the Outcomes

A total of 34 outcomes was reported in the 18 studies that assessed the effectiveness of universal FASD-prevention approaches. The types of outcome were examined in these studies are listed in Table 3.7.

The universal prevention approaches were evaluated mainly through an analysis of immediate outcomes (25 outcomes) related to knowledge about and attitudes towards drinking alcohol during pregnancy. Less frequently reported were intermediate outcomes (eight outcomes) related to behavioral changes, as well as ultimate outcomes (one outcome).

The most frequently reported outcomes were those related to knowledge about alcohol use during pregnancy and FASD (15 outcomes), followed by self-reported measures of alcohol intake (six outcomes), and attitudes toward alcohol use during pregnancy (five outcomes). Outcomes related to the effects of alcohol use on the mother, alcohol abstinence, and binge drinking were less frequently evaluated (one outcome each). The effects of the universal prevention approaches on the incidence of FASD were not evaluated in any of the studies.

3.5.1.6 Types of Result Reported in the Individual Studies

The types of result described in the 18 studies that evaluated the effects of universal prevention approaches are displayed in Table 3.8. The results are described in

Table 3.7 Types of outcome measure examined in studies on universal prevention approaches to FASD.

Type of outcome		Number of outcomes assessed at different follow-up periods					
		≤3 months	>3 months and ≤6 months	>6 months and ≤9 months	>9 months and ≤1 year	>1 year	Total number of outcomes
Immediate	Knowledge about alcohol use during pregnancy/FASD	7	1	3	2	2	15
	Attitudes toward alcohol use during pregnancy	5	–	–	1	–	6
	Awareness of risk of alcohol use during pregnancy	–	1	–	–	1	2
	Perceptions about alcohol use during pregnancy	1	–	–	1	–	2
Intermediate	Alcohol intake	–	2	1	2	1	6
	Alcohol abstinence	–	–	–	–	1	1
	Binge drinking	–	–	–	–	1	1
Ultimate	Maternal outcomes	–	–	–	–	1	1
Total		13	4	4	6	7	34

FASD = fetal alcohol spectrum disorder.

Table 3.8 Types of results reported in the individual studies assessing the effectiveness of universal prevention approaches to FASD.

Report of statistically significant differences in the results	Study conclusion				Total number of studies
	No support of the effectiveness of the intervention (number of studies)	No conclusions regarding the effectiveness of the intervention (number of studies)	Partial support of the effectiveness of the intervention (number of studies)	Support of the effectiveness of the intervention (number of studies)	
Study did not provide data on statistical testing of the differences	2 ☺	6 ☺	–	–	8
Study did not find statistically significant differences	1 ☺	3 ☺	–	1 ☹	5
Study reported statistically significant differences	–	–	1 ☹	4 ☺	5
Total number of studies	3	9	1	5	18

☺ = an appropriate conclusion based on study results; ☹ = an inappropriate conclusion based on study results; ☺ = an appropriate partial conclusion based on study results.

terms of the finding of statistically significant differences in the outcomes of interest, and the support of the approach under the study conclusions.

Among the 18 studies that provided evidence on the effectiveness of universal prevention approaches to FASD, five [29, 32, 50, 58, 72] reported statistically significant differences in the results, whereas five [30, 41, 46, 59, 73] did not find statistically significant differences in the analysis of outcome data. Eight studies [27, 31, 48, 49, 54, 55, 62, 65, 73] did not report the use of statistical tests to analyze whether statistically significant differences existed among the groups or study periods for the outcomes of interest.

In interpreting the results of their studies, the primary authors in nine cases [27, 31, 46, 48, 49, 54, 55, 59, 73] did not state definite conclusions regarding the effectiveness of the intervention, whereas the authors of five studies [29, 30, 32, 58, 72] claimed that the intervention was effective. Three studies [41, 62, 65] did not support the effectiveness of the intervention under study. One study [50] gave a partial endorsement to the universal approach, based on the interpretation of secondary outcome data.

Only one study [30] yielded to conclusions that were not supported by the analysis of the outcome data. The study concluded that the preventive intervention was effective, although no statistically significant differences were found. Four studies that did not find any statistically significant differences in the analysis of outcome data correctly either concluded that the intervention was not effective [41], or did not draw conclusions regarding the effectiveness of the intervention [46, 59, 73]. The five studies that gave full [29, 32, 58, 72] or partial [50] support to the effectiveness of the intervention reported statistically significant differences in the analysis of the outcomes.

3.5.2
Methodological Quality of the Studies

Seventeen out of 18 studies that evaluated the effectiveness of FASD universal prevention approaches were considered of poor methodological quality (i.e., rated as "weak"), and only one study [50] was rated as "moderate."

An overview of how well the studies on universal prevention approaches were able to control for methodological issues related to selection bias, allocation bias, confounding, blinding of outcome assessors, validity and reliability of data collection methods, and management of withdrawals and dropouts is provided in Table 3.9.

The majority of the studies were consistently rated as weak in all the domains of methodological quality that were assessed. The most common methodological weaknesses were related to the lack of control for confounders, the description of withdrawals and dropouts, and the methods for data collection. A detailed description of the methodological quality of the individual studies that assessed the effectiveness of universal prevention approaches is provided in Table 3.G.1 in Appendix 3.G.

Methodological aspects that go beyond the internal validity of the studies were also evaluated. Overall, the reporting of dates for starting and stopping accession

Table 3.9 Methodological quality of studies assessing the effectiveness of universal prevention approaches to FASD.

Domains of Methodological Quality	Number of studies rated as Weak	Number of studies rated as Moderate	Number of studies rated as Strong
Methods to control for selection bias	10	6	2
Methods to control for allocation bias	–	15	3
Methods to control for confounders	17	–	1
Methods of blinding	11	7	–
Data collection methods	14	1	3
Methods to handle withdrawals and dropouts	15	–	3
Global methodological quality	17	1	–

to participants was adequate. Only three studies [49, 50, 54] failed to report the study enrollment dates. The majority of the studies provided information on how well the sample represented the selection criteria for enrolling participants. Only four studies [27, 31, 55, 58] failed to describe the set of inclusion and exclusion criteria used to enroll participants in their studies, while only three studies [46, 59, 65] reported the number of ineligible patients before intervention allocation took place.

The quality of reporting of the characteristics and conditions under which the interventions operated was poor. Only one study [30] reported the use of a systematic mechanism to monitor the fidelity of the universal preventive intervention that was implemented. For eight studies [27, 31, 46, 49, 50, 54, 65, 73], it was unknown whether the study participants received an unintended intervention that may have influenced the results. It is likely that participants in eight of the studies [29, 32, 41, 48, 55, 58, 59, 62] received an unintended cointervention. Only two studies [30, 72] provided some description of how the effect of potential cointerventions was controlled for.

Four studies [32, 50, 72, 73] described the frequency of the universal intervention delivered, while another four [32, 49, 50, 62] reported on the duration of the intervention.

Some issues related to data analysis in the individual studies were evaluated. Only one study [30] reported that an ITT approach was used. Finally, more than one-third of the studies [27, 48, 55, 58, 59, 62, 77] had unit-of-analysis errors; that is to say, participants were allocated to the interventions in clusters, but individuals were used as the unit of analysis.

3.5.3
Results of Qualitative Synthesis of the Evidence

The large heterogeneity of the study designs and characteristics of interventions precluded a meta-analysis of the data to assess the effectiveness of FASD universal interventions. However, a qualitative review was conducted in order to identify patterns across individual study results. The following variables were systematically examined to shed light on reasons for the findings: study design; duration of follow-up; sample size; population characteristics; comparison; and outcomes. The following is an overview of the qualitative review of universal preventive interventions for FASD based on the data provided in 18 studies (three clinical trials and 15 observational studies). The presentation of the studies and their results are arranged by study design, from clinical trials to observational studies.

3.5.3.1 Clinical Trials

LaChausse [50] conducted a clinical trial that evaluated the effectiveness of a multimedia program to prevent FAS among youth from a suburban population in southern California (USA). A total of 114 high-school students of both sexes, the majority of whom (68%) were Hispanic, were enrolled in the study. The authors described the study as an RCT; however, it was classified in this review as a CCT, because the methods of intervention allocation and generation of the randomization sequence were not described. Study participants were assigned to one of two groups: one group was subjected to the Fetal Alcohol Spectrum Teaching and Research Awareness Campaign (FASTRAC), while a second comparison group received no intervention. FASTRAC was a peer-delivered educational multimedia program which consisted of a 35-slide PowerPoint presentation that included information on the history of FAS, how alcohol damages the fetus, the characteristics of FAS, and the social and economic impact of FAS. Immediate outcome measures, such as knowledge about FAS, attitudes toward alcohol use during pregnancy, intention to use alcohol during pregnancy, and perceived severity of alcohol use during pregnancy, were assessed at two weeks of follow-up. The results showed that, whilst FASTRAC significantly increased the students' knowledge of FAS, the program did not affect the participants' attitudes toward drinking during pregnancy. The FASTRAC program did not make participants less likely to use alcohol during pregnancy, nor did it increase the perceived severity of using alcohol during pregnancy. The authors gave partial support to the effectiveness of the intervention for its efficacy in increasing knowledge, but no behavioral correlates of knowledge increase were identified as a result of the intervention. The methodological quality of this study was rated as moderate.

Calabro et al. [30] conducted a clinical trial that evaluated whether health education materials written at a lower, rather than a higher, reading level were more effective at producing changes in knowledge, attitudes, and behavioral intention to use alcohol among pregnant women. The study was conducted in public health clinics in the southwestern region of the USA between July and December of 1993. The study population consisted of 252 pregnant women (youth and adults) attending the clinics for their first prenatal visit. Both, English- and Spanish-speaking participants were enrolled. The authors mentioned that the allocation to intervention groups was random, but no descriptions of the method of allocation and generation of the randomization sequence were provided. Thus, the study was classified in this review as a CCT. The study tested the effectiveness of health education materials written at two different reading levels (grades 3 and 10). The materials were designed to influence three immediate outcome variables: knowledge; attitude; and behavioral intention to avoid alcohol consumption while pregnant. Overall, the authors did not find any statistically significant differences between the two reading levels; however, the materials written at the lower reading level seemed to be more effective among English-speaking women. Despite a lack of statistically significant results, the authors endorsed the effectiveness of the intervention. The methodological quality of this study was rated as weak.

Waterson [73] conducted a controlled clinical trial that compared three methods of imparting basic information and advice about the risks of alcohol in pregnancy at the first visit to an antenatal clinic. The study was conducted between May 1982 and October 1983, and consisted of a sample of 2100 pregnant women attending an antenatal clinic in London (UK). Two trials were conducted. In the first trial, 1036 women were allocated to one of two groups: (1) prenatal educative intervention delivered in a written format only; and (2) prenatal education combining written information and physician advice. The second trial was conducted in 1064 women, and compared a group that received prenatal written information with a group that received prenatal education combining written information, physician advice and a four-minute video. Outcomes of interest were alcohol intake and knowledge about "safe" daily alcohol intake and "safe" daily drinking when planning a pregnancy, or at 28 weeks of pregnancy. There were no statistically significant differences among the groups in the percentage of women that consumed less than seven units of alcohol per week during pregnancy. There were also no significant differences among the groups in the number of women who considered that less than one unit of daily alcohol was safe during pregnancy, or when planning a pregnancy. The authors made no conclusions regarding the effectiveness of the interventions. The methodological quality of this study was rated as weak.

3.5.3.2 Observational Studies

Mengel *et al.* [62] conducted a prospective analytical cohort study that evaluated the effectiveness of a targeted media campaign to increase FASD knowledge. The study was conducted in a community sample of African-American women of childbearing age residing in the city of Saint Louis, Missouri (USA), between October 2002 and March 2004. The intervention was a social marketing campaign that was built around four FAS-prevention messages: (1) A description of the birth defects associated with FASD; (2) No "safe level" of drinking during pregnancy exists; (3) Sexually active women should not drink if they are at risk of becoming pregnant; and (4) Women who feel their alcohol use may put them at risk of delivering an infant with FASD should seek medical care. The campaign was delivered through visual, audio and print advertisements, direct marketing to the community, displays at community events, and educational videos for high-school students. A group of 418 women of childbearing age were surveyed before and after the campaign was implemented, and compared to a group of women from another community (Kansas City) that had not been exposed to the intervention. The outcomes of interest were message recall and level of knowledge about alcohol intake during pregnancy. When comparing the post-intervention and pre-intervention results, the authors found there to be a small – but statistically significant – decline in knowledge scores in the population exposed to the prevention messages. Moreover, the knowledge scores increased in direct proportion to the number of times that the respondents heard the message. In general, the FAS intervention messages had to be heard 10 or more times in order to improve FAS-prevention knowledge. The authors concluded that the targeted media campaign was ineffective in improving knowledge of FAS. The methodological quality of this study was rated as weak.

Mazis et al. [59] conducted a retrospective analytical cohort study that evaluated the impact of alcohol beverage warning labels in community samples (59% females) from across the USA. The study analyzed data from 1020 participants who were surveyed in May 1990, following exposure to beverage warning labels. These data were then compared with data from a historical cohort of 1008 individuals surveyed in 1989, who had not been exposed to beverage warning labels. The outcome of interest was change in the perception of risk associated with consuming alcohol. The data showed that the perception of risk associated with alcohol use increased, but the results were of only marginal statistical significance. No definite conclusions were made regarding the effectiveness of alcohol beverage warning labels, and no behavioral correlates of risk perception were evaluated. The methodological quality of this study was rated as weak.

Casiro et al. [32] conducted a retrospective analytical cohort study to evaluate the effectiveness of a television public awareness campaign on the risks of drinking alcohol during pregnancy. The study was conducted between June 1991 and September 1991 in a study population that consisted of 3900 women of childbearing age attending health facilities in Manitoba (Canada). At 10 weeks after the implementation of the awareness campaign, the women were surveyed about their knowledge of the risks of drinking alcohol during pregnancy, and their responses compared to those of a group of women who were surveyed before the campaign took place. The study found statistically significant differences in the level of knowledge regarding mental, physical, and behavioral abnormalities in infants whose mothers drink alcohol during pregnancy. The authors supported the effectiveness of the intervention; however, a cause–effect relationship could not be established, and it was unknown whether changes in knowledge led to behavioral changes. The methodological quality of this study was rated as weak.

Bowerman [29] conducted a retrospective analytical cohort study to analyze the effect of a community-initiated FAS intervention in an Aboriginal community. An alcohol ban was implemented from November 1994 to March 1995 in the community of Barrow, Alaska (USA). Regional rates of prenatal alcohol consumption were measured at five months after the ban was implemented, and compared with the rates of prenatal alcohol consumption in a similar group of women who lived in the community prior to the ban (January 1992 to April 1994). The study found a substantial reduction in prenatal alcohol consumption during the initial period of the alcohol ban, with both second- and third-trimester consumption rates falling, but not at significant levels. The methodological quality of this study was rated as weak.

Olsen *et al.* [65] conducted a retrospective analytical cohort study that evaluated the effectiveness of a comprehensive health campaign to reduce the use of alcohol and tobacco during pregnancy. The study was conducted between April 1984 and April 1987 among pregnant women attending midwifery centers in two cities in Denmark (Odense and Aalborg). The health campaign started in Odense in April 1985 and ended in April 1987. The city of Aalborg did not receive the health campaign, which was entitled "Healthy Habits for Two" and consisted of a brochure about smoking and drinking during pregnancy; stickers on shopping bags; as well as television, cinema, radio, and newspaper advertisements. There was no modification of the usual prenatal care that pregnant women received. Women in both cities were surveyed before and after the intervention period regarding their health behavior during pregnancy. The results showed alcohol consumption during pregnancy to be the same in both groups, with no statistically significant differences being reported in the number of teetotalers, the number of drinks per week during pregnancy, and the frequency of binge episodes. The methodological quality of this study was rated as weak.

Hankin *et al.* [46] conducted an interrupted time series study to evaluate the impact of alcohol beverage warning labels on drinking during pregnancy. The study was conducted between September 1986 and September 1993 in a prenatal clinic in Detroit, Michigan (USA). The study population consisted of 17 632 pregnant African American women (mean age 23.7 years) attending their first prenatal visit. An alcohol beverage warning label campaign was implemented in November 1989, urging women not to drink during pregnancy because of the risk of birth defects in the infant. Time series analyses were constructed for the six-year study period, examining trends in monthly means of periconceptional self-reported drinking scores among the study population. The results showed that multiparous women did not seem to be affected by the warning label, whereas the warning label had a significant, albeit small, impact on nulliparous women. The authors made no definite conclusions regarding the effectiveness of the intervention. The methodological quality of this study was rated as weak.

Awopetu *et al.* [27] was a before-and-after study that evaluated the impact of a multimedia public education campaign implemented in the broad community. The study was conducted in Essex and Atlantic counties in New Jersey (USA) between July 2006 and December 2007. The study population consisted of the entire communities of the two counties. The "Be in the kNOw" advertisement campaign urged women of childbearing age not to drink alcohol, take drugs, or smoke cigarettes if they were pregnant, and to avoid these substances if they became pregnant. Methods of delivery included the use of printed materials distributed in churches, community centers and grocery stores; public service announcements for radio broadcast; and billboard posters on city buses. Campaign materials also included the website address for the New Jersey FASD Diagnostic Centers, where information about the effects of prenatal exposure to alcohol was provided. A key feature of the campaign was the availability of a 24-hour toll-free number that referred individuals to the FASD diagnostic centers. The authors measured the number of FAS-related telephone calls that were received during a six-month follow-up period, but no other measures of clinical or social relevance were provided. No baseline information was provided regarding the average number of calls received before the intervention was implemented, and the authors drew no conclusions about the effectiveness of the intervention. The methodological quality of this study was rated as weak.

Carr and Brand [31] conducted a before-and-after study with no comparison group in order to evaluate the impact of a multimedia FASD-prevention campaign on the public's knowledge of FASD. The study was conducted in Saskatchewan, Canada, between 2005 and 2006, and the study population consisted of a representative geographical distribution of Saskatchewan residents over 19 years of age. The characteristics and delivery methods of the campaign were not described in detail. The authors measured the proportion of individuals in the community who perceived that the messages were effective, and their acquisition of knowledge. The authors suggested that the campaign may have had an impact on the public's knowledge about FASD, but drew no conclusions regarding the effectiveness of the intervention. The methodological quality of this study was rated as weak.

Ma et al. [54] conducted a before-and-after study with no comparison group to evaluate a prevention strategy that targeted Native American youth at the highest risk of engaging in behaviors that lead to FAS births. The intervention was part of a multiphased project that involved the participation of prevention specialists and gatekeepers from six states in the USA with large Native American populations. The intervention was evaluated in a sample of 90 sixth- to eighth-grade Native American students of both sexes, and consisted of a culturally appropriate multimedia presentation ("Faces Yet to Come") that was used in conjunction with activities in a curriculum guide to provide comprehensive information on the general concepts of FAS. This information was linked to concepts relevant to Native American youth. The prevention content emphasized the importance of healthy decision-making regarding the use of alcohol, and linked sexual activities to pregnancy, with the objective of stressing that FAS prevention is the shared responsibility of males and females. Measures of knowledge and attitudes about FAS prevention were evaluated at two weeks of follow-up. The authors reported that there was a significant increase in knowledge about FAS prevention, but the tests of statistical significance were not reported. The authors did not draw any definite conclusions regarding the effectiveness of the intervention. The methodological quality of this study was rated as weak.

The study conducted by Marin [55] was a before-and-after study with no comparison group, that was used to investigate the self-reported awareness of product-warning messages among independent random samples of Hispanics residing in San Francisco, California (USA). The study was conducted between 1989 and 1992, and analyzed the survey responses of a group of 4661 individuals of Hispanic background from the general population (57% females; mean age 37 years). The study objective was to evaluate changes over time in the level of awareness of various product-warning messages, including those about the use of alcohol during pregnancy. Four surveys were conducted: the first survey was conducted three months before the implementation of alcohol beverage warning labels, and the other surveys were conducted yearly after the implementation of labeling. The outcome of interest was change in the level of awareness regarding the risk of drinking alcohol during pregnancy. The authors did not report any measures of statistical significance used to assess the changes over time, and made no conclusions regarding the effectiveness of the use of alcohol warning labels in this population. No other behavior-change outcomes were evaluated in this study. The methodological quality of this study was rated as weak.

May and Hymbaugh [58] conducted a before-and-after study with no comparison group to evaluate the impact of a comprehensive, macro-level FASD-prevention program for Native Americans in Arizona, Montana and Alaska (USA). The evaluation was part of the National Indian Fetal Alcohol Syndrome Prevention Program, an initiative that aimed to provide Native American communities with the knowledge and skills to implement FASD-prevention programs targeting four populations: the community; students at both elementary and secondary schools; and women in their first pregnancy. The intervention consisted of a series of pamphlets, posters, fact sheets, curricula changes, and educational sessions that were culturally sensitive to the particular Aboriginal groups that were targeted (Plains tribes, Navajo, Alaska natives, Pueblo tribes, and acculturated Native Americans). The study analyzed the responses of 215 individuals from the community and school samples in order to assess their gain in knowledge regarding alcohol use and FASD. Overall, the study found statistically significant gains in knowledge of FASD in both the school and community samples. No outcomes related to behavioral change were evaluated in this study. The authors concluded that a macro-level health education program that targets Native American populations can be effective in increasing knowledge of FASD. The methodological quality of this study was rated as weak.

Glik *et al.* [41] conducted a before-and-after study with no comparison group to evaluate the effectiveness of a social marketing intervention to raise awareness of FAS among Hispanic and African American youth. The study was conducted between April 1998 and January 1999. The study population consisted of 971 female African American youth (mean age 15.1 years) recruited from high schools in Los Angeles, the Crenshaw area, and the northeastern San Fernando Valley area in California (USA). The campaign was aimed at increasing awareness among young females of the risks of drinking, and consisted of framed posters for message delivery accompanied by small, informational tear-off cards with similar messages. Messages were posted in public and private spaces (e.g., restrooms, waiting areas at physicians' offices, beauty parlors). The campaign was conducted during a nine-month period, and levels of knowledge about alcohol and pregnancy were evaluated at the end of a follow-up period. The results showed that exposure to the campaign was not correlated with any statistically significant increase in knowledge about the effects of alcohol during pregnancy. The authors suggested that the campaign information may have been processed peripherally, but not centrally, by the respondents, and they made no claims of effectiveness of the intervention in the study conclusions. The methodological quality of this study was rated as weak.

Walker *et al.* [72] conducted a before-and-after study with no comparison group to evaluate the impact of a brief intervention to increase knowledge about FASD among women of childbearing age (mean age 23.8 years) who had requested emergency contraception or a pregnancy test. A sample of 50 participants attending two community clinics in southeastern Michigan (USA) were enrolled for study. Participants were asked to read a short brochure ("The Facts About Fetal Alcohol Syndrome") that described FASD and fetal alcohol effects. The brochure also offered information on how to prevent FASD, and recommended abstinence from alcohol while pregnant. When measures of knowledge of alcohol use were assessed immediately afterwards, the authors found the changes in knowledge to be statistically significant, and concluded that the intervention was effective in communicating knowledge about FASD. The methodological quality of this study was rated as weak.

Kaskutas *et al.* [48] conducted a before-and-after study with no comparison group to evaluate the effects of a series of health messages, including alcohol beverage warning labels, in a cross-national community sample of pregnant women and women of childbearing age in the USA. Several methods were used to communicate the risk of drinking alcohol during pregnancy: point-of-sale warning signs; warning labels on beverage containers; and media messages delivered through television, radio, print media, and billboards. The study analyzed self-reported data from 365 women aged under 40 years who were surveyed between 1989 and 1994, about changes in the maximum number of drinks consumed while pregnant. The authors reported that most drinking women reduced their consumption during pregnancy, and over half abstained completely. A causal relationship with the exposure to the health messages was not established, however. The level of statistical significance of the results was not reported, and the authors did not draw any conclusions regarding the effectiveness of using alcohol beverage warning labels to reduce alcohol use during pregnancy. The methodological quality of this study was rated as weak.

Kinzie *et al.* [49] conducted a before-and-after study with no comparison group to evaluate the impact of a computer-based multimedia prenatal alcohol education program ("The Healthy Touch") for low-income rural women. The study population consisted of 59 women (mean age 23.5 years) presenting for prenatal care at a public clinic. The multimedia intervention provided factual and culturally relevant information about the effects of alcohol in pregnancy. Alcohol preferences were evaluated before and immediately after the intervention. The results showed that all participants indicated that they would not drink alcoholic beverages in a social situation during pregnancy. The authors suggested that the program may have influenced the participants' intentions to abstain from alcohol while pregnant, but made no final conclusions regarding the effectiveness of the intervention. The methodological quality of this study was rated as weak.

3.5.4
Summary of the Overall Results

3.5.4.1 General Characteristics

- Eighteen studies, including two Canadian studies [31 32], provided evidence regarding the effectiveness of universal prevention approaches for FASD.
- Half of the studies were published more than 13 years ago (the median year of publication was 1997).
- The majority of studies that evaluated universal preventive interventions used a before-and-after design. No RCTs were identified.
- Studies were conducted mainly in urban health facilities, or in the community.

3.5.4.2 Populations

- The majority of the studies targeted pregnant women and the broad general public. Three studies targeted youth only.

- The studies were conducted mainly in non-Caucasian populations. Three studies evaluated the impact of a universal preventive intervention in Native American populations, while the others combined the results for participants of other ethnicities.

3.5.4.3 Interventions

- The majority of universal preventive approaches targeted entire populations within the community. Social marketing activities were the most frequently implemented universal interventions, followed by health education activities.

- Individual components of the interventions included education (audiovisual materials, mass media strategies, motivational messages, computer-based education) and legal/system activities (alcohol beverage warning labels or an alcohol ban in the community).

3.5.4.4 Outcomes

- Most of the studies evaluated knowledge acquisition regarding alcohol use during pregnancy and FASD, self-reported measures of alcohol intake, and attitudes toward alcohol use during pregnancy.

- Five studies reported statistically significant differences in the results, whereas five studies did not find statistically significant differences in the analysis of outcome data. Eight studies did not test whether statistically significant differences existed between intervention groups or study periods for the outcomes of interest.

3.5.4.5 Methodological Quality of the Studies

- Only one study was considered of moderate methodological quality, while the other 17 studies were rated as weak.

3.5.4.6 Evidence on the Effectiveness of Universal Prevention Approaches

- A qualitative synthesis of individual study results (Table 3.10) showed that the best available evidence regarding the effectiveness of universal prevention approaches for FASD is for a multimedia education program aimed at youth in a suburban high-school setting. A non-randomized clinical trial [50] of moderate quality found that the program significantly increased the students' knowledge about FASD after two weeks. No information is available on whether participants sustained these knowledge gains over time.

- Two Canadian studies [31, 32] evaluated the effectiveness of universal prevention approaches implemented in Saskatchewan and Manitoba, respectively. The Saskatchewan study [31] evaluated the effects of a multimedia FASD-prevention campaign conducted between 2005 and 2006 on the negative effects of drinking alcohol during pregnancy. The study did not yield conclusions regarding the effectiveness of the intervention in increasing knowledge. The Manitoba study [32] evaluated the effectiveness of a television public awareness campaign focused on the risks of drinking alcohol during pregnancy that was conducted between June and September of 1991. The authors concluded that the intervention increased the public's knowledge of alcohol-related birth defects. The methodological quality of both studies was rated as weak.

- The evidence for the effectiveness of other universal interventions, such as alcohol-related warning messages, health education activities, and alcohol bans, is based on studies of poor methodological quality. Overall, the studies did not provide evidence that these interventions produce significant modifications over time in knowledge of FASD, attitudes toward drinking during pregnancy, and perception of the risks associated with this behavior. Only a few studies evaluated behavioral changes in alcohol intake. None of the interventions significantly modified self-reported measures of alcohol intake.

- Only five studies [27, 31, 50, 62, 72] assessing the effectiveness of universal preventive interventions have been published in the past five years. It is unknown whether universal interventions that were evaluated 15–20 years ago are still relevant and sensitive to our societal and media-technological changes.

Table 3.10 Synthesis of individual study results on the effectiveness of universal prevention approaches to FASD.

Study	Intervention	Brief description of the intervention	Study design	Study population	Results regarding the effectiveness of the intervention	Methodological quality
LaChausse [50]	Multimedia education program – FASTRAC	Multimedia, peer-delivered educational PowerPoint presentation that included information on the history of FASD, FAS and the effects of alcohol on the fetus	CCT	Broad public (Youth from a suburban high school)	The intervention significantly increased knowledge regarding FAS. However, it did not affect attitudes toward drinking during pregnancy, make participants less likely to use alcohol during pregnancy or increase the perceived severity of using alcohol during pregnancy. Partial support given for the effectiveness of the intervention in increasing knowledge.	Moderate
Calabro *et al.* [30]	Written health education materials – third-grade reading level	Health education materials written at a third-grade reading level delivered at the first prenatal visit, aimed to influence knowledge, attitude and behavioral intention to avoid alcohol while pregnant	CCT	Pregnant women	The intervention did not significantly improve knowledge, attitude and behavioral intention to avoid alcohol during pregnancy	Weak

(Continued)

Table 3.10 (Continued)

Study	Intervention	Brief description of the intervention	Study design	Study population	Results regarding the effectiveness of the intervention	Methodological quality
Waterson [73]	Health education materials	Written information about the risks of alcohol in pregnancy; personal advice and reinforcement given by a doctor; educational video	CCT	Pregnant women	The intervention did not produce significant changes in the percentage of women that consumed less than seven units of alcohol per week during pregnancy, or in the number of women who considered that less than one unit of daily alcohol was safe during, or when planning, a pregnancy.	Weak
Mengel et al. [62]	Public education campaign	Media campaign built around four FASD-prevention messages delivered through visual, audio and print advertisements, direct marketing to the community, public relations/media interviews, displays at community events, educational videos for high-school students	Prospective analytical cohort study	Women of childbearing age	The intervention was ineffective in improving knowledge of FAS.	Weak

Mazis et al. [59]	Alcohol beverage warning label	Warning label on alcohol beverages about drinking during pregnancy	Retrospective analytical cohort study	Broad public	The intervention marginally modified the perception of risks associated with alcohol use during pregnancy.	Weak
Casiro et al. [32]	Television public awareness campaign	Thirty-second television public service announcement with a message on alcohol and pregnancy, broadcast during both prime time and non-prime time viewing hours.	Retrospective analytical cohort study	Women of childbearing age	The intervention significantly improved the level of knowledge regarding newborn abnormalities caused by alcohol drinking during pregnancy.	Weak
Bowerman [29]	Alcohol ban	Prohibition of alcohol possession in the community	Retrospective analytical cohort study	Pregnant women	The intervention significantly helped to reduce regional prenatal alcohol consumption rates and fetal alcohol exposure.	Weak
Olsen et al. [65]	Health campaign – Healthy Habits for Two	Brochure about smoking and drinking during pregnancy; stickers on shopping bags; television, cinema, radio and newspaper advertisements	Retrospective analytical cohort study	Pregnant women	The intervention did not significantly increase the number of teetotalers or significantly decrease the self-reported number of drinks per week during pregnancy or the frequency of binge episodes	Weak

(Continued)

Table 3.10 (*Continued*)

Study	Intervention	Brief description of the intervention	Study design	Study population	Results regarding the effectiveness of the intervention	Methodological quality
Hankin *et al.* [46]	Alcohol beverage warning label	Federal alcohol beverage warning label urging women not to drink during pregnancy because of the risk of birth defects	Interrupted time series	Pregnant women	No conclusions about the effectiveness of the intervention. The intervention seemed to have a significant, albeit small, impact on self-reported perinatal drinking in nulliparous women.	Weak
Awopetu *et al.* [27]	Multimedia public education campaign – "Be in the kNOw"	Public education through mass media advertisement on billboard and transit posters, local newspapers, radio public service announcements, website. Content on negative consequences associated with alcohol consumption in pregnancy. Provision of resources for women who have alcohol dependency.	Before-and-after study	Broad public	No conclusions about the effectiveness of the intervention.	Weak
Carr and Brand [31]	Multimedia public education campaign	Campaign was not described in detail	Before-and-after study	Broad public	No conclusions about the effectiveness of the intervention.	Weak

Ma [54]	Educational FAS prevention program	Multimedia FAS prevention package. videos, computer-assisted technology, videotape to accompany a curriculum guide featuring 19 lessons with specific goals, project flyers, program brochure, website page	Before-and-after study	Broad public (Native American youth)	No conclusions about the effectiveness of the intervention	Weak
Marin [55]	Alcohol-related warning messages	Warning label on alcohol beverages about drinking during pregnancy	Before-and-after study	Broad public	No conclusions about the effectiveness of the intervention.	Weak
May and Hymbaugh [58]	Macro-level FAS education program – National Indian Fetal Alcohol Syndrome Prevention Program	Macro-level FAS prevention program aimed to provide communities with comprehensive knowledge, skills and materials to carry out prevention and intervention on their own	Before-and-after study	Broad public	The intervention significantly increased the level of FASD knowledge.	Weak
Glik *et al.* [41]	Public education campaign – Social marketing campaign	Social marketing intervention using a "narrowcasting" approach to raise awareness of the risks of drinking during pregnancy. Small posters and tear-off cards put in places frequented by female youth.	Before-and-after study	Women of childbearing age (African American and Hispanic youth)	The intervention did not significantly increase the level of knowledge about the effects of drinking alcohol during pregnancy.	Weak

(Continued)

Table 3.10 (*Continued*)

Study	Intervention	Brief description of the intervention	Study design	Study population	Results regarding the effectiveness of the intervention	Methodological quality
Walker *et al.* [72]	Brief intervention for prenatal alcohol use	Education brochure ("Facts About Fetal Alcohol Syndrome")	Before-and-after study	Women of childbearing age	The intervention was significantly effective in communicating knowledge about FASD.	Weak
Kaskutas *et al.* [48]	Alcohol beverage warning label	Health messages on drinking during pregnancy (labels on alcohol beverage containers, point-of-sale signs, advertisements)	Before-and-after study	Pregnant women and women of childbearing age	No conclusions about the effectiveness of the intervention.	Weak
Kinzie *et al.* [49]	Interactive multimedia education program – The Healthy Touch	Computer-based multimedia educational program addressing alcohol use in pregnancy	Before-and-after study	Pregnant women	No conclusions about the effectiveness of the intervention.	Weak

CCT = controlled clinical trial; FAS = fetal alcohol syndrome; FASD = fetal alcohol spectrum disorder; FASTRAC = The Fetal Alcohol Spectrum Teaching and Research Awareness Campaign.

3.6

Evidence on the Effectiveness of Selective Prevention Approaches for FASD

3.6.1

Characteristics of Included Studies

3.6.1.1 General Characteristics

Twenty-three studies [26, 28, 33–40, 44, 47, 51, 52, 60, 61, 63, 64, 66, 67, 69, 71, 75] provided evidence on the effectiveness of selective prevention approaches for FASD. The characteristics of studies that evaluated selective prevention approaches are summarized in Table 3.E.2 of Appendix 3.E.

The studies were published between 1983 and 2010, with a median year of publication of 2000 (IQR: 1995, 2007). All of the studies except for two dissertations [36, 38] were published as journal articles. The majority of studies (n = 19) originated in the USA, the exceptions being two studies conducted in Sweden [51, 63], one in Norway [60], and one multicenter study [28] that involved four Latin American countries (Argentina, Brazil, Cuba, and Mexico). Of the 23 studies, 14 were clinical trials (six RCTs [26, 33, 34, 36, 39, 40] and eight CCTs [28, 38, 44, 47, 64, 66, 67, 69]), three were prospective observational analytical cohort studies [37, 60, 61], one study was a retrospective analytical cohort study [63], and five [35, 51, 52, 71, 75] were before-and-after studies with no comparison group.

Eighteen studies reported their sources of funding. Sixteen studies [26, 28, 33, 34, 37, 39, 40, 44, 51, 52, 61, 63, 64, 66, 69, 75] were funded by government agencies, and one study [60] received funding from a society. One study [47] used internal as well as government and society funds.

Twenty studies [26, 28, 33–39, 44, 51, 52, 60, 61, 63, 64, 67, 69, 71, 75] were conducted in health facilities, and one study [47] was conducted in a school setting. Two studies combined settings: community, health facilities and an urban jail [40], and community, schools, and health facilities [66], respectively.

3.6.1.2 Characteristics of the Populations

The populations most frequently targeted in the studies were women at risk of an AEP (evaluated in 11 studies [26, 33–35, 37, 39, 44, 64, 67, 71, 75]) and pregnant women (nine studies [28, 36, 38, 51, 52, 60, 61, 63, 69]). Participants in three studies [40, 47, 66] were women of childbearing age who consumed alcohol. Two studies [28, 34] involved partners or support persons in the study sampling. The residential settings of the target populations were urban in 11 studies [28, 33, 34, 38, 44, 47, 51, 60, 64, 66, 75], suburban city areas in four studies [35, 36, 69, 71], and a mix of urban and rural areas in five studies [39, 40, 52, 61, 67]. Three studies [26, 37, 63] did not report the residential setting of the study population.

Overall, the studies had large sample sizes, the median number of participants per study being 265 (IQR: 119, 652; data from 22 studies that reported the number of enrolled participants). All of the studies except one [34] involved female populations only. The median chronological age of participants in the studies was 24.7 years (IQR: 22.1, 27.9; data from 16 studies). Half of the studies included adult populations only (13 studies [33, 34, 37–40, 44, 47, 60, 61, 63, 64, 75]), whereas three studies [28, 66, 69] included youth populations only. Six studies [26, 35, 36, 51, 67, 71] included both adult and youth populations, and one study [52] did not report the age range of study participants.

Seventeen studies [26, 33–40, 44, 47, 64, 66, 67, 69, 71, 75] included participants of miscellaneous races, whereas two studies [28, 61] focused on non-Caucasian populations (i.e., Native Americans and Hispanics). Four studies [51, 52, 60, 63] did not report the race of study participants. Only two studies that included participants of various races [39, 67] reported separate results by race. One study that included both Native Americans and Hispanics [61] did not conduct a subgroup analysis by race. It is unknown whether the study populations had past or current exposure to similar or other FASD prevention approaches.

3.6.1.3 Characteristics of the Interventions

The vast majority of selective preventive approaches evaluated in the studies were directed at the individual level (22 studies [26, 28, 33–40, 44, 47, 51, 60, 61, 63, 64, 66, 67, 69, 71, 75]). One study [52] implemented the intervention at the community and system-wide level. The types of public health intervention implemented in the selective preventive approaches for FASD are described in Figure 3.6. Some

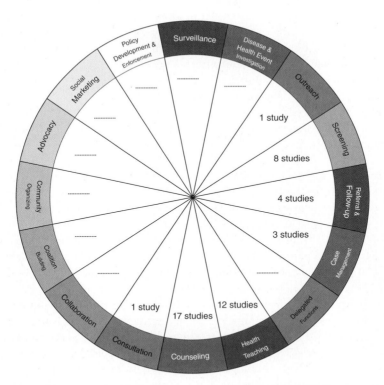

Figure 3.6 Types of public health intervention implemented in selective prevention approaches for FASD. Adapted from the Minnesota Department of Health Division of Community Health Services [76].

studies implemented more than one intervention and, therefore, the number of interventions does not match the number of studies.

Counseling activities were the most frequently implemented interventions in the studies (17 studies [26, 33–35, 37, 39, 40, 44, 47, 51, 52, 60, 63, 64, 66, 71, 75]), followed by health teaching (12 studies [28, 33, 35, 36, 38, 52, 61, 64, 66, 67, 69, 71]), referrals and follow-up (four studies [35, 37, 51, 52]), screening and case-finding activities (six studies [35, 37, 51, 52, 64, 71]), case management (three studies [35, 37, 66]), consultation (one study [60]), and outreach (one study [35]).

The FASD selective prevention approaches examined in the individual studies, according to the type of population targeted, are described in Table 3.11. The studies have been arranged by study design, from clinical trials to observational analytical designs.

3.5.1.4 Components of the Interventions

Nine studies described their underlying theoretical frameworks; these included social cognitive theory [38, 64, 67], an activated health education model [36], an ecological model of social support [28], a cognitive behavioral approach [39, 66, 75], social marketing theory [61], and a transtheoretical model that was not further specified [40].

While the majority of selective preventive interventions were implemented in healthcare facilities (16 studies [26, 33, 34, 36, 38–40, 51, 60, 61, 63, 64, 66, 69, 71, 75]), a few were implemented in other settings, such as the community [37, 52], homes [28, 35], or schools [47]. In two studies [44, 67], the interventions were implemented both at health facilities and in homes.

The individual components of the interventions fell into two main categories: brief interventions; and education. Brief interventions included individual counseling (16 studies [26, 33–35, 37, 39, 40, 44, 47, 51, 52, 60, 63, 64, 71, 75]), referral to available services (five studies [35, 37, 51, 52, 66]), case management (four studies [35, 37, 51, 66]), skills training (two studies [36, 66]), support groups (two studies [37, 52]), and alcohol-intake testing and counseling (one study [33]). Educational activities included educational sessions (five studies [36, 61, 66, 67, 69]), the use of motivational messages (five studies [33, 36, 61, 67, 69]), the distribution of printed educational materials [28, 52], audiovisual materials [38], and mass media strategies [52].

The interventions required the participation of a variety of providers, such as midwives [60, 63], health educators [36, 61, 67], counselors [40], physicians [33], nurses [34], nutritionists [64], public health nurses [71] and multidisciplinary teams (i.e., nurses and certified alcoholism therapists [52]; nurses and medical students [75]; obstetric nurses and research staff [39]; public health nurses, substance-abuse counselors, and other members of interdisciplinary teams not further specified [35]; social workers and health educators [66]; social workers and obstetric nurses [28]; social workers and substance-abuse treatment providers [26]; and midwives and social workers [51]). Two studies [38, 69] delivered the interventions through media or printed materials, and therefore no providers or other personnel were required. Three studies [37, 44, 47] did not describe the type of provider.

Table 3.11 FASD selective prevention approaches examined in individual studies.

Study	Study design	Intervention	Population
Floyd *et al.* [40]	RCT	Counseling (motivational interview)	Women of childbearing age who consume alcohol
Armstrong *et al.* [26]	RCT	Brief intervention	Women at risk of an AEP
Chang *et al.* [33]	RCT	Assessment and brief intervention	Women at risk of an AEP
Chang *et al.* [34]	RCT	Brief intervention	Women at risk of an AEP, and their partners/support persons
Fleming [39]	RCT	Brief intervention	Women at risk of an AEP
Crosby [36]	RCT	Health education program	Pregnant women
Ingersoll *et al.* [47]	CCT	Counseling (motivational interview)	Women of childbearing age who consume alcohol
Palinkas *et al.* [66]	CCT	Counseling (cognitive behavioral approach)	Women of childbearing age who consume alcohol
O'Connor and Whaley [64]	CCT	Counseling	Women at risk of an AEP
Reynolds *et al.* [67]	CCT	Health education program	Women at risk of an AEP
Belizan *et al.* [28]	CCT	Health education program	Pregnant women and their partners/support persons
Eustace [38]	CCT	Health education program	Pregnant women
Sarvela and Ford [69]	CCT	Health education program	Pregnant women
Handmaker *et al.* [44]	CCT	Counseling (motivational interview)	Women at risk of an AEP
Eisen *et al.* [37]	Prospective analytical cohort study	Counseling (case management and referral to services)	Women at risk of an AEP
Meberg [60]	Prospective analytical cohort study	Counseling	Pregnant women
Mehl-Madrona [61]	Prospective analytical cohort study	Health education program	Pregnant women
Nilsen [63]	Retrospective analytical cohort study	Counseling	Pregnant women
Corrarino *et al.* [35]	Before-and-after study	Assessment and brief intervention	Women at risk of an AEP

Table 3.11 (*Continued*)

Study	Study design	Intervention	Population
Tavris [71]	Before-and-after study	Assessment and brief intervention	Women at risk of an AEP
Yonkers [75]	Before-and-after study	Motivational interview and therapy	Women at risk of an AEP
Larsson [51]	Before-and-after study	Assessment and brief intervention	Pregnant women
Little *et al.* [52]	Before-and-after study	Counseling	Pregnant women

AEP = alcohol-exposed pregnancy; CCT = controlled clinical trial; RCT = randomized controlled trial.

Eleven studies [28, 34, 36. 39, 40, 47, 61, 64, 66, 67, 75] reported that the providers received training prior to implementing the intervention. Seven studies [28, 33, 36, 39, 47, 64, 67] used a manual to guarantee the integrity of the implementation. A detailed description of the characteristics of the selective preventive approaches that were evaluated in the individual studies is provided in Table 3.F.2 of Appendix 3.F.

3.6.1.5 Characteristics of the Outcomes

A total of 75 outcomes was reported in the 23 studies that assessed the effectiveness of FASD selective prevention approaches. The types of outcome measure that were examined in the studies are listed in Table 3.12.

The effects of selective FASD-prevention approaches were evaluated mainly through intermediate outcomes (45 outcomes) related to changes in patterns of drinking behavior, followed by ultimate outcomes related to maternal, neonatal and infant-related outcomes (25 outcomes). Immediate outcomes related to knowledge about and perception of alcohol use during pregnancy were less frequently examined (five outcomes).

The most frequently studied outcomes were those of self-reported alcohol intake (36 outcomes), followed by neonatal and infant outcomes (16 outcomes), maternal outcomes (five outcomes). alcohol abstinence (four outcomes), and binge drinking (three outcomes).

3.6.1.6 Types of Result Reported in the Individual Studies

The types of result described in the 23 studies on selective prevention approaches to FASD are displayed in Table 3.13. They are described in terms of the report of statistically significant differences in the outcomes of interest and the support of the selective approach under the study conclusions.

Among the 23 studies that provided evidence on the effectiveness of selective prevention approaches to FASD, ten studies [26, 37–40, 47, 52, 61, 64, 67] reported

Table 3.12 Types of outcome measure examined in studies on selective prevention approaches to FASD.

Type of outcome		Number of outcomes assessed at different follow-up periods					
		≤3 months	>3 months and ≤6 months	>6 months and ≤9 months	>9 months and ≤1 year	>1 year	Total number of outcomes
Immediate	Attitudes toward alcohol use during pregnancy	–	1	–	1	–	2
	Knowledge about alcohol use during pregnancy/FASD	1	1	–	–	–	2
	Awareness of risk of alcohol use during pregnancy	–	–	–	1	–	1
	Perceptions about alcohol use during pregnancy	–	–	–	–	–	–
Intermediate	Alcohol intake	12	10	3	11	–	36
	Alcohol abstinence	2	–	1	1	–	4
	Binge drinking	1	–	1	1	–	3
	AEP	1	–	1	–	–	2
Ultimate	Neonatal and infant outcome	–	–	1	14	1	16
	FASD outcome	–	–	–	2	–	2
	Legal outcome	–	–	–	1	–	1
	Maternal outcome	–	–	2	3	–	5
	Economic and healthcare utilization outcome	–	–	–	1	–	1
	Family outcome	–	–	–	–	–	–
Total		17	12	9	36	1	75

AEP = alcohol-exposed pregnancy; FASD = fetal alcohol spectrum disorder.

Table 3.13 Types of results reported in the individual studies assessing the effectiveness of selective prevention approaches to FASD.

Report of statistically significant differences in the results	Study conclusion				Total number of studies
	No support of the effectiveness of the intervention (number of studies)	No conclusions regarding the effectiveness of the intervention (number of studies)	Partial support of the effectiveness of the intervention (number of studies)	Support of the effectiveness of the intervention (number of studies)	
Study did not provide data on statistical testing of the differences	–	1 ☺	–	2 ☹	3
Study did not find statistically significant differences	7 ☺	–	1 ☹	2 ☹	10
Study reported statistically significant differences	–	1 ☹	2 ☺	7 ☺	10
Total number of studies	7	2	3	11	23

☺ = an appropriate conclusion based on study results; ☹ = an inappropriate conclusion based on study results; ☺ = an appropriate partial conclusion based on study results.

statistically significant differences in the results, whereas another ten [28, 33, 34, 36, 44, 51, 60, 63, 66, 69] reported that they found no statistically significant differences in the analysis of outcome data. Three studies [35, 71, 75] did not describe the use of statistical tests to analyze whether statistically significant differences existed among the groups or study periods for the outcomes of interest.

In interpreting the results of their studies, the primary authors of 11 studies [34, 35, 37, 39, 40, 44, 47, 61, 64, 67, 71] claimed that the intervention under study was effective, whereas the authors of eight studies [28, 33, 36, 52, 60, 63, 66, 69] did not support the effectiveness of the intervention. Three studies [26, 38, 51] gave partial endorsement to the effectiveness of the selective approach under study, based on the interpretation of secondary outcomes in the studies. Two studies [52, 75] did not state definite conclusions regarding the effectiveness of the intervention.

Six studies yielded to conclusions regarding the effectiveness of the FASD selective prevention approach that were not supported by the analysis of the outcome data. Two studies [35, 71] that did not provide information on the statistical significance of the differences in the results concluded that the intervention was effective. Among the studies that reported no statistically significant differences in the data analysis, two [34, 44] supported the effectiveness of the intervention, and one study [51] gave partial support. Seven studies [28, 33, 36, 60, 63, 66, 69] that did not find statistically significant differences in the analysis of outcome data correctly concluded that the intervention was not effective. Among the ten studies that found statistically significant differences in the results, nine studies gave full [37, 39, 40, 47, 61, 64, 67] or partial [26, 38] support to the effectiveness of the selective approach, and one study [52] made no conclusions regarding the effectiveness of the intervention.

3.6.2
Methodological Quality of the Studies

Twelve studies [26, 34, 35, 37, 44, 51, 52, 60, 67, 69, 71, 75] that evaluated the effectiveness of selective FASD-prevention approaches were rated as weak in their methodological quality, while ten [33, 36, 38, 40, 47, 61, 63, 64, 66, 78] were considered to be of moderate quality. Only one study [39] was rated as strong in methodological quality.

An overview of how well the studies controlled for methodological issues related to selection bias, allocation bias, confounding, blinding of outcome assessors, validity and reliability of data collection methods, and management of withdrawals and dropouts is provided in Table 3.14.

There was a large variation across the studies in the ratings of the individual quality components. Overall, the majority of the studies were able to control for the effect of confounders in the allocation of interventions and the analysis of data. The most common methodological weaknesses were related to the methods used to select the study samples, and the blinding of outcome assessors. A detailed description of the methodological quality of the individual studies that assessed

Table 3.14 Methodological quality of studies assessing the effectiveness of selective prevention approaches to FASD.

Domains of Methodological Quality	Number of studies rated as Weak	Number of studies rated as Moderate	Number of studies rated as Strong
Methods to control for selection bias	13	8	2
Methods to control for allocation bias	–	10	13
Methods to control for confounders	7	2	14
Methods of blinding	14	8	1
Data collection methods	10	3	10
Methods to handle withdrawals and dropouts	5	7	11
Global methodological quality	12	10	1

the effectiveness of selective prevention approaches is provided in Table 3.G.2 of Appendix 3.G.

Methodological aspects that go beyond the internal validity of the studies were also evaluated. Ten studies [34, 35, 38, 44, 47, 60, 61, 66, 67, 75] failed to report the dates for starting and stopping accession of participants. The majority of the studies mentioned how representative the sample was of the selection criteria for enrolling participants. Only two studies [52, 63] failed to describe the inclusion and exclusion criteria used. One-third of the studies [26, 28, 33, 34, 36, 40, 64, 67] reported the number of eligible participants before intervention allocation took place.

The quality of the reporting of the characteristics of interventions, and the conditions under which the interventions operated, was poor. Four studies [34, 36, 64, 67] monitored the fidelity of the intervention. For most of the studies ($n = 21$) it was unknown whether the study participants received another, unintended intervention. It is likely that participants in the other two studies [38, 52] received an unintended cointervention that may have influenced the results.

Sixteen studies [26, 28, 33–36, 38–40, 47, 60, 61, 63, 66, 69, 75] described the frequency of delivery of the intervention, whereas ten studies [26, 33, 34, 38–40, 63, 64, 67, 75] reported on the duration of the intervention.

Some issues related to the data analysis in the individual studies were evaluated. Four studies [34, 39, 60, 61] reported that an ITT approach was used in the analysis of the results. Finally, three studies [26, 52, 64] had unit-of-analysis errors; that is to say, the groups were the unit of allocation, but individuals were used as the unit of analysis.

3.6.3
Results of Qualitative Synthesis of the Evidence

The large clinical heterogeneity of the individual interventions implemented in the studies that assessed the effectiveness of selective FASD-prevention approaches precluded a meta-analysis of the data. However, a qualitative review was conducted to identify patterns across individual study results. The variables that were systematically examined to shed light on reasons for the findings were study design, duration of follow-up, sample size, population characteristics, comparison, and outcomes. The following is an overview of the qualitative review of selective preventive interventions for FASD based on the data provided in 23 studies. The presentation of the studies and their results is by study design, from clinical trials to observational studies.

3.6.3.1 Clinical Trials

Floyd *et al.* [40] conducted an RCT that evaluated the effectiveness of a brief motivational intervention to reduce the risk of an AEP among women of childbearing age (mean age 29.6 years) who consumed alcohol. The study was part of the Project CHOICES, a multisite collaborative study conducted in six community settings (jails, drug and alcohol treatment centers, suburban primary care practices, and other health facilities) in Florida, Texas, and Virginia (USA). A total of 830 non-pregnant women (mean age 29.6 years) was randomized to two intervention groups: Project CHOICES (counseling and information regarding the risks of alcohol abuse during pregnancy); and a group that received information only. The study included African American and non-Hispanic participants, but did not conduct an analysis of the results by race. The CHOICES intervention delivered counseling through a motivational interview intended to encourage women to change the target behavior of risky drinking. Previously trained counselors delivered the intervention; however, the authors of the study did not mention the use of a manual to guarantee intervention fidelity. Self-reported alcohol intake was measured, and the risk of AEP was evaluated, at three, six, and nine months of follow-up. The results showed a statistically significant reduction in risk of an AEP in the CHOICES Project group at three months (unadjusted odds ratio [OR] = 2.0; 95% CI = 1.5, 2.80), six months (unadjusted OR = 1.9; 95% CI = 1.4, 2.6) and nine months (unadjusted OR = 1.9; 95% CI = 1.3, 2.6) of follow-up. The results remained significant after the study results had been adjusted for confounders in the analysis. The women in the CHOICES Project group were also more likely to reduce alcohol consumption to below risk levels (OR = 1.5; 95% CI = 1.1, 2.2). The authors supported the effectiveness of the CHOICES Project intervention in reducing the risk of an AEP among women of childbearing age. The methodological quality of this study was rated as moderate.

Armstrong *et al.* [26] conducted an RCT to evaluate the effect of two brief interventions (Early Start Plus and Early Start) implemented in the prenatal care clinics of Kaiser Permanente Northern California (USA) between May 2000 and June 2004. The study participants included 908 pregnant women aged 15 to 44 years, who screened positive for alcohol drinking. The participants were randomized to one of three groups: (1) Early Start Plus, which incorporated a computerized drink-size assessment tool and a prenatal care focused on drinking reduction; (2) Early Start intervention, which consisted of substance-abuse screening and a treatment program integrated with prenatal care focused on abstention; and (3) A control group of untreated alcohol users. The intervention was delivered by licensed clinical social workers and other trained substance-abuse treatment providers. Neonatal outcomes, such as assisted ventilation, birth weight, preterm delivery, admission in the neonatal intensive care unit and rehospitalizations, were assessed at the postpartum period. Compared to the control group, women in the Early Start Plus group were less likely to initiate preterm labor (OR = 0.44 (95% CI = 0.20, 0.97). Likewise, the infants of women assigned to the Early Start group were less likely to have a low birth weight than infants of the untreated (control) women. The authors concluded that Early Start Plus and Early Start were potentially helpful in reducing the incidence of preterm events. The methodological quality of this study was rated as moderate.

Chang *et al.* [33] conducted an RCT to evaluate the impact of a brief intervention on antepartum alcohol consumption. The study was conducted in an urban obstetric practice in Boston, Massachusetts (USA), in 1994. The study population consisted of 250 adult women (mean age 30.7 years) at risk of an AEP. The study included participants of diverse races, but did not analyze the results by race. Patients were randomized either to a group receiving a brief intervention for prenatal alcohol use, or to an assessment-only group. The brief intervention was structured as follows: (1) Review of the participant's general health; (2) Review of lifestyle changes made since pregnancy; (3) Articulation of drinking goals and pregnancy; (4) Identification of circumstances that may tempt her to drink; (5) Identification of alternatives to drinking; and (6) Summary of the session. The intervention was delivered by physicians, but no description of any previous training in the intervention, or the use of a manual to ensure intervention fidelity, was provided. Self-reported measures of alcohol intake were evaluated at 22 weeks of follow-up and at the postpartum period; neonatal outcomes were also evaluated. The study results showed no statistically significant differences between the groups in the net decrease of drinks per drinking day at 22 weeks, in the mean number of antepartum drinking episodes, and in neonatal measures such as infant birth weight and 1-minute Apgar scores. The authors concluded that both interventions helped to reduce antepartum alcohol consumption. The methodological quality of this study was rated as moderate.

Chang *et al.* [34] conducted an RCT to evaluate the effectiveness of a brief single-session intervention in the reduction of prenatal alcohol consumption. The study was conducted in an urban obstetric practice in Boston, Massachusetts (USA). The study dates are unclear, but the study population consisted of 304 adult women (mean age 31.3 years) at risk of an AEP, and their partners. The study included participants of diverse races, but did not conduct an analysis of the results by race. Patients were randomized to a group that received a single-session intervention, or to a group that received assessment of their alcohol status only. The brief intervention included: (1) Knowledge assessment with feedback; (2) Contracting and goal setting; (3) Behavioral modification; and (4) Summary of the intervention. Previously trained nurse practitioners delivered the intervention to study participants; however, the study did not mention whether a manual was used to ensure implementation fidelity. Self-reported measures of alcohol intake were evaluated between nine months and one year of follow-up. The study results showed no statistically significant differences between the groups in the mean percentage of drinking days at the end of the follow-up period, nor in the percentage of participants who consumed less than half a drink per episode in the postpartum period. Effectiveness of the intervention was demonstrated only for the group of women who drank more prenatally. The authors supported the effectiveness of the intervention in the conclusions. The methodological quality of this study was rated as moderate. Although the study used a method of randomization which ensured that no imbalances existed at baseline, there was bias in the selection of participants for the study before randomization took place, and a lack of blinding in the outcome assessment.

Fleming [39] conducted an RCT to evaluate the effectiveness of a brief intervention among postpartum women. The study was conducted in community clinics in southcentral and southeastern Wisconsin (USA) from 2002 to 2005. The study population consisted of 235 postpartum adult women (mean age 28 years) who screened positive for high-risk alcohol use. The participants were randomized either to a group that received a two-session brief intervention, or to a control group that received standard postnatal care. The intervention was delivered by clinic nurses, who used a workbook to ask scripted questions and provide feedback on current health behaviors, problem drinking, and the adverse effects of alcohol, particularly focused on women and pregnancy. Self-reported measures of alcohol intake were evaluated at six months of follow-up. The authors found that the intervention produced statistically significant reductions in the number of drinks consumed in the previous month, the number of drinking days, and the number of heavy drinking days. The authors concluded that the brief intervention was effective at reducing alcohol use in postpartum women. The methodological quality of this study was strong, and it is the study that provides the best evidence regarding the effectiveness of a selective intervention approach to FASD.

Crosby [36] conducted an RCT to evaluate the effects of a prenatal alcohol-education intervention in a convenience sample of 80 women (mean age 27.7 years) receiving prenatal care at the early stages of pregnancy in an urban health facility in West Seneca, New York (USA). The study included participants of diverse races, but did not conduct a subgroup analysis by race. Patients were randomized to one of three interventions: a cognitive-based prenatal alcohol education program; a program of information only; and usual prenatal care. The prenatal alcohol education program was integrated into a class that addressed such topics as prenatal exercises, prenatal nutrition, and alcohol education. Two methods of presentation were compared: (i) a program that used a modified activated method of participation; and (ii) a program that provided only information on alcohol use during pregnancy. Both groups were compared with a group that received usual prenatal care. Previously trained health educators delivered the intervention, and a manual was used to guarantee intervention fidelity. Measures of attitudes and knowledge about alcohol use during pregnancy, alcohol intake, and risk of FASD were evaluated at five months of follow-up. The study results showed that alcohol intake before pregnancy and in early and late pregnancy were greatly reduced in all three groups. The two experimental groups reported a higher alcohol intake before pregnancy, and showed a greater reduction in the amount of alcohol ingested in the period from before pregnancy to early pregnancy than did the group that received usual prenatal care. The change in alcohol intake in the period from early to late pregnancy did not vary among the groups. The study did not report any statistically significant results among the groups, and the authors did not support the effectiveness of the interventions in their conclusions. The methodological quality of this study was rated as moderate.

Ingersoll et al. [47] conducted a clinical trial that evaluated a motivational interview-based intervention to reduce the risk of AEP in a sample of 228 female students (mean age 20.4 years) from a mid-Atlantic urban university who consumed alcohol. The authors described the study as an RCT; however, in this review it was classified as a CCT because the methods of intervention allocation and generation of the randomization sequence were not described. Study participants received one of two interventions: (i) a session called Birth Control and Alcohol Awareness: Negotiating Choices Effectively (BALANCE); or (ii) health information delivered in a pamphlet. The BALANCE intervention was based on the principles of Project CHOICES [40], and included a single session of personalized feedback and motivational interviewing. Counselors with previous training delivered the intervention, and a manual was available to guarantee the integrity of the intervention. Measures of alcohol intake (use, binge drinking) and the risk of AEP were evaluated at one month of follow-up. The study results showed that the BALANCE intervention was efficacious in reducing the risk of AEP in the short term (one-month follow-up). The methodological quality of this study was rated as moderate.

Palinkas et al. [66] conducted a clinical trial to evaluate the effectiveness of social skills training and social network restructuring in the prevention of drug use among high-risk females (i.e., youth who were pregnant or at-risk for pregnancy, and who were using drugs or at-risk for using drugs). The study participants were 296 youth (mean age 16 years) who had been recruited from health facilities and schools in the San Diego, California (USA) area. The authors stated that participants' allocation to the intervention was random; however, the study was classified as a CCT in this review because the methods of intervention allocation and generation of the randomization sequence were not described. Study participants were allocated to one of two interventions: (i) a normative education intervention (Facts of Life), combined with a social skills training program (Positive Adolescent Life Skills, or PALS); or (ii) Facts of Life only. The PALS program consisted of cognitive and behavioral training to improve social skills and restructure the youth's social network. The goals of the program were to enable youth to: (1) assertively refuse requests to engage in high-risk behaviors (i.e., drug and alcohol use); (2) assertively handle fair and aggressive criticism from parents and other authority figures; (3) increase positive social support; (4) decrease negative social support; and (5) develop assertive problem-solving skills. The intervention was delivered by a multidisciplinary team of social workers and health educators. No description of previous training, nor the use of a manual to guarantee intervention integrity were provided. When self-reported measures of alcohol intake were assessed at three months post-intervention, the authors found that alcohol intake was increased significantly in the PALS group. They concluded that the PALS skills training intervention may be ineffective and possibly even counterproductive as a preventive intervention in high-risk youth. An alternative explanation for the failure of the PALS intervention was that the implementation lacked cultural sensitivity in a setting in which African-Americans and Mexican-Americans made up 80% of the study group. The methodological quality of this study was rated as moderate.

O'Connor and Whaley [64] conducted a clinical trial that evaluated the efficacy of a brief intervention for alcohol use by pregnant women. The study was conducted between June 2001 and March 2004 among attendees of the Public Health Foundation Enterprises Management Solutions Special Supplemental Nutrition Program for Women, Infants and Children (PHFE-WIC) in Los Angeles and Orange Counties, California (USA). The study participants were 345 women (mean age 28.1 years) who were at risk of an AEP. The authors described the study as an RCT, but in this review it was classified as a CCT because the methods of intervention allocation and generation of the randomization sequence were not described. Study participants received one of two interventions: (i) a comprehensive assessment of alcohol use; or (ii) a standardized workbook-driven brief intervention consisting of education and feedback, cognitive-behavioral procedures and a therapeutic contract. Self-reported alcohol intake during the third trimester and neonatal outcomes at birth were assessed. The study results showed that women who received the brief intervention were fivefold more likely to report abstinence after the intervention than women in the assessment-only group. However, a large confidence interval around the effect estimate indicates a large uncertainty about the true value of this parameter. The study also found that newborns whose mothers received the brief intervention had higher birth weights, while the fetal mortality rates were threefold lower than newborns in the assessment-only group. The authors concluded that the brief intervention was more effective than the assessment alone in reducing alcohol drinking and improving neonatal outcomes. The methodological quality of this study was rated as moderate.

Reynolds et al. [67] conducted a clinical trial that evaluated the effects of a cognitive-behavioral intervention for reducing alcohol consumption among economically disadvantaged pregnant women. The study included 78 pregnant women (mean age 22.4 years) who reported drinking during the previous month. The participants were predominantly African Americans (67%), but no subgroup analyses were made by race. The authors stated that the participants' allocation to intervention was made at random; however, in this review the study was classified as a CCT because the methods of intervention allocation and generation of the randomization sequence were not provided. Participants were assigned to one of two groups: a cognitive-behavioral self-help intervention; or the usual prenatal care. The self-help intervention consisted of a 10-minute educational session coupled with a nine-step self-help manual to be completed at home. Measures of alcohol intake at two months post-intervention showed that the self-help intervention produced a higher rate of alcohol cessation and greater reductions in alcohol consumption than did the usual prenatal care. The authors concluded that a cognitive-behavioral self-help intervention was more effective than usual prenatal care to reduce alcohol consumption among pregnant women. The methodological quality of this study was rated as moderate.

Belizan *et al.* [28] conducted a clinical trial to evaluate the impact of health education during pregnancy on behavior and the utilization of health resources. The study was conducted in Argentina, Brazil, Cuba, and Mexico between January 1989 and March 1991. The study population consisted of 2235 pregnant women (mean age 24.4 years), who initiated prenatal care between the 15th and 22nd weeks of pregnancy. The authors stated that allocation to intervention groups was random; however, in this review the study was classified as a CCT because the methods of intervention allocation and generation of the randomization sequence were not described. Study participants were allocated to one of two interventions: health education delivered through home visits; and the usual prenatal care. The health education intervention was delivered by trained female social workers or obstetric nurses, and consisted of four home visits at weeks 22, 26, 30, and 34 of gestation. During the home visits, the participants and their support person or partner were encouraged to discuss healthy choices during pregnancy, and the woman was provided with direct emotional support and assistance in resolving problems related to the implementation of medical recommendations or prenatal care attendance. Self-reported measures of alcohol intake and maternal morbidity at week 36 were evaluated. No statistically significant differences were found between the groups in either alcohol use or in maternal or perinatal outcomes, such as the premature rupture of membranes, intrauterine growth retardation, and preterm labor. The authors did not support the effectiveness of the intervention. The methodological quality of this study was rated as moderate.

The study conducted by Eustace [38] was a CCT that evaluated the effects of a nurse supportive-educative intervention on alcohol consumption during pregnancy. The study, which was conducted in a large southern city in the USA, included 281 pregnant women (mean age 23 years) who attended prenatal clinics at less than 30 weeks of gestation. The study participants were mainly African-American and Caucasian. The participants were assigned (by the day of their clinic attendance) to one of three intervention groups, using a biased method for intervention allocation. One intervention group viewed a supportive-educative video that provided positive reinforcement, while another group viewed a supportive-educative video that provided negative reinforcement. These two groups were compared with a control group that viewed a video with neutral information. The interventions were media-based, and therefore no provider was required. Measures of alcohol intake and knowledge about alcohol use during pregnancy were evaluated at a maximum follow-up period of 12 weeks. The study results showed that the interventions with positive and negative reinforcements significantly increased knowledge about the effects of alcohol use during pregnancy. This knowledge gain, however, did not reflect in reductions in alcohol intake during pregnancy. The authors gave partial support to the effectiveness of the interventions because of the increase in knowledge. The methodological quality of this study was rated as moderate.

Sarvela and Ford [69] conducted a CCT that evaluated the effectiveness of a prenatal substance-abuse education program for pregnant youth. The study enrolled 212 pregnant African-American and Caucasian youth who were seeking prenatal care in health facilities in southern Illinois counties (USA). They were allocated to one of the following two intervention groups by county of residence: (i) the Adolescent Substance Prevention Education Network (ASPEN) prenatal health education program; or (ii) the usual prenatal care. The ASPEN program was a series of eight self-administered educational modules concerning the use of alcohol and other drugs during pregnancy. Each module included an educational page and an activity page that were culturally sensitive to the target population. No intervention provider was required, as the participants completed the modules while waiting to see a physician for prenatal care. Measures of alcohol intake during the postpartum period, as well as neonatal outcome, were evaluated. The study results showed that both the ASPEN program and the usual prenatal care interventions decreased the frequency of alcohol use at postpartum. The incidence of birth defects, infant complications, and positive meconium testing were similar between the groups, and there were no statistically significant differences between the groups in terms of infant birth weights. The authors did not support the effectiveness of the intervention over usual prenatal care, and concluded that both programs may be effective. The methodological quality of this study was rated as weak.

Handmaker *et al.* [44] conducted a clinical trial that evaluated the efficacy of motivational interviewing as a preventive intervention to reduce alcohol use in pregnant women. The study participants included 42 urban women (mean age 24 years) enrolled from the University of Mexico (USA) medical center obstetric clinics, who had reported consuming at least one drink during the past month. The authors described the study as an RCT; however, it was classified in this review as a CCT because the methods of intervention allocation and generation of the randomization sequence were not described. Study participants received one of two interventions: a motivational interview; or a control condition consisting of the provision of information about the potential risks of drinking during pregnancy. The motivational interview was a 1-hour session in which a healthcare provider discussed issues related to the woman's drinking behavior and knowledge of alcohol use during pregnancy. The training of the provider was not described, and it is unknown whether a manual was available to guarantee the integrity of the intervention. Self-reported measures of alcohol intake (total drinks, total number of abstinent days) were evaluated at two months of follow-up. No statistically significant results were reported for the main outcomes evaluated in the study; however, the authors supported the effectiveness of the intervention based on within-group measures of change. The authors concluded that motivational interviewing shows promise as a specific intervention for initiating a reduction in drinking among pregnant women who are at greatest risk. The methodological quality of this study was rated as weak.

3.6.3.2 Observational Studies

Eisen *et al.* [37] conducted a prospective analytical cohort study that evaluated the impact of a community-based drug-prevention, education, and treatment project for pregnant and postpartum women and their infants. The study was conducted in health facilities in the USA, but it is unknown whether the geographic setting was rural or urban. The study population consisted of 658 adult pregnant women of various races, who had used alcohol or other drugs during pregnancy. Two cohorts were compared: the first group was exposed to Pregnant and Postpartum Women and their Infants (PPWI) programs; the second group received an alternative or no intervention. The PPWI programs employed either case management and provision or referral to individual or group counseling or day treatment with direct provision of counseling services. It is unknown what type of providers delivered the intervention, and whether measures to guarantee the fidelity of the intervention (i.e., procedures manual, training of providers) were implemented. Self-reported measures of alcohol intake were evaluated at 30 days and six months of follow-up. There were some important differences in the groups at baseline: women in the PPWI group were more likely to have drunk from one end of the spectrum all the way to alcohol intoxication. The study results showed that, compared to baseline, participants in the intervention group had a significantly reduced alcohol intake at 30 days, but the results were not maintained at six months after delivery. Other outcome measures – such as alcohol use during the last month measured at 30 days and six months of follow-up – were similar between the intervention groups. The authors supported the effectiveness of the intervention in the conclusions. The methodological quality of this study was rated as weak.

Meberg [60] conducted a prospective analytical cohort study which evaluated supportive counseling that focused on the reduction of alcohol consumption in pregnancy. The study was conducted in healthcare facilities in Norway (study dates not specified), with a study population of 132 pregnant women. Two cohorts were compared: one group was exposed to supportive counseling that focused on the reduction of alcohol consumption and its potential benefits to the fetus, while a second group received usual prenatal care. The supportive intervention was delivered by midwives. It is unknown whether measures to guarantee the fidelity of the intervention (i.e., procedures manual, training) were implemented. Self-reported measures of alcohol use (including abstinence) were evaluated at postpartum. The study found that drinking patterns in both groups changed during pregnancy, and that any differences were not statistically significant. The authors did not support the effectiveness of the intervention. The methodological quality of this study was rated as weak.

Mehl-Madrona [61] conducted a prospective analytical cohort study that evaluated the impact of a psychosocial prenatal intervention to reduce substance use among Native American and Hispanic populations in both urban and rural communities of Tucson, Arizona, and Albuquerque, New Mexico (USA). The study population consisted of 640 pregnant women attending prenatal clinics. The group exposed to the psychosocial intervention was compared to a group that was assembled from data collected during the five years prior to the intervention. The two groups were matched for important psychosocial variables, except that there was a trend toward more Cesarean deliveries and a greater use of analgesia and anesthesia in the intervention group. The psychosocial prenatal intervention was culturally appropriate to the particular setting in which it was implemented (e.g., Native American methods of communication, such as a Talking Circle, were used where appropriate). The intervention focused on the following topics: (1) addressing fears; (2) getting support; (3) coping with stress; (4) attaching to the unborn child; (5) preparing for birth; and (6) environmental awareness. The information was delivered by previously trained health educators, but it is not known whether a manual was available to guarantee the integrity of the intervention. Self-reported measures of alcohol intake and maternal and neonatal outcomes were evaluated between 36 and 40 weeks of gestation. The intervention significantly increased the number of normal spontaneous vaginal deliveries; reduced the number of Cesarean deliveries; improved neonatal outcomes; and significantly reduced alcohol consumption among heavy drinkers. The authors supported the effectiveness of the intervention in the conclusions. The methodological quality of this study was rated as moderate.

Nilsen *et al.* [63] conducted a retrospective analytical cohort study that compared the current standard provision of alcohol advice during pregnancy with a more comprehensive counseling model. The study was conducted in Linköping, Sweden, in a sample of pregnant women who were registered at a maternity care center from 2005 to 2007, and whose pregnancies resulted in liveborn infants without birth defects. The study measured patterns of drinking during pregnancy in one cohort that received comprehensive questionnaire-based counseling, and in another cohort that had received standard counseling without a questionnaire. The questionnaire-based counseling intervention was based on motivational interviewing techniques about the harmful effects of alcohol consumption during pregnancy. The authors found that questionnaire-based counseling was no more effective than existing standard counseling in its impact on the proportion of women who abstained from drinking during pregnancy. The methodological quality of this study was rated as moderate.

Corrarino *et al.* [35] conducted a before-and-after study with no comparison group to evaluate a pilot program that linked substance-abusing pregnant women with treatment. The study was conducted in health facilities in an underserved suburban community in Suffolk County, New York (USA). The study dates are unknown. The study population consisted of 10 pregnant substance-abusing women (mean age 22 years) who were not receiving drug treatment upon entry into prenatal care. The intervention was delivered by a multidisciplinary team through a Perinatal Outreach Project that consisted of the following activities: (1) Assignment of a primary public health nurse for case management; (2) A flexible home visit plan; (3) Health education concerning pregnancy-related preventive health care; (4) Services of a substance-abuse counselor; (5) Referral to community and social services as needed; and (6) Availability of a medical social worker for social needs. No description of any previous training in the intervention, nor the use of a manual to ensure intervention fidelity was provided. Self-reported measures of alcohol intake were evaluated at six months of follow-up, and legal outcomes related to custody retention were assessed during the postpartum period. The study showed that the severity of participants' substance addiction was reduced at six months after the intervention, and that nine out of 10 mothers were able to retain custody of their infants. There was no reporting of the statistical significance of the results, but the authors supported the effectiveness of the Perinatal Outreach Project interventions to improve the health of pregnant women. The methodological quality of this study was rated as weak, while the sample size was too small to draw reliable conclusions on the effectiveness of the intervention.

Tavris [71] conducted a before-and-after trial with no comparison group to evaluate the effectiveness of a prenatal care program in reducing self-reported risk factors for adverse pregnancy outcomes among predominantly Caucasian women (mean age 21.7 years) at risk of an AEP. The study was conducted in 1997 in the health facilities of Waukesha County, Wisconsin (USA). The intervention—a program called the Prenatal Care Coordination Program (PNCC)—consisted of an assessment of risk factors for adverse pregnancy outcomes, followed by preventive counseling and follow-up. The intervention was delivered by a public health nurse. No description of previous training in the intervention, nor the use of a manual to ensure intervention fidelity was provided. Measures of alcohol intake at 38 weeks were assessed. Based on their findings of "large and statistically significant" improvements in several prenatal risk factors known to have substantial effects on pregnancy outcomes, the authors concluded that the intervention was efficacious. However, no values of statistical significance were reported in the analysis of the results. The methodological quality of this study was rated as weak.

Yonkers [75] conducted a before-and-after trial with no comparison group to evaluate a motivational interviewing and cognitive behavioral therapy intervention delivered in an obstetric setting in Connecticut, USA. The study participants were 14 adult women (mean age 27.4 years) at risk of an AEP. The intervention was delivered in six sessions over the term of pregnancy, and consisted of motivational interviews and cognitive therapy delivered by primary healthcare personnel. Measures of alcohol use and depression were evaluated at the postpartum period. The authors suggested that the intervention delivered by non-behavioral health professionals has the potential to promote a reduction in hazardous substance use in pregnant women; however, the study did not yield any final conclusions regarding the effectiveness of the intervention. The methodological quality of this study was rated as weak.

Larsson [51] conducted a before-and-after trial with no comparison group to evaluate the impact of a prenatal program for early detection of pregnancies at risk. The study was conducted in 1979 among 464 women attending four urban antenatal clinics in Stockholm, Sweden. The intervention was delivered by a multidisciplinary team (i.e., one midwife and two social workers), and consisted of evaluating the participants' alcohol-drinking habits and identifying excessive drinkers. Excessive drinkers were offered various types of support, such as more frequent visits for prenatal care, counseling, and psychosocial support. No description of previous training in the intervention, nor the use of a manual to ensure intervention fidelity was provided. The outcomes assessed were self-reported measures of alcohol intake in the postpartum period and the incidence of FAS. No statistically significant changes from baseline were reported for alcohol intake. However, the study reported differences in the reduction of alcohol intake among three groups of participants that were identified at baseline as occasional drinkers, excessive drinkers, or alcohol abusers. The changes were significantly higher for excessive drinkers ($p < 0.01$) and alcohol abusers ($p < 0.001$) when compared with occasional drinkers. Two infants were born with FAS and partial FAS (one each in the groups of alcohol abusers and excessive drinkers). The overall results were not statistically significant, and the authors gave partial support to the effectiveness of the intervention. The methodological quality of this study was rated as weak.

Little et al. [52] conducted a before-and-after study with no comparison group that evaluated the impact of the Pregnancy and Health Program (PHP), an intervention offered to an urban community in King County in the state of Washington (USA). The program was established to reduce maternal alcohol abuse during pregnancy. The study was conducted between 1979 and 1981 in a study population of 688 pregnant women of various races. The PHP program consisted of five clinical components: (1) Public education; (2) Professional training; (3) Volunteer services; (4) Adult treatment and education services; and (5) Child assessment services. The program was delivered by a multidisciplinary team of nurses and certified alcoholism therapists. It is not known whether measures to guarantee the fidelity of the intervention (i.e., procedures manual, training of providers) were implemented. Measures of the participants' beliefs regarding alcohol use during pregnancy were evaluated before and after the implementation of PHP. An analysis of the results showed statistically significant changes in the participants' belief in alcohol abstinence as a beneficial behavior during pregnancy. Nevertheless, as beliefs do not necessarily reflect behavioral changes, the authors did not draw any conclusions regarding the effectiveness of the intervention in reducing maternal alcohol abuse during pregnancy. The methodological quality of this study was rated as weak.

3.6.4
Summary of the Overall Results

3.6.4.1 General Characteristics

- Twenty-three studies provided evidence regarding the effectiveness of selective prevention approaches for FASD.
- Half of the studies were published after the year 2000.
- No Canadian studies on selective prevention approaches to FASD were identified.
- Six RCTs and eight CCTs that evaluated a selective prevention approach for FASD were identified.
- The majority of the studies were conducted in urban health facilities.

3.6.4.2 Populations

- The majority of the studies targeted pregnant women and women at risk of an AEP. Only three studies were conducted exclusively in youth populations.
- Two studies focused exclusively on non-Caucasian populations (i.e., Native Americans and Hispanics).

3.6.4.3 Interventions

- Counseling was the most frequently implemented intervention, followed by health teaching, referrals and follow-up, and screening and case-finding activities.
- Individual components of the interventions included brief interventions (counseling) and educational activities.

3.6.4.4 Outcomes

- The effects of selective prevention approaches to FASD were evaluated mainly through the analysis of intermediate outcomes related to changes in drinking behavior, followed by ultimate outcomes related to maternal and neonatal and infant-related outcomes. Immediate outcomes, such as knowledge and perception of alcohol drinking during pregnancy, were less frequently examined.
- Ten studies reported statistically significant differences in the results, whereas another ten reported no statistically significant differences in the analysis of outcome data. Three studies did not test whether statistically significant differences between intervention groups or study periods existed for the outcomes of interest.

3.6.4.5 Methodological Quality of the Studies

- Only one study was considered of strong methodological quality, whereas ten were considered of moderate quality and 12 were rated as weak.

3.6.4.6 Evidence on the Effectiveness of Selective Prevention Approaches

- A qualitative synthesis of results reported in the individual studies (Table 3.15) showed that, compared to universal preventive interventions, some selective preventive interventions have a better evidence base on which to make inferences regarding their effectiveness. The best evidence (*strong and moderate quality*) regarding the effectiveness of selective prevention approaches for FASD is available for counseling activities and health education programs directed to women of childbearing age who consume alcohol, pregnant women and women at risk of an alcohol-exposed pregnancy. This evidence is as follows:

  - One RCT of strong methodological quality [39] found that a brief *counseling* intervention delivered to women at high risk of an AEP was effective at reducing the number of drinking days and the frequency of alcohol use during pregnancy.

Table 3.15 Synthesis of individual study results on the effectiveness of selective prevention approaches to FASD.

Study	Intervention	Brief description of the intervention	Study design	Study population	Results regarding the effectiveness of the intervention	Methodological quality
Floyd et al. [40]	Counseling (motivational interview) – Project CHOICES	Brief motivational interviewing intervention, counseling sessions and contraception consultation and services visit and information	RCT	Women of childbearing age who consume alcohol	The intervention significantly reduced the risk of an alcohol-exposed pregnancy.	Moderate
Armstrong et al. [26]	Brief intervention for prenatal alcohol use (Early Start Plus)	Alcohol counseling, psychological support and prenatal care; computerized drink-size assessment tool and intervention focused on drinking reduction	RCT	Women at risk of an AEP	Early Start Plus appears to be helpful in reducing the incidence of preterm events	Moderate
Chang et al. [33]	Brief intervention for prenatal alcohol use, including the partner	Comprehensive assessment of alcohol use and a brief intervention; patient education and a self-help manual	RCT	Women at risk of an AEP	The effectiveness of the intervention on self-reported measures of alcohol intake was demonstrated only for the group of women that drank more prenatally.	Moderate
Chang et al. [34]	Brief intervention for prenatal alcohol use	Single-session brief intervention enhanced by including a partner chosen by the pregnant woman. Structure of the session: (1) knowledge assessment with feedback; (2) contracting and goal setting; (3) behavioral modification; (4) summary	RCT	Women at risk of an alcohol-exposed pregnancy and their partners	The intervention did not significantly decrease self-reported measures of alcohol use during pregnancy. The intervention did not produce significant improvement in neonatal measures.	Moderate

Study	Intervention	Description	Design	Target population	Outcome	Evidence
Fleming [39]	Brief intervention for prenatal alcohol use	Two-session brief intervention that included a workbook with scripted questions and feedback regarding current health behaviors, problem drinking, and adverse effects of alcohol, focused on women and pregnancy	RCT	Women at risk of an AEP, and their partners	A brief intervention significantly reduced alcohol use in postpartum women	Strong
Crosby [36]	Health education program – Cognitive-based health education	Activated health education: behavioral instructional model focused on participants' attitude, knowledge and behavior towards alcohol use during pregnancy	RCT	Pregnant women	The intervention did not significantly change attitudes toward and knowledge of alcohol use or self-reported alcohol use during pregnancy.	Moderate
Ingersoll et al. [47]	Counseling (motivational interview) – BALANCE	Motivational interviewing brief intervention. Personalized feedback and counseling on drinking and contraception.	CCT	Women of childbearing age who consume alcohol	The intervention significantly reduced the risk of AEP in the short term.	Moderate
Palinkas et al. [66]	Counseling (cognitive behavioral approach) – Project PALS	Cognitive and behavioral techniques to improve social skills and restructure social networks; a normative education program that included information on the hazards of drug use; teaching sessions (group format) and individual case sessions	CCT	Women of childbearing age who consume alcohol	Alcohol intake increased significantly after the intervention. The intervention may be ineffective and possibly counterproductive as a preventive intervention in high-risk youth.	Moderate

(Continued)

Table 3.15 *(Continued)*

Study	Intervention	Brief description of the intervention	Study design	Study population	Results regarding the effectiveness of the intervention	Methodological quality
O'Connor and Whaley [64]	Counseling	Counseling aimed at increasing awareness of the negative consequences of drinking, advice on identifying risky situations and taking actions to reduce consumption, and assistance with formulating drinking reduction goals. Education, feedback, cognitive behavioral procedures, goal setting and therapeutic contract.	CCT	Women at risk of an AEP	The intervention was effective at reducing alcohol drinking and improving neonatal outcomes (birth weight and mortality rate).	Moderate
Reynolds et al. [67]	Health education program – Cognitive-behavioral self-help materials	Self-help program to reduce alcohol consumption among pregnant women (10-minute educational session and a nine-step self-help manual)	CCT	Women at risk of an AEP	The intervention produced greater alcohol cessation and greater reductions in the amount of alcohol consumed at two months of follow-up.	Moderate
Belizan et al. [28]	Health education – Home visits	Health education consisting of reinforcement of social support network, knowledge about pregnancy and delivery, and reinforcement of adequate utilization of health services	CCT	Pregnant women	The intervention did not produce significant changes in self-reported alcohol use and maternal or perinatal outcomes.	Moderate

Eustace [38]	Health education program – Positive teaching reinforcement (video)	Positive teaching reinforcement education intervention about the dangers of alcohol consumption during pregnancy	CCT	Pregnant women	The interventions significantly increased knowledge about the effects of drinking alcohol during pregnancy. The knowledge increase remained stable during a 12-week period, but did not translate into reductions in alcohol intake during pregnancy.	Moderate
Sarvela and Ford [69]	Health education program – ASPEN prenatal health education program	Self-administered series of eight educational modules completed by pregnant women while they waited to see a physician at the participating clinics; one module completed at each prenatal visit.	CCT	Pregnant women (youth)	The intervention did not significantly decrease the frequency of alcohol use at postpartum, nor produce significant changes in neonatal outcomes (birth defects, infant complications and presence of meconium stool).	Weak
Handmaker et al. [44]	Counseling – Motivational interview	Motivational interviewing; brief intervention	CCT	Women at risk of an AEP	The intervention did not significantly reduce self-reported measures of alcohol intake (i.e., total drinks, total number of abstinent days) at two months follow-up.	Weak

(Continued)

Table 3.15 (Continued)

Study	Intervention	Brief description of the intervention	Study design	Study population	Results regarding the effectiveness of the intervention	Methodological quality
Eisen et al. [37]	Counseling (case management and referral to services) – PPWI treatment programs	a) Case management with provision or referral to individual and group counseling; or b) day treatment with direct provision of individual and group counseling	Prospective analytical cohort study	Women at risk of an AEP	The intervention significantly reduced alcohol use at 30 days of follow-up, but the results were not maintained at six months postpartum.	Weak
Meberg [60]	Counseling	Structured interviews during pregnancy, including counseling focused on reduction of alcohol consumption and potential benefits to the fetus, and interview after delivery	Prospective analytical cohort study	Pregnant women	The intervention did not produce significant reductions in postpartum alcohol use.	Weak
Mehl-Madrona [61]	Health education program	Psychosocial prenatal intervention for reducing substance use and perceived life stress (seven sessions dedicated to addressing fears, getting support, reducing stress, attaching to the unborn child, preparing for birth, and environmental awareness)	Prospective analytical cohort study	Pregnant women	The intervention significantly increased the number of normal spontaneous vaginal deliveries; improved neonatal outcomes; and decreased the number of Cesarean births. Alcohol reductions were significant for heavy drinkers.	Moderate

Nilsen et al. [63]	Questionnaire-based alcohol counseling	Alcohol counseling based on questionnaire and motivational interview about the harmful effects of alcohol consumption during pregnancy	Retrospective analytical cohort study	Pregnant women	Questionnaire-based counseling was not more effective than standard counseling in increasing the proportion of women who abstained from drinking during pregnancy.	Moderate
Corrarino et al. [35]	Assessment and brief intervention – Perinatal Outreach Project	Identification of women with untreated alcohol or drug problem; home visits, health education on pregnancy-related health care, services of a substance-abuse counselor, follow-up of needs; referral to community and social services as needed, referral to substance-abuse treatment when the woman was ready; interdisciplinary team case follow-up and evaluation	Before-and-after study	Women at risk of an AEP	No conclusions about the effectiveness of the intervention.	Weak
Tavris [71]	Assessment and brief intervention – PNCC program	Assessment, preventive counseling and follow-up	Before-and-after study	Women at risk of an AEP	No conclusions about the effectiveness of the intervention.	Weak
Yonkers [75]	Motivational interview and cognitive behavioral therapy	Motivational interviewing and cognitive behavioral therapy intervention delivered by non-behavioral health practitioners	Before-and-after study	Women at risk of an AEP	No conclusions about the effectiveness of the intervention.	Weak

(Continued)

Table 3.15 (*Continued*)

Study	Intervention	Brief description of the intervention	Study design	Study population	Results regarding the effectiveness of the intervention	Methodological quality
Larsson [51]	Assessment and brief intervention – Antenatal program for early detection of pregnancies at risk	Structured interview for early detection of maternal alcohol abuse and referral to treatment for women with excessive alcohol consumption	Before-and-after study	Pregnant women	The intervention did not significantly reduce the level of alcohol intake. However, the changes in alcohol use were significantly higher for excessive drinkers and alcohol abusers when compared with occasional drinkers.	Weak
Little *et al.* [52]	Counseling – PHP program	Public education, professional training, telephone information service, screening and counseling services, pregnancy outcome assessment	Before-and-after study	Pregnant women	The intervention significantly changed beliefs about alcohol abstinence as a beneficial behavior during pregnancy. Behavioral change was not evaluated and no conclusions were made on effectiveness of the intervention in reducing maternal alcohol abuse during pregnancy.	Weak

AEP = alcohol-exposed pregnancy; ASPEN = Adolescent Substance Prevention Education Network; BALANCE = Birth Control and Alcohol Awareness: Negotiating Choices Effectively; CBT = cognitive behavioral therapy; CCT = controlled clinical trial; ESP = Early Start Plus; MI = motivational interviewing; PALS = Positive Adolescent Life Skills; PHP = Pregnancy and Health Program; PNCC = Prenatal Care Coordination Program; PPWI = Pregnant and Postpartum Women and their Infant; RCT = randomized controlled trial.

- Evidence from clinical trials of moderate methodological quality indicated that *counseling* was effective at reducing the risk of an AEP [40, 47] and the frequency of alcohol drinking [64].

- Evidence from a clinical trial of moderate quality indicated that *counseling* had a positive effect on neonatal outcomes, such as birth weight and infant mortality rates [64].

- Evidence from a clinical trial of moderate quality indicated that a *counseling intervention* that used a cognitive behavioral approach had a negative effect on (i.e., increased) the rate of alcohol intake among high-risk youth [66].

- Different types of *health education programs* directed at pregnant women were reported in three studies [38, 61, 67]. The studies found that health education increased knowledge about the effects of alcohol use during pregnancy [38] and also reduced alcohol use [67] in the short term (less than three months of follow-up). There is no evidence that these effects were sustained over time. One study of moderate quality [61] provided evidence that a health education intervention was effective in increasing the number of normal spontaneous vaginal deliveries (no other maternal outcomes related with alcohol exposure were evaluated). This study found significant reductions in alcohol use by heavy drinkers.

- Two studies (one of moderate [34] and one of weak methodological quality [37]) did not find that counseling and health educational interventions significantly reduced alcohol use during pregnancy.

• The positive results associated with counseling and health educational programs as selective FASD-prevention interventions that were found in this qualitative analysis of the evidence should be interpreted with caution. Of interest, the majority of the studies of moderate quality were conducted in the past five years. Compared to the universal and indicated preventive approaches evaluated in this review, the selective interventions under study might be more applicable to the current times and needs.

3.7
Evidence on the Effectiveness of Indicated Prevention Approaches for FASD

3.7.1
Characteristics of Included Studies

3.7.1.1 General Characteristics
Nine studies [42, 43, 45, 53, 56, 57, 68, 70, 74] provided evidence on the effectiveness of indicated prevention approaches for FASD. The characteristics of studies that evaluated indicated prevention approaches for FASD are summarized in Table 3.E.3 of Appendix 3.E.

The studies were published between 1983 and 2008, the median year of publication being 1999 (IQR: 1989, 2004). All of the studies except for one abstract from a scientific conference [45] were published as journal articles. All of the studies except for one Finnish study [43] were conducted in the USA. Of the 10 studies, five were before-and-after studies with no comparison group, two [45, 53] were CCTs, and two were observational analytical cohort studies (one prospective [74] and one retrospective [70]). No RCTs were identified that evaluated the effectiveness of indicated prevention approaches for FASD.

Six studies reported their sources of funding. Three studies [56, 57, 74] were funded by government agencies, and one study each obtained internal funds [70], government and society funding [68], and government, society, and internal funds [42].

All of the studies were conducted in health facilities, except for one [42] that was conducted in both the community and a health facility.

3.7.1.2 Characteristics of the Populations

The population targeted most frequently in the studies was women at risk of an AEP. This population was evaluated in all of the studies except one [53], in which women of childbearing age were targeted. None of the studies included partners or support persons in the study sample. The residential setting of the target population was urban in three studies [42, 70, 74]; other residential settings included suburban areas [68], rural areas [56, 57], and a mix of urban and rural areas [53]. Two studies [43, 45] did not describe the residential setting of the study population.

The median number of participants per study was 129 (IQR: 81, 183; data from six studies that reported the number of enrolled participants). All of the studies involved females only. The median chronological age of participants in the studies was 26.2 years (IQR: 24.8, 28.2; data from six studies). Six studies [42, 45, 56, 57, 70, 74] included adult populations (i.e., older than 18 years of age) only. None of the studies was conducted in youth, and three studies [43, 53, 68] did not report the age range of the participants.

Five studies [42, 45, 68, 70, 74] included participants of miscellaneous races, two studies [56, 57] focused exclusively on non-Caucasian populations (i.e., Native Americans), and two studies [43, 53] did not report on study participants' race. Only one study that included participants of various races [68] reported separate results by race. It is unknown whether study participants had past or current exposure to similar or other FASD-prevention approaches.

3.7.1.3 Characteristics of the Interventions

All of the indicated preventive approaches were directed at the individual level. The types of public health intervention that were implemented in the indicated FASD-prevention approaches are described in Figure 3.7. Some studies implemented more than one intervention; therefore, the number of interventions does not match the number of studies.

Counseling interventions were the most frequently implemented (eight studies [43, 45, 53, 56, 57, 68, 70, 74]), followed by case management (five studies [42, 53, 56, 57, 68]), referrals and follow-up (four studies [42, 53, 56, 74]), consultation

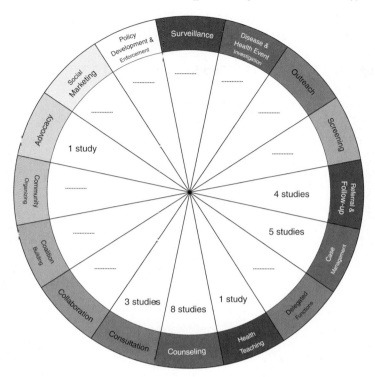

Figure 3.7 Types of public health intervention implemented in indicated prevention approaches for FASD. Adapted from the Minnesota Department of Health Division of Community Health Services [76].

(three studies [53, 56, 74]), advocacy (one study [42]), and health teaching (one study [74]).

The indicated FASD-prevention approaches examined in the individual studies, according to the type of population of targeted, are described in Table 3.16. The studies have been arranged by study design, from clinical trials to observational analytical designs.

3.7.1.4 Components of the Interventions

Four studies on indicated preventive interventions described their underlying theoretical framework. These included a cognitive behavioral approach [45], a health belief model [53], a home visitation model [42], and Miller's self-in-relation theory [74].

Seven studies [43, 45, 56, 57, 68, 70, 74] implemented the interventions in health facilities, and one study [42] was implemented at participants' homes. One study [53] was undertaken either at a health facility or at participants' homes.

The individual components of the interventions fell mainly within the category of counseling and brief interventions. Individual counseling was delivered in seven studies [43, 45, 53, 56, 57, 68, 74], case management in five [42, 53, 56, 57, 68], skills training in four [42, 53, 70, 74], referral to available services in four [42,

Table 3.16 FASD indicated prevention approaches examined in individual studies.

Study	Study design	Intervention	Population
Loudenburg [53]	CCT	Multifaceted intervention	Women of childbearing age
Hankin [45]	CCT	Counseling	Women at risk of an AEP
Whiteside-Mansell et al. [74]	Prospective analytical cohort study	Intensive outpatient program	Women at risk of an AEP
Svikis et al. [70]	Retrospective analytical cohort study	Counseling	Women at risk of an AEP
Grant et al. [42]	Before-and-after study	Outpatient program	Women at risk of an AEP
Halmesmaki [43]	Before-and-after study	Counseling	Women at risk of an AEP
Masis and May [56]	Before-and-after study	Counseling (case management)	Women at risk of an AEP
May et al. [57]	Before-and-after study	Counseling (case management and motivational interview)	Women at risk of an AEP
Rosett et al. [68]	Before-and-after study	Counseling	Women at risk of an AEP

AEP = alcohol-exposed pregnancy; CCT = controlled clinical trial.

53, 56, 74], and support groups in three [53, 70, 74]. One study [74] delivered educational sessions as part of the indicated preventive approach.

All of the studies required the participation of a variety of providers, such as physicians [43], public health nurses [42], social workers [45], substance-abuse counselors [70] and multidisciplinary teams (i.e., prevention and case managers [57]; psychiatrists and counselors [68]; and a team of social worker, nurse practitioner, case managers, and consultants in medicine, addictions, psychology, and law/ethics [74]). It was unclear what types of professional delivered the interventions in two studies [53, 56].

Three studies [42, 53, 57] stated that providers received training prior to implementing the intervention. None of the studies used a manual to guarantee the integrity of the implementation of the intervention. A detailed description of the characteristics of the indicated preventive approaches that were evaluated in the individual studies are provided in Table 3.F.3 of Appendix 3.F.

3.7.1.5 Characteristics of the Outcomes

A total of 34 outcomes was reported in the nine studies that assessed the effectiveness of indicated FASD-prevention approaches. The types of outcome measure that were examined in the studies are displayed in Table 3.17.

The effects of indicated FASD-prevention approaches were evaluated mainly through ultimate outcomes (21 outcomes) related to maternal, neonatal and infant-related outcomes, and through intermediate outcomes related to patterns

Table 3.17 Types of outcome measure examined in studies on indicated prevention approaches to FASD.

Type of outcome		Number of outcomes assessed at different follow-up periods					
		≤3 months	>3 months and ≤6 months	>6 months and ≤9 months	>9 months and ≤1 year	>1 year	Total number of outcomes
Immediate	Perceptions about alcohol use during pregnancy	–	1	–	–	–	1
	Attitudes toward alcohol use during pregnancy	–	–	–	–	–	–
	Awareness of risk of alcohol use during pregnancy	–	–	–	–	–	–
	Knowledge about alcohol use during pregnancy/FASD	–	–	–	–	–	–
Intermediate	Alcohol intake	–	–	–	7	1	8
	Alcohol abstinence	–	–	1	1	2	4
	Binge drinking	–	–	–	–	–	–
	AEP	–	–	–	–	–	–
Ultimate	Neonatal and infant outcomes	–	–	–	7	5	12
	Maternal outcomes	–	–	–	1	3	4
	Economic and healthcare utilization outcomes	–	–	–	1	–	1
	Family outcomes	–	–	–	–	1	1
	FASD outcomes	–	–	–	2	1[a]	3
	Legal outcomes	–	–	–	–	–	–
Total		–	1	1	19	13	34

a) The study did not report the maximum follow-up period for FASD outcome assessment.
AEP = alcohol-exposed pregnancy; FASD = fetal alcohol spectrum disorder.

of drinking behavior during pregnancy (10 outcomes). Immediate outcomes related to the perception of alcohol drinking during pregnancy were seldom examined (one outcome).

The most frequently studied outcomes were neonatal and infant outcomes (12 outcomes), followed by alcohol intake (eight outcomes) and alcohol abstinence and maternal outcomes (four outcomes each).

3.7.1.6   Types of Result Reported in the Individual Studies

The types of result that were described in the studies, in terms of the report of statistically significant differences in the outcomes of interest and the support of the indicated approach in the study conclusions, are displayed in Table 3.18.

Among the 10 studies that provided evidence on the effectiveness of indicated prevention approaches for FASD, three [45, 70, 74] reported statistically significant differences in the results, whereas one study [57] reported that no statistically significant differences were found in the analysis of outcome data. Five studies [42, 43, 53, 56, 68] did not report the results of statistical tests to analyze whether statistically significant differences existed among the groups or study periods for the outcomes of interest.

In interpreting the study results, the primary authors of four studies [42, 45, 70, 74] claimed that the intervention under study was effective. None of the studies concluded that the intervention was ineffective. One study [57] gave a partial endorsement to the indicated approach under study, based on the interpretation of secondary outcome data. Four studies [43, 53, 56, 68] did not state any definite conclusions regarding the effectiveness of the intervention.

Two studies yielded to conclusions that were not supported by the analysis of the outcome data. One study [57] partially supported the effectiveness of the intervention when the statistical analysis showed no significant differences in the outcome. Among the studies that did not conduct a statistical analysis of the data, one [42] supported the effectiveness of the intervention.

3.7.2
Methodological Quality of the Studies

Eight studies [42, 43, 45, 56, 57, 68, 70, 74] that evaluated the effectiveness of indicated FASD-prevention approaches were rated as weak in their methodological quality, whereas one study [53] was considered to be of moderate quality.

An overview of how well the studies on indicated prevention approaches were able to control for methodological issues related to selection bias, allocation bias, confounding, blinding of outcome assessors, validity and reliability of data collection methods, and management of withdrawals and dropouts, is provided in Table 3.19.

Overall, the studies rated poor in most of the quality components, particularly in the domains of blinding and data-collection methods. A detailed description of the methodological quality of the individual studies that assessed the effectiveness of indicated prevention approaches is provided in Table 3.G.3 of Appendix 3.G.

Table 3.18 Types of result reported in the individual studies assessing the effectiveness of indicated prevention approaches to FASD.

Report of statistically significant differences in the results	Study conclusion				Total number of studies
	No support of the effectiveness of the intervention (number of studies)	No conclusions regarding the effectiveness of the intervention (number of studies)	Partial support of the effectiveness of the intervention (number of studies)	Support of the effectiveness of the intervention (number of studies)	
Study did not provide data on statistical testing of differences	–	4 ☺	–	1 ☹	5
Study did not find statistically significant differences	–	–	1 ☹	–	1
Study reported statistically significant differences	–	–	–	3 ☺	3
Total number of studies	–	4	1	4	9

☺ = an appropriate conclusion based on study results; ☹ = an inappropriate conclusion based on study results; ☺ = an appropriate partial conclusion based on study results.

Table 3.19 Methodological quality of studies assessing the effectiveness of indicated prevention approaches to FASD.

Domains of Methodological Quality	Number of studies rated as Weak	Number of studies rated as Moderate	Number of studies rated as Strong
Methods to control for selection bias	5	4	–
Methods to control for allocation bias	–	7	2
Methods to control for confounders	5	–	4
Methods of blinding	7	2	–
Data collection methods	6	–	3
Methods to handle withdrawals and dropouts	5	3	1
Global methodological quality	8	1	–

Methodological aspects that go beyond the internal validity of the studies were also evaluated. Five of the studies [42, 45, 56, 68, 70] reported the dates for starting and stopping accession to participants. The majority of the studies mentioned how well the sample represented the selection criteria for enrolling participants. Three studies [53, 56, 74] failed to describe the set of inclusion and exclusion criteria used to enroll the participants. Fewer than half of the studies [42, 56, 57, 68] provided a description of the number of ineligible participants before intervention allocation took place.

The quality of reporting of the characteristics of the interventions and conditions in which the interventions operated was poor. None of the studies reported the use of a systematic mechanism to monitor the fidelity of the intervention. In seven of the nine studies, it was unknown whether the study participants received an unintended intervention that may have influenced the results. It is likely that participants in the other two studies [53, 70] received a cointervention.

Five studies [43, 45, 68, 70, 74] described the frequency with which the intervention was delivered, whereas two studies [42, 68] reported the duration of the intervention.

Some issues related to the data analysis in the individual studies were evaluated. None of the studies reported that an ITT approach was used in the analysis of the results. Finally, none of the studies had unit-analysis errors.

3.7.3
Results of Qualitative Synthesis of the Evidence

The large clinical heterogeneity of the characteristics of individual interventions precluded a meta-analysis of the data to assess the effectiveness of indicated FASD-interventions. However, a qualitative review of studies that assessed the effectiveness of indicated approaches was conducted to identify patterns across individual study results. Variables that were examined systematically to shed light on the reasons for the findings were: study design; duration of follow-up; sample size; population characteristics; comparison; and outcomes. The following is an overview of the qualitative review of indicated preventive interventions for FASD based on the data provided in nine studies (two CCTs and seven observational studies). The presentation of the individual studies is arranged by study design, from clinical trials to observational studies.

3 7.3.1 Clinical Trials

Loudenburg [53] conducted a CCT to evaluate the impact of a multifaceted intervention to reduce substance use among high-risk women of childbearing age. The study was conducted as part of the Four-State FAS Consortium initiative, in which a series of interventions to reduce and ameliorate the risk factors for FAS were implemented and evaluated in the states of North Dakota, South Dakota, Minnesota, and Montana. The participants received one of two interventions: interventions under the Four-State FAS Consortium program (e.g., home visits, parent education, counseling, referral to specialized services); or the usual prenatal care. The interventions under the Four-State FAS Consortium program were delivered by multidisciplinary teams (not further described). The intervention providers were trained in order to guarantee the integrity of the intervention. Data from 302 participants were analyzed to assess changes in perception regarding alcohol use, well-being, family functioning, and mental health status. The authors did not report the statistical significance of the results, and did not make any firm conclusions regarding the effectiveness of the interventions under the program. The methodological quality of this study was rated as moderate.

The study by Hankin [45] was a clinical trial that evaluated the effect of a brief intervention designed to prevent drinking during the next pregnancy among adult women who drank heavily during an index pregnancy. The study was conducted at the postpartum unit of an academic hospital in Detroit, Michigan (USA). The participants were women consuming at least four drinks per week at the time they conceived an index pregnancy, or women who had delivered an infant of low birth weight. The authors described the study as an RCT, but it was classified in this review as a CCT because the methods of intervention allocation and generation of the randomization sequence were not described. Study participants were assigned to one of two interventions: (i) a brief intervention for prenatal alcohol use; or (ii) a control group that received assessment and basic information. The brief intervention began one month after delivery and continued through 13 months postpartum. The intervention was delivered by a social worker. It is unknown whether a manual was available to guarantee the integrity of the intervention. The brief intervention used a cognitive-behavioral approach in which women were helped to set a goal of abstention from alcohol or reduction of alcohol use to established limits. Data from 96 women were analyzed regarding the developmental outcome (mean score in the Bailey Developmental Scales) of the index infants and the subsequent infants at five years of follow-up. The authors found that the brief intervention significantly protected not only the women's subsequent infants but also their index infant from mental and psychomotor delays. However, the sample size was small and the authors recommended caution in interpreting these results. The methodological quality of this study was rated as weak.

3.7.3.2 Observational Studies

Whiteside-Mansell *et al.* [74] conducted a prospective analytical cohort study to evaluate the impact of a comprehensive substance-use prevention and treatment program for low-income pregnant and parenting women. The study examined the evolution of the Arkansas Center for Addictions Research, Education and Services (AR-CARES) program over a follow-up period of five years. This program provides residential and outpatient substance-abuse prevention services to women at risk of an alcohol-exposed pregnancy. The services include day treatment, assessment of alcohol and drug use, education, individual counseling, parenting support, and coordination with other services. The program was evaluated with a sample of 72 participants and compared to a nonparticipating group of 23 women. Data were analyzed for 27 and 10 women of the groups, respectively, on the following outcomes of interest: alcohol use at postpartum; obstetric complications; neonatal outcomes (fetal distress, meconium staining, infant weight and length, head circumference, Apgar scores); and hospitalization outcomes (number of maternal and infant hospital days). Infant outcomes (infant weight and length, head circumference, and Bailey scales score) were evaluated at 6, 12, and 18 months. The authors found that there was a significant reduction in the proportion of alcohol users in the intervention group. Children from women in the participating group reached normal ranges in both growth and development. Program participation was associated with a significant reduction in alcohol use during the time before the birth of the target child. The authors concluded that there are indications that the AR-CARES program may have had an impact on later child development. The methodological quality of this study was rated as weak.

Svikis *et al.* [70] conducted a retrospective analytical cohort study that evaluated the clinical and economic efficacy of an on-site support group for drug-abusing pregnant women. The study population consisted of 121 women attending an urban, academic hospital obstetric clinic from 1989 to 1990, who screened positive for alcohol and drug use based on clinician interview or urinalysis at their first prenatal visit. Women in need of treatment for substance abuse were referred to a once-a-week support group led by a substance-abuse counselor. Topics covered in the sessions included how to avoid alcohol relapse, the establishment of social support networks, and behavioral contracting. Treatment compliance was monitored. The outcomes of interest were alcohol use (self-reported and by urinalysis) at postpartum, neonatal outcomes (meconium staining and birth weight), and medical costs (maternal and infant) after delivery. Participants who attended two or more group meetings were compared with a cohort of women who attended none or only one session during the follow-up period. The authors reported a statistically significant improvement in neonatal (birth weight and Apgar scores) and economic outcomes. The authors endorsed the utility of support groups for pregnant, substance-abusing women in obstetric clinic settings. The methodological quality of this study was rated as weak.

Grant *et al.* [42] conducted a before-and-after study with no comparison group that evaluated the impact of a home visitation intervention delivered to high-risk women (mean age 28.4 years) who abused alcohol and drugs during pregnancy. A cohort of 249 pregnant or postpartum women who self-reported heavy use of alcohol or illicit drugs were selected for the study. The intervention – the Parent-Child Assistance Program – consisted of case management aimed at assisting women in obtaining alcohol and drug treatment and staying sober and linking them with community services. Measures of severity of addiction, abstinence, and the frequency of subsequent pregnancies unexposed to alcohol or drugs were evaluated after a follow-up period of three years. Results were reported for three samples: the original demonstration project conducted between July 1991 and December 1992; and two replication studies conducted in Seattle and Tacoma, Washington (USA) between July 1994 and December 1995. Although the authors did not report the statistical significance of the results, they supported the effectiveness of the intervention. The methodological quality of this study was rated as weak.

The study by Halmesmaki [43] was a before-and-after study with no comparison group, conducted in Finland, that evaluated the effectiveness of a treatment program consisting of counseling, psychological support, and prenatal care delivered to pregnant alcoholic women in their 8th to 12th gestational week. The study setting and characteristics of the participants and the intervention were poorly reported. Self-reported measures of alcohol use and perinatal and neonatal mortality rates in the postpartum period were evaluated. The authors found that two out of three drinkers could reduce their alcohol consumption in the treatment program, and this decreased the risk of fetal damage. The authors did not report on the statistical significance of the results, and did not yield to any firm conclusions regarding the effectiveness of the intervention. The methodological quality of this study was rated as weak.

Masis and May [56] conducted a before-and-after study with no comparison group that evaluated the impact of a hospital-based, comprehensive approach to the prevention of FAS among women defined as high-risk for an AEP. The study was conducted among 48 Native American women (mean age 27.2 years) referred to the FAS Prevention Project program at the Tuba City Indian Medical Center in Tuba City, Arizona (USA), between January 1988 and July 1989. The program implemented a variety of preventive methods that included the use of media advertisements, screening and case management, and social services. It is unclear what type of providers delivered the intervention, and whether a manual was used to guarantee the fidelity of the interventions. The outcome of interest in the study was the rate of abstinence at 18 months of follow-up (which was calculated as 56.3%). The authors did not report the statistical significance of the results, and did not make any firm conclusions regarding the effectiveness of the interventions under the FAS Prevention Project program. The methodological quality of this study was rated as weak.

May *et al.* [57] conducted a before-and-after study with no comparison group that evaluated the impact of a case management approach to prevent FAS in four Native American communities in the USA. The selected participants were 137 Native American women who were identified for second-level screening for risk of alcohol abuse during pregnancy. Participants were offered a case management intervention delivered by a previously trained multidisciplinary team. Measures of alcohol use (abstinence, number of drinks consumed in the past 30 days, peak blood alcohol content) were assessed at 6 and 12 months of follow-up. Changes in measures of alcohol use at 6 and 12 months were not statistically significant. The number of FASD cases per births was also evaluated postpartum, with two of 149 infants being diagnosed as FASD cases. The authors gave partial support to the effectiveness of the intervention in their conclusions. The methodological quality of this study was rated as weak.

Rosett *et al.* [68] conducted a before-and-after study with no comparison group that evaluated the effect of integrating alcohol screening and supportive counseling for heavy drinking into routine prenatal care. The study was conducted in a women's clinic in Boston (USA) between 1974 and May 1979. The study participants were 162 pregnant women (mean age 25.2 years; almost 60% were African-American) identified as heavy drinkers (i.e., women who consumed a minimum of 45 drinks per month, and at least five drinks on some occasions). The intervention was delivered by a multidisciplinary team, and consisted of counseling sessions focused on reduction of alcohol use. It is unclear whether the study implemented control mechanisms to guarantee the integrity of the intervention among all the participants. The outcome of interest was abstinence or a reduction of alcohol consumption at the end of the third trimester. Data for only 49 women were analyzed. No statistically significant results were reported and the authors did not make any conclusions regarding the effectiveness of the intervention. The methodological quality of this study was rated as weak.

3.7.4
Summary of the Overall Results

- Nine studies provided evidence regarding the effectiveness of indicated prevention approaches for FASD.

3.7.4.1 General Characteristics

- No Canadian studies evaluating indicated prevention approaches to FASD were identified.

- More than half of the studies were before-and-after studies with no comparison group. No RCTs were identified to assess the effectiveness of indicated prevention approaches for FASD.

- Studies were conducted mainly in urban health facilities.

3.7.4.2 Populations

- The majority of the studies targeted women at high risk of an AEP, because of their level of alcohol consumption.
- Two studies focused exclusively on Native American populations.

3 7.4.3 Interventions

- Counseling was the most frequent intervention, followed by case management, referrals, and follow-up activities.

3.7.4.4 Outcomes

- The effects of indicated FASD-prevention approaches were evaluated mainly through ultimate outcomes related to maternal, neonatal and infant-related outcomes, and intermediate outcomes related to patterns of drinking behavior during pregnancy. Immediate outcomes related to perception of alcohol drinking during pregnancy were seldom examined.

- The most frequently studied outcomes were neonatal and infant outcomes, followed by self reported-measures of alcohol intake and abstinence.

- Three studies reported statistically significant differences in the results, whereas one study reported that no statistically significant differences were found in the analysis of outcome data. Five studies did not report on the use of statistical tests to analyze whether statistically significant differences existed among the groups or study periods for the outcomes of interest. Two studies yielded to conclusions that were not supported by the analysis of the outcome data.

3.7.4.5 Methodological Quality of the Studies

- Eight studies that evaluated the effectiveness of indicated FASD-prevention approaches were considered of poor methodological quality (i.e., rated as "weak"), and one study was considered of moderate quality.

3.7.4.6 Evidence on the Effectiveness of Indicated Prevention Approaches

- A qualitative synthesis of individual results in the studies (Table 3.20) showed that the methodological quality of the studies which evaluated indicated preventive interventions was poor (i.e., rated as "weak"), precluding the application of their results to inform the practice. Only one study assessing a multifaceted intervention (i.e., the Four-State FAS Consortium initiative [53]) was considered of moderate quality, but it is unknown whether the intervention was effective in modifying such outcomes as perceptions of alcohol use, well-being, family functioning and mental health status. The evidence base to support the effectiveness of indicated preventive approaches is weak.

Table 3.20 Synthesis of individual study results on the effectiveness of indicated prevention approaches to FASD.

Study	Intervention	Brief description of the intervention	Study design	Study population	Results regarding the effectiveness of the intervention	Methodological quality
Loudenburg [53]	Multifaceted intervention – Four-State FAS Consortium	Multifaceted intervention including an intensive case-management and home visit program and motivational interviewing.	CCT	Women of childbearing age	No conclusions about the effectiveness of the intervention.	Moderate
Hankin [45]	Counseling	Intensive brief intervention: counseling sessions that reviewed the definition of a standard drink, helped participants set a goal of abstention or reduction of alcohol use, established limits on consumption, and taught ways to reduce drinking.	CCT	Women at risk of an AEP	The intervention significantly protected women's subsequent infants as well as the target child from mental and psychomotor delays.	Weak
Whiteside-Mansell et al. [74]	Intensive outpatient program – AR-CARES	Intensive outpatient program: day treatment, alcohol and drug use assessment, education and treatment, mental health assessment and referral, life skills assessment and development, group and individual counseling, assistance in locating child care, parenting education and support, health services, health education, service coordination.	Prospective analytical cohort study	Women at risk of an AEP	The intervention significantly reduced alcohol use during the time before the birth of the target child.	Weak

Study	Intervention	Description	Study design	Population	Outcome	Rating
Svikis et al. [70]	Counseling	Support group for drug-abusing pregnant women. Sessions included discussion of how to avoid relapse, dangers of drugs to the fetus, mother's health needs, establishment of social support networks to avoid drug use, behavioral contracting for attendance to the sessions.	Retrospective analytical cohort study	Women at risk of an AEP	The intervention produced significant improvement in neonatal outcomes (birth weight and Apgar scores) and economic outcomes (maternal and infant delivery costs).	Weak
Grant et al. [42]	Outpatient program – PCAP	Home visitation, advocacy and case management to help participants obtain alcohol and drug treatment and to stay in recovery; linking with comprehensive community resources.	Before-and-after study	Women at risk of an AEP	No conclusions about the effectiveness of the intervention.	Weak
Halmesmaki [43]	Counseling – Counseling, psychological support and prenatal care	Alcohol-use counseling, psychological support and prenatal care.	Before-and-after study	Women at risk of an AEP	No conclusions about the effectiveness of the intervention.	Weak
Masis and May [56]	Counseling (case management) – FAS Prevention Project	Clinical assessment, community outreach, case management and support of women at risk of having a FASD/FAE child. Case management included counseling, detoxification, individual and group alcohol treatment, follow-up, voluntary birth control.	Before-and-after study	Women at risk of an AEP	No conclusions about the effectiveness of the intervention.	Weak

(Continued)

Table 3.20 (*Continued*)

Study	Intervention	Brief description of the intervention	Study design	Study population	Results regarding the effectiveness of the intervention	Methodological quality
May et al. [57]	Counseling – Case management and motivational interview	Case management and motivational interviewing	Before-and-after study	Women at risk of an AEP	The intervention did not produce significant changes in measures of alcohol use at 6 and 12 months follow-up.	Weak
Rosett et al. [68]	Counseling	Counseling and treatment for pregnant problem drinkers: assess drinking patterns, evaluate psychopathology and strengths, explain effects of alcohol on the fetus, recognize pregnancy as a normal crisis, use mother's concern for the unborn child to engage her in supportive psychotherapy, assist with social problems, avoid use of potential teratogens, withdraw alcohol gradually if tolerance was developed, plan aftercare before delivery.	Before-and-after study	Women at risk of an AEP	No conclusions about the effectiveness of the intervention.	Weak

AEP = alcohol-exposed pregnancy; AR-CARES = Arkansas Center for Addictions Research, Education, and Services; CCT = controlled clinical trial; FASD = fetal alcohol spectrum disorder; FAE = fetal alcohol effects; FAS = fetal alcohol syndrome; FASD = fetal alcohol spectrum disorder; PCAP = Parent-Child Assistance Program.

3.7.5
Analysis of Publication Bias

Due to the very small number of trials available for each category of intervention, the statistical tests lacked the power to detect publication bias. Therefore, an analysis of the effect of publication bias was not conducted.

3.8
Discussion

This systematic review summarized the evidence from 50 studies on the effectiveness of a variety of FASD-prevention approaches. The majority of the studies were conducted in the United States and published as journal articles. Half of the studies were published at least a decade ago. A careful consideration of the characteristics of the populations, interventions and outcomes evaluated in these studies is crucial to understanding the extent to which research in this field has been conducted in representative settings, and how research findings can be translated to practice.

3.8.1
Characteristics of the Study Populations

Most research on the potential benefits of FASD-prevention strategies has been conducted in clinical and community settings in the United States, and has examined the effects of interventions in adult women considered to be at risk of an AEP because alcohol use was either suspected, or confirmed. Only two Canadian studies met the inclusion criteria for the review; these studies evaluated the effectiveness of universal FASD-prevention approaches that targeted communities in Manitoba and Saskatchewan, respectively. Comprehensive searches of the published literature revealed that Canadian studies evaluating the effects of selective and indicated FASD-prevention approaches are scarce in the mainstream scientific literature. The lack of Canadian research in this area has been identified previously in reviews assessing interventions aimed at supporting women to reduce their use of alcohol in the childbearing years and during pregnancy [79].

As most of the studies on FASD-prevention strategies have specifically targeted adult women, it is not possible to apply their results more generally. For example, studies evaluating the effect of universal FASD-prevention strategies in female youths are scarce compared to those that have targeted adult women. Similarly, studies assessing the effectiveness of preventive approaches to FASD have largely overlooked the role of a woman's partner and other support persons as determinants of her drinking behavior during pregnancy. Whilst it is well established that a mother's drinking during pregnancy is the direct cause of FASD [7], the biological role that a father's drinking plays in producing the disorder remains an open question. Yet, it is expected that the partner has a strong influence on the mother's drinking pattern during pregnancy. Women with partners who drink are themselves more likely to drink, and having a partner who drinks can make it difficult for a woman to avoid drinking while she is pregnant. Likewise, the role of other family members and friends is a factor to take into account, particularly in cultural groups in which extensive support networks are created around maternity and childrearing. The research and implementation of FASD-prevention interventions should consider the strong influence of these and other environmental and cultural factors when formulating the objectives and potential targets of their interventions.

During the past three decades, FASD has emerged as an important health concern for Aboriginal people in Canada. It has been suggested that the incidence of FASD in the Aboriginal population is higher than in the general population [80], based on indirect evidence from studies that have reported higher numbers of binge drinking episodes during pregnancy among Aboriginal women than among their counterparts in the general population [81, 82]. However, because there is insufficient information about the prevalence of FASD in both the Aboriginal and the general Canadian populations [83], no comparison of FASD rates is possible. Furthermore, Canadian studies examining FASD rates among Aboriginals have been criticized for a lack of standardized diagnostic criteria and a failure to blind examiners to maternal alcohol use [84]. Likewise, statistics on the prevalence of alcohol abuse among Aboriginal peoples in Canada are generally not available.

No studies conducted in Canadian Aboriginal populations that met the selection criteria of the review were identified. This finding is similar to that of Parkes et al. [79], in their review of interventions aimed at supporting women to reduce their use of alcohol in the childbearing years and during pregnancy. Three studies [29, 54, 58] evaluated the impact of a universal preventive intervention (i.e., alcohol ban, educational initiatives to the broad community) in Native American populations, but the methodological quality of these studies was rated as weak and consequently no definite conclusions regarding the effectiveness of the interventions were made. In the best scenario, the interventions helped to improve the immediate outcomes, such as an increased knowledge about FASD, although no change in FASD frequency was reported. Likewise, two studies [56, 57] of poor methodological quality that assessed the effectiveness of indicated preventive approaches in Native American women at high risk of an AEP failed to show any benefits in maternal or neonatal/infant outcomes.

May [85] conducted a systematic review of the scientific literature published from 1982 through 1994 on interventions to prevent alcohol misuse among Native Americans. Of the 29 studies included in this review, only three addressed the effects of universal interventions for FASD. The review described the types of preventive approach that had been implemented in the studies, but did not provide any data on the effectiveness of the interventions.

Maternal alcohol abuse and FASD among Aboriginal people in Canada varies, and should be recognized as a problem of certain individuals and subpopulations, rather than as a problem of all Aboriginal people [86]. The results of this review have suggested that programming and services for the prevention of FASD among

Aboriginal people should target particular subgroups who are at risk, rather than target all groups regardless of their level of alcohol use. There is also a need to incorporate Aboriginal concepts of health and healing [87] into prevention initiatives that are implemented among Aboriginal populations. Likewise, research in this group should include outcomes that are culturally sensitive and relevant to the study populations involved.

It may be argued that the choice of appropriate populations for studies on the effects of FASD-prevention approaches is an overlooked area of research. However, an open discussion among research groups in the field would surely help to establish a consensus of priorities for the research agenda in FASD prevention.

3.8.2
Characteristics of the Interventions

A relatively heterogeneous group of preventive approaches to FASD was evaluated in the studies. While the interventions varied widely, for the purposes of this review they were classified into three categories (i.e., universal, selective, and indicated), and organized along a targeted-audience continuum that takes into account the breadth of the target group, the risk of having a child with the disorder, and the cost–benefit ratio of committing resources to the prevention strategy. Indicated prevention approaches, which targeted individuals who exhibit the highest risk of AEP, were less frequently evaluated than universal and selective prevention approaches.

Overall, the studies in this review poorly reported details about the implementation of the interventions. Assessing the implementation of an intervention is important to understanding which components are critical to intervention success, and how feasible it is to implement the intervention [88, 89]. Also of importance is the integrity of the interventions implemented in the studies. Systematically monitoring the integrity with which interventions are implemented provides an insight into the effectiveness of the programs [90]. For example, a program may have been ineffective because it was poorly conceptualized; however, it is equally possible that it was ineffective because the components of the program were not implemented as intended.

A major challenge in designing and researching interventions tailored to prevent FASD by reducing alcohol consumption during pregnancy is to provide a clear description of the essential components of a given intervention. Since only a few studies reported the use of a manual or described training for providers, it is unknown whether the interventions within each category were equivalent in their components, characteristics and methods of implementation.

3.8.3
Characteristics of Study Outcomes

The majority of studies presented in this review assessed the effectiveness of the FASD-prevention approach by evaluating the impact of the intervention on intermediate outcomes; that is, changes in maternal drinking behavior, such as alcohol intake and abstinence rates during pregnancy. The studies provided little or no information about how the interventions might ultimately affect the incidence of FASD and related disorders.

Evaluating how a preventive intervention can reduce the incidence of FASD poses several challenges. The specific assessment techniques used to make a definitive diagnosis of FASD remain matters of debate [91]. Furthermore, studies assessing the incidence of FASD are limited in number, vary widely in their methodology [3], and may lead to further questions about the true pattern and frequency of FASD and related disorders. The evaluation of immediate and intermediate outcomes of preventive interventions is an important step in understanding whether changes in knowledge, perceptions and behaviors related to alcohol drinking may ultimately lead to changes in the frequency of FASD. However, more effort should be directed to refining methods of directly evaluating the frequency of FASD, so that such methods can be implemented in studies that assess the effectiveness of preventive approaches to reduce or eliminate this disorder. The results of research into the effectiveness of preventive approaches for FASD should be situated within a framework in which immediate and intermediate outcomes constitute logical steps towards the ultimate goal of reducing the incidence of FASD and related disorders.

3.8.4
Methodological Quality of the Studies

Consistent with a previous review conducted by Elliott *et al.* [12] on FASD-prevention research, we found no differences in quality among the three categories of interventions. The majority of the studies were considered of poor methodological quality. Of the 50 studies included in the review, 37 were rated as weak, 12 as moderate, and only one study was rated as strong.

The methodological quality of the studies was assessed by evaluating indicators in a variety of domains related to their internal and external validity. This approach revealed important potential methodological weaknesses in this field of research that both temper the conclusions which may be drawn from the individual studies and highlight areas for improving future research. For example, observational cohort studies and before-and-after studies without a control group accounted for over 60% of the studies in the review. These types of study are subject to several forms of systematic error, such as selection bias, detection bias, and attrition bias. Therefore, caution should be exerted when interpreting their results as evidence of the effectiveness of FASD-prevention strategies. This is particularly true for the before-and-after studies included in this review, as the lack of a control group generally leads to an exaggerated estimate of the treatment benefit [92].

Another issue of concern is the general lack of rigorous reporting of the methods used in the original studies. Characteristics of the populations, settings, definitions of outcomes, and intervention procedures were not systematically described in the majority of the studies included in the review. This poor and heterogeneous reporting prevented any quantitative synthesis, and therefore any overall clinical evaluation of the comparative effectiveness of the interventions.

3 8.5
Main Findings

The interpretation and generalization of the results from this exhaustive review of prevention approaches for FASD is complicated by a number of factors. First, the majority of the studies evaluated the impact of a variety of prevention strategies to reduce maternal drinking during pregnancy, rather than the direct effect of the intervention on the incidence of FASD. Only a few studies reported on the incidence of FASD after implementing the prevention intervention (three outcomes in total). Although a strong correlation between alcohol abuse during pregnancy and the risk of having a child with FASD has been reported in the literature [4, 7], there is no consensus in the scientific community regarding the noxious effects of low to moderate prenatal alcohol exposure, or whether there is a clear threshold below which alcohol is nonteratogenic [12, 13]. Furthermore, other factors, such as poverty, smoking, and the stage of fetal development at which alcohol exposure occurs, may interact to mediate the relationship between alcohol consumption during pregnancy and FASD. With all of these considerations in mind, general conclusions about the effectiveness of FASD-prevention approaches that target the reduction of maternal drinking during pregnancy need to be made cautiously where direct measurements of FASD incidence are lacking.

The interventions evaluated in the studies were complex and multifaceted, implemented in different ways, in different settings, and by different people, including both professionals and lay people. This body of literature needs to be interpreted in light of how the intervention was implemented, and how it will be applied in reality.

The following is a brief synthesis of the main findings of the review, and how our results compare with syntheses of the evidence.

3.8.6
Universal Prevention Approaches

The evidence on the effectiveness of universal interventions, such as alcohol-related warning messages, health educational activities, and alcohol bans targeting entire populations, is based on studies of poor quality. Likewise, the studies did not generally provide evidence that these interventions produce significant modifications over time in knowledge of FASD, attitudes toward drinking during pregnancy, and the perception of risks associated with this behavior. Only a few studies evaluated changes in drinking behavior, and none of the interventions significantly modified self-reported measures of alcohol intake. An increase in knowledge about the risks of drinking during pregnancy does not necessarily translate into reductions in alcohol use during pregnancy, or the incidence of FASD. Changes in the knowledge of FASD and attitudes towards drinking during pregnancy may be necessary, but are not sufficient conditions for reducing alcohol consumption during pregnancy and, ultimately, the number of children born with FASD.

These results agree with those of similar systematic reviews. Murphy-Brennan and Oei [93] reviewed the effectiveness of primary-prevention programs in lowering the incidence of FAS, based on the evidence reported in five studies that were also included in our review. The authors concluded that FASD-prevention programs have been successful in raising awareness of FASD; however, this awareness has not been translated into behavioral changes and thus has had minimal or no impact in lowering the incidence of FASD. Likewise, Elliot *et al.* [12] conducted a systematic review of the scientific literature published from 1966 to July 2008 pertaining to the relative effectiveness of various FASD screening and prevention approaches. Prevention strategies were categorized as primary (six studies), secondary (13 studies) and tertiary prevention (13 studies). All of the primary studies in the review by Elliot *et al.* were also included in our review, except for four case studies that were excluded due to study design considerations. Conversely, the Elliot *et al.* review did not include publications that evaluated changes in knowledge about the danger of alcohol consumption during pregnancy.

Universal preventive approaches are important components of health intervention strategies designed to alter risky behaviors through education and persuasion. Public messages have the potential to influence many individuals; however, the evidence to support the effectiveness of these approaches is incomplete and seldom adequate.

3.8.7
Selective Prevention Approaches

Compared to universal preventive interventions, some selective preventive interventions have a better evidence base with which to make inferences regarding their effectiveness. The best evidence (moderate quality) regarding the effectiveness of selective prevention approaches for FASD is available for counseling activities and health education programs directed at women of childbearing age who consume alcohol, pregnant women, and women at risk of an AEP. Similar results were reported by Schorling [20], who critically reviewed five studies on prenatal education and counseling interventions aimed at reducing alcohol use in pregnancy. These five studies were also included in our review. The authors found that all of the studies except one were of poor methodological quality. Schorling concluded that no intervention has proven to be superior to the usual care provided to pregnant women, and that interventions to prevent or modify patterns of alcohol use and abuse during pregnancy have not been rigorously evaluated. Similar results were reported by Elliot *et al.* [12], in a systematic review on secondary prevention strategies for FASD. The authors found that, although some secondary prevention strategies can be effective in reducing alcohol use during pregnancy, there is insufficient evidence to determine which intervention components are most effective.

3.8.8
Indicated Prevention Approaches

The evidence base supporting the effectiveness of indicated preventive approaches was found to be weak, with only a few studies of poor methodological quality having evaluated the effectiveness of indicated FASD-prevention approaches. One study assessing a multifaceted intervention (i.e., the Four-State FAS Consortium initiative) was considered of moderate quality, but it is unknown whether the intervention was effective in modifying outcomes such as perceptions of alcohol use, well-being, family functioning, and mental health status. The analysis of Elliot *et al.* [12] on the effectiveness of tertiary FASD-prevention strategies, is in tune with the findings of our review: the studies are generally of weak to moderate methodological quality, and only a few showed a reduction in alcohol consumption during pregnancy.

3.8.9
Strengths and Limitations

The strengths of this systematic review pertain to its rigor in searching the literature, the criteria-based selection of relevant evidence, the rigorous appraisal of validity, and the evidence-based inferences. The search strategy is likely to have identified most of the available literature on the effectiveness of prevention approaches to FASD. Although various criteria to assess the methodological quality of studies are available in the scientific literature [94, 95], and there is no consensus on which quality-assessment tool can be recommended without reservation [96], we adopted a comprehensive strategy that focused mainly on the assessment of the internal validity of the studies, as recommended by several research groups [94, 96, 97]. We used a standard quality-rating tool (i.e., developed by the Public Health Research Education and Development Program (PHRED) and the Effective Public Health Practice Project [EPHPP]) [98] that has been examined and approved by experts in the field and has received positive ratings [99]. We also evaluated other methodological aspects related to the external validity of the findings (i.e., study selection criteria, type of intervention providers, and treatment fidelity).

Another important asset of this systematic review is that we controlled for the impact of multiple-publication bias in the analysis of the results. In total, 17 studies were identified as multiple publications of unique studies included in the review. The production of multiple publications from single studies can bias a review in a number of ways. Studies with significant results are more likely to lead to multiple publications and presentations [100], which makes it more likely that they will be located in literature searches. Including them in a meta-analysis can lead to an overestimation of the intervention effects [23, 24]. The identification of multiple publications is this review avoided the inclusion of duplicate publication of data that may have skewed the evidence base in the analysis of the study results.

One potential limitation of this review is its restriction to English-language publications. Some studies have documented the exclusion of non-English studies in the meta-analysis of RCTs as yielding conflicting results [101, 102]. Ideally, a systematic review with a meta-analysis of studies published in many different languages would increase the precision, generalizability, and applicability of findings; however, the potential impact of studies published in languages other than English in a meta-analysis is thought to be minimal [102]. Currently, there is no evidence on the impact of the language of publication on the results of systematic reviews that do not incorporate a meta-analysis. Therefore, it is difficult to predict how the exclusion of non-English studies may bias the results of this review.

3.8.10
Methodological Issues and Research Directions in the Evaluation of FASD Prevention Interventions

In light of the recognition that drinking alcohol during pregnancy constitutes a major public health problem because of its association with FASD and other birth and developmental problems, it is necessary for the research community and health services providers to join in collective efforts and formal partnerships to support the ongoing evaluation of FASD-prevention programs. Likewise, it is important to identify and evaluate approaches by which community partnerships may disseminate and implement evidence-based FASD-prevention programs.

More research should be focused on multilevel and multicomponent community-based interventions in multiple settings (e.g., schools, healthcare, home, community, public policy, social marketing) that can be incorporated into existing healthcare and community infrastructures to maximize effectiveness and minimize costs. Preventive interventions that use technology (e.g., Internet, media, novel electronic approaches) to influence behavior should be further assessed, and implemented if their effectiveness is proven.

In research on FASD prevention, more attention needs to be devoted to examining the range of possible prevention goals and their implications. Prevention goals can range from immediate outcomes such as an increase in knowledge of the danger of drinking alcohol during pregnancy, to intermediate outcomes such as the modification of drinking behavior during pregnancy, to ultimate outcomes such as the reduction of the incidence of FASD. Studies assessing FASD prevention interventions must clearly specify the goals and targets of the interventions, in order to substantially increase the amount of useful information that can be derived from these studies. Authors of these studies must also clearly explain why they expect that the preventive interventions will achieve the selected goals.

The majority of studies in this review on the effectiveness of FASD-prevention interventions did not specify the underlying theoretical model. The theoretical models and conceptual frameworks that were reported in a few studies included social marketing theory, social cognitive theory, activated health education model, ecological model of social support, health belief model, health communication process model, Miller's self-in-relation theory, reasoned action, and social learning theory. An important step in the further development of FASD prevention as an area of scientific inquiry is that studies on the effectiveness of prevention approaches make explicit the theoretical foundation underlying the intervention under evaluation. An explicit theoretical model affords an understanding of the key components of a prevention intervention and the causal mechanisms that are proposed to explain why it works. Theoretical models also have important methodological implications for the design of prevention interventions. They help researchers to explore which independent variables might be manipulated through the intervention, moderator variables that might enhance or reduce the effects of the intervention on certain individuals or populations, and outcome variables that might be modified as a result of the prevention intervention. Further research is needed to assess the potential of various theoretical models to contribute to FASD prevention in appropriate settings and target populations.

FASD-prevention research will benefit from advances in other disciplines, such as basic science research, behavioral research, and epidemiological and etiological research. Observational and experimental research on the factors that influence women's drinking behavior during pregnancy–including environmental, social (family and partner), psychological, biological, and genetic factors–is particularly needed to evaluate potentially promising interventions and their incorporation into clinical and public health practice. Such studies can help to define the subgroups of the population most at risk of alcohol use during pregnancy–information that is useful in the design and content of prevention programs targeted to specific populations. In some instances–and depending on the research question–interdisciplinary methodological perspectives (e.g., statistics, biostatistics, psychometrics, education, economics, and qualitative methods) should be supported. Collaboration between methodologists and prevention scientists in methodological research within the context of FASD-prevention research should be encouraged.

FASD-prevention research findings have demonstrated inconsistencies related to differences in study design and methodological rigor among studies, and appropriate research designs and analytic approaches should, therefore, be supported. The Standards of Evidence developed by the Society for Prevention Research are good examples of criteria that should be set in studies evaluating the efficacy, effectiveness, and dissemination of FASD-prevention interventions [103, 104]. Likewise, standards for reporting the results of studies on the effectiveness of FASD interventions should be endorsed [105, 106].

Research assessing the effectiveness of FASD-preventive approaches will improve substantially if more effort is made to explore what are the most effective components, duration, intensity, and settings of interventions. Likewise, it is important to understand the factors (individual and combined) that determine whether changes in behavior resulting from interventions will be maintained over time. Investigators conducting research on FASD-prevention interventions should carefully consider their outcome measures, and standardize the use of such outcome measures in order to improve the comparability of studies.

There is a need for more research to inform population-based approaches to the prevention of FASD and maternal drinking in high-risk populations. Research on individually tailored strategies to prevent maternal drinking in the most disproportionately affected populations is crucial; however, interventions at the individual level without companion interventions at the family or community level may not be effective. Research areas of particular interest are the development of effective strategies for community engagement in maternal drinking-prevention programs in high-risk populations, and an expansion of the paradigms used to develop FASD research so that prevention approaches take into consideration core family and community values. The role of women's partners and other family members also warrants further study, and should be incorporated into interventions designed to change women's drinking behavior during pregnancy.

Additional emphasis should be placed on expanding research on the prevention of FASD and maternal drinking among certain subgroups, such as low-income, ethnically, and socio-economically diverse populations, pregnant women in rural communities, and immigrant minorities. Alcohol use and FASD can have a devastating impact on these groups, yet we know little about the types of prevention program and initiatives that are effective in reducing the incidence and prevalence of these problems in these groups. Various methods to increase the participation of high-risk subgroups in FASD-prevention research studies should be explored, particularly fostering community engagement in study design and implementation and bidirectional partnerships between researchers and communities.

3.9
Conclusions

Considering the importance of – and demand for – interventions to prevent FASD, and the current rising trend in new programs, a rigorous synthesis of high-quality evidence regarding the effectiveness of the spectrum of preventive interventions for FASD was undertaken to provide much-needed information for the clinical community, policy makers, researchers, and families. In spite of the published studies on the subject, there remains deep controversy and no definitive answer regarding the "best" approach to prevent the occurrence of FASD.

There is today a substantial gap in our knowledge regarding the effectiveness of preventive approaches for FASD. The evidence base to support decisions related to preventive interventions for FASD is weak, and particularly in the case of universal and indicated approaches. Moderate evidence supporting selective prevention activities such as counseling and health education for pregnant women and women at risk of an AEP was identified, although these results should be interpreted with caution. Many studies of preventive programs suffer from significant methodological problems that make definitive conclusions regarding the effectiveness of the programs tenuous.

There is a clear mandate for researchers, policy makers, and healthcare providers to continue monitoring evidence-based preventive interventions to determine their success for individual women, their partners, and their babies. Management decisions should be guided by the needs of the community and the availability of resources for implementation of the intervention. Research on new prevention strategies is recommended, as the majority of the studies that were summarized in this review were conducted before the year 2000, and the conditions in which they were evaluated may have changed over time. Future studies on the effectiveness of these interventions need to be more rigorous. It is critical to evaluate comprehensive, practical and community-responsive interventions to expand the FASD prevention literature base. Although two Canadian studies were identified with the systematic review methods that we used, greater efforts should be made to publish and disseminate the results of research on prevention programs that may have been implemented in Canada, as this body of evidence remains mostly unpublished and unknown to the public.

Acknowledgments

The Institute of Health Economics (IHE) is most grateful to the persons that reviewed and provided information and comments on this chapter. The following individuals acted as member of a technical panel of experts that provided feedback and guidance during its development:

- Sterling K. Clarren, MD, FAAP; CEO and Scientific Director, Canada NW FASD Research Network; Clinical Professor of Paediatrics, University of British Columbia, Vancouver, BC, Canada; Clinical Professor of Pediatrics, University of Washington, Seattle, WA, USA.

- Suzanne Tough, PhD; Professor, Departments of Paediatrics and Community Health Sciences, Faculty of Medicine, University of Calgary. Calgary, AB, Canada; Health Scholar, Alberta Heritage Foundation for Medical Research; Scientific Director, Alberta Center for Child, Family and Community Research, Edmonton, AB, Canada.

The following individuals acted as peer-reviewers and provided feedback and comments to the final draft of this report:

- June Bergman, MD, CCFP, FCFP; Medical Director, Primary Care Initiative, Calgary Health Region; Assistant Professor, Department of Family Medicine, University of Calgary, Calgary, AB, Canada.

- Nancy Poole, PhD; Director, Research and Knowledge Translation, BC Centre of Excellence for Women's Health; Vancouver, BC, Canada.

Thanks to Mr Dough Stich, BSc; Program Director, Towards Optimized practice Alberta, Edmonton, AB, Canada, for his comments and feedback to the study protocol of the review.

The following individual(s) and institution(s) are acknowledged for provision of information regarding published/unpublished studies:

- Michael Fleming, MD, MPH; Department of Family Medicine, University of Wisconsin-Madison, Madison, WI, USA.

- Lewis Ball Holmes, MD; Unit Chief, Genetics and Teratology, Pediatric Service; Director, Genetic Counseling & Screening Services, Perinatal Diagnostic Unit, Obstetrics Program, MassGeneral Hospital for Children, Boston, MA, USA.

- Fiona Julian; Senior Policy Analyst, National Drug Policy Minimizing Harm Group, Population Health Directorate, New Zealand Ministry of Health, Auckland, New Zealand.

- Linda Sobell, Ph.D.; Center for Psychological Studies, Nova Southeastern University, Fort Lauderdale-Davie, FL, USA.

- Mark Sobell, Ph.D.; Center for Psychological Studies, Nova Southeastern University, Fort Lauderdale-Davie, FL, USA.

Competing Interest

Competing interest is considered to be financial interest, either direct or indirect, that would be affected by the research contained in this report, or the creation of a situation where an author's and/or external reviewer's judgment could be unduly influenced by a secondary interest such as personal advancement.

Based on the statement above, no competing interest exists with the author(s) and/or external reviewer(s) of this report.

This research has been made possible by a financial contribution from Health Canada and Alberta Health and Wellness. The views expressed herein do not necessary represent the official policy of Health Canada and Alberta Health and Wellness.

Appendix 3.A: Methodology

Search Strategy

Comprehensive searches of psychological, sociological and biomedical electronic databases, as listed in Table 3.A.1, were conducted for the period from 1970 (or database inception) to March 2010 to identify reports evaluating interventions to prevent FASD. The search strategy was designed by an Information Specialist at the IHE, and comprised both controlled vocabulary and keywords. In addition, reference lists of reviews and retrieved articles were browsed for relevant studies. Gray literature searches were conducted to identify literature from nontraditional sources, including proceedings from relevant scientific meetings, government documents, theses and dissertations, unpublished studies, and ongoing studies. Finally, primary authors and experts in the area were contacted to identify other potentially relevant studies. The search was limited to English-language articles.

Table 3.A.1 Databases searched for relevant studies.

Database	Edition or date searched	Search terms
The Cochrane Library	1996–March 2010	fetal alcohol in Title, Abstract or Keywords or (alcohol* AND (pregnancy OR fetus OR prenatal)) in Title, Abstract or Keywords
MEDLINE (Ovid Interface)	1970–March 2010	1) fetal alcohol syndrome/ 2) fetal alcohol.tw. 3) ((alcohol* or ethanol) adj3 (birth defects or congenital malformations or neurodevelopmental)).tw. 4) fasd.tw. 5) fae.tw. 6) arbd.tw. 7) arnd.tw. 8) or/1–7 9) Alcoholism/ 10) Alcoholic Intoxication/ 11) Alcohol-Induced Disorders/ 12) Alcohol-Related Disorders/ 13) Substance-Related Disorders/ and (alcohol* or ethanol).tw. 14) exp Alcoholic Beverages/ 15) Alcohol Drinking/ 16) Ethanol/ 17) or/9–16 18) fetus/ 19) pregnancy/ 20) pregnancy, high-risk/ 21) exp pregnancy outcome/ 22) prenatal injuries/ 23) prenatal exposure delayed effects/ 24) pregnancy complications/ 25) maternal exposure/ 26) or/18–25 27) 17 and 26 28) ((alcohol* or ethanol or (drinking not drinking water)) and (pregnan* or fetus or fetal or prenatal or in utero or intrauterine)).tw. 29) limit 28 to ("in data review" or in process or "pubmed not medline") 30) 8 or 27 or 29 31) Fetal Alcohol Syndrome/pc 32) Preventive Health Services/ 33) primary prevention/ 34) secondary prevention/ 35) tertiary prevention/ 36) public policy/ 37) health policy/

(*Continued*)

Table 3.A.1 (*Continued*)

Database	Edition or date searched	Search terms
		38) house calls/
		39) risk reduction behavior/
		40) prevent*.tw.
		41) ((reduc* or lower or decrease* or smaller) adj3 risk*).tw.
		42) protect*.tw.
		43) best practice*.tw.
		44) exp Communications Media/
		45) Social Marketing/
		46) Product Labeling/
		47) campaign$.mp.
		48) counseling/
		49) government programs/
		50) Community Health Services/
		51) health promotion/
		52) exp Health education/
		53) Social Control Policies/
		54) Prenatal Care/ and ((intervention* or trial).ti. or ((reduc* or lower) adj3 (alcohol or drinking or substance)).tw.)
		55) program evaluation/
		56) or/32–55
		57) (30 and 56) or 31
		58) limit 57 to animals
		59) 57 not 58
		60) limit 59 to english language
EMBASE (Ovid Interface)	1980–March 2010	1) exp Fetal Alcohol Syndrome/
		2) fetal alcohol.tw.
		3) (alcohol* adj3 (birth defects or congenital malformations or neurodevelopmental)).tw.
		4) (alcohol* adj4 prenatal).tw.
		5) (fasd or fae or arbd or arnd).tw.
		6) or/1–5
		7) alcohol/
		8) alcoholism/
		9) alcohol abuse/
		10) alcohol drinking patterns/
		11) alcohol intoxication/
		12) exp alcoholic beverages/
		13) alcohol consumption/
		14) drinking patterns/
		15) or/7–14
		16) pregnancy/
		17) fetus/
		18) prenatal exposure/

Table 3.A.1 (*Continued*)

Database	Edition or date searched	Search terms
		19) or/16–18
		20) 15 and 19
		21) 6 or 20
		22) Fetal Alcohol Syndrome/pc
		23) "prevention and control"/
		24) protection/
		25) primary prevention/
		26) secondary prevention/
		27) tertiary prevention.mp.
		28) health education/
		29) prevention/
		30) health promotion/
		31) policy/
		32) social marketing/
		33) health care policy/
		34) health program/
		35) harm reduction/
		36) risk reduction/
		37) best practice*.tw.
		38) ((reduc* or lower or decrease* or smaller) adj3 risk*).tw.
		39) prenatal care/
		40) or/23–39
		41) (21 and 40) or 22
		42) limit 41 to english language
		43) (exp vertebrate/ or animal/ or exp experimental animal/ or nonhuman/ or animal.hw.) not exp human/
		44) 42 not 43
CRD Databases (DARE, HTA & NHS EED)	1995–March 2010	#1 fetal AND alcohol OR fetal AND alcohol
		#2 alcohol* AND (pregnancy OR fetus OR prenatal)
		#1 OR #2
CINAHL (Ebsco Interface)	1970–March 2010	S1: fetal alcohol
		S2: ((MH "Alcoholic Intoxication") or (MH "Alcohol Abuse") or (MH "Alcohol Drinking") or (MH "Alcoholic Beverages+") or (MH "Alcoholism")) and ((MH "Fetus") or (MH "Pregnancy") or Prenatal)
		S3: S1 OR S2
		S4: (MH "Fetal Alcohol Syndrome/PC")
		S5: prevent* or protect* or policy or policies or education or program or health promotion or marketing or best practice* or identifying or identification
		S6: (S3 AND S5) OR S4
		Limiters – Publication Year from: 1970–2010; Language: English

(*Continued*)

Table 3.A.1 (*Continued*)

Database	Edition or date searched	Search terms
Web of Science (ISI Interface)	1970–March 2010	#1 : TI=((fetal alcohol) OR ((pregnan* OR fetus OR prenatal) AND alcohol*)) AND TS=(screening or prevent* or protect* or policy or policies or education or program or health promotion or marketing or identifying OR identification or label*)
		#2 : TS=((fetal alcohol) OR ((pregnan* OR fetus OR prenatal) AND alcohol*)) AND TI=(screening or prevent* or protect* or policy or policies or education or program or health promotion or marketing or identifying OR identification or label*)
		#3 #1 OR #2 AND Language=(English)
		#4 TS=(mouse OR mice OR murine OR rat OR rats OR pig OR pigs OR porcine OR sheep)
		#5 #3 NOT #4
PsycINFO (Ovid Interface)	1970–March 2010	1) exp Fetal Alcohol Syndrome/
		2) fetal alcohol.tw.
		3) (alcohol* adj3 (birth defects or congenital malformations)).tw.
		4) (alcohol* adj3 neurodevelopmental).tw.
		5) fasd.tw.
		6) fae.tw.
		7) arbd.tw.
		8) arnd.tw.
		9) or/1–8
		10) alcoholism/ or alcohol abuse/ or alcohol drinking patterns/ or alcohol intoxication/
		11) exp alcoholic beverages/
		12) 10 or 11
		13) pregnancy/
		14) fetus/
		15) prenatal exposure/
		16) or/13–15
		17) 12 and 16
		18) health education/
		19) prevention/
		20) health promotion/
		21) social marketing/
		22) health screening/
		23) screening/
		24) risk management/ or risk assessment/
		25) ((reduc* or lower or decrease* or smaller) adj3 risk*).tw.
		26) prevent*.tw.
		27) health care policy/ or policy making/ or government policy making/
		28) protect*.tw.

Table 3.A.1 (*Continued*)

Database	Edition or date searched	Search terms
		29) or/18–28 30) (9 or 17) and 29 31) limit 30 to English language 32) limit 31 to animal 33) 31 not 32
Sociological Abstracts (CSA Interface)	1970–March 2010	KW=((fetal alcohol) OR ((pregnancy OR fetus OR prenatal) AND alcohol)) AND KW=(prevent* or protect* or policy or policies or education or program or health promotion or marketing or identifying or identification or label*)
SocINDEX with Full Text (EBSCO Interface)	1970–March 2010	S1: fetal alcohol OR fetal alcohol S2: DE "ALCOHOLISM" or DE "ALCOHOLIC beverages" or DE "ALCOHOLICS" or DE "DRINKING of alcoholic beverages" S3: DE "PREGNANCY" or DE "PREGNANT women" or DE "TEENAGE pregnancy" S4: S1 OR (S2 AND S3) S5: prevent* or protect* or policy or policies or education or program or health promotion or marketing or best practice or identifying or identification S6: S4 AND S5
Social Services Abstracts (CSA Interface)	1970–March 2010	KW=((fetal alcohol) OR ((pregnancy OR fetus OR prenatal) AND alcohol)) AND KW=(prevent* or protect* or policy or policies or education or program or health promotion or marketing or identifying or identification or label*)
CBCA Reference (Proquest Interface)	1982–March 2010	(fetal alcohol) OR ((pregnancy OR fetus OR prenatal) AND alcohol) AND prevent* or protect* or policy or policies or education or program or health promotion or marketing or best practice or identifying or identification or label*
CPI.Q. Canadian Periodicals Index (Gale Interface)	1988–March 2010	(ke (fetal alcohol OR fetal alcohol)) And (ke ((pregnancy or fetus or prenatal) AND alcohol))
Canadian Research Index (MicroLog) (Proquest Interface)	1970–March 2010	(fetal alcohol) OR ((pregnancy OR fetus OR prenatal) AND alcohol) AND (prevent* or protect* or policy or policies or education or program or health promotion or marketing or identifying or identification or label*)
AMA Clinical Practice Guidelines	March 2010	Browsed list
CMA Infobase	March 2010	Fetal alcohol

(*Continued*)

Table 3.A.1 (*Continued*)

Database	Edition or date searched	Search terms
National Guideline Clearinghouse	March 2010	"Fetal alcohol" (browsed through list); pregnancy AND alcohol (browsed through list) (0 relevant results)
Clinical Trials		
ClinicalTrials.gov (US)	March 8, 2010	FASD; fetal alcohol; alcohol AND pregnancy
Granting Agencies		
CIHR funded research database	March 8, 2010	FASD; fetal alcohol; alcohol pregnancy; alcohol pregnant
Alberta Innovates (Health Solutions) Formerly Alberta Heritage Foundation for Medical Research (AHFMR)	March 8, 2010	Browsed through "Independent investigator awards" and "Interdisciplinary team grant" in the funding decisions section 2006–2009
Alberta Center for Child Family and Community Research	March 8, 2010	Browsed research section of Fetal Alcohol Spectrum Disorder Also looked at ACCFCR Funded research projects on FASD
PHAC page on FASD	March 8, 2010	Browsed pages
HTA resources		
AETMIS	2001–March 2010	Browsed publications
CADTH	March 2010	Fetal alcohol; pregnancy alcohol; pregnant alcohol
Institute for Clinical and Evaluative Sciences (ICES)	March 2010	Fetal alcohol; pregnancy alcohol
Health Technology Assessment Unit At McGill	2001–March 2009	Browsed publications
Medical Advisory Secretariat	2001–March 2009	Browsed publications
NZHTA	1999–2007	Browsed publications
NICE	March 2010	Fetal alcohol; fetal alcohol; pregnancy AND alcohol; pregnant AND alcohol
Internet searching		
Google	March 2010	Fetal alcohol prevention

Study Selection Process

Two reviewers independently examined the titles and abstracts generated from the search strategies to identify articles potentially relevant to the topic of study. The full text of all articles deemed relevant was retrieved for a closer inspection. Two reviewers independently appraised the full manuscripts of potentially relevant studies to determine their eligibility for the review. Disagreements about eligibility were resolved through discussions between reviewers until consensus was reached. The eligibility criteria for the review are summarized in Table 3.A.2.

Studies considered for inclusion were prospective and retrospective studies with a control group (i.e., RCTs, CCTs), case-control studies, prospective and retrospective cohort studies with comparison groups, interrupted time series studies, and before-and-after studies. Studies had to report numeric data on at least one study outcome. Outcomes that were examined included the following: incidence of FASD; alcohol consumption during pregnancy; neonatal and infant outcomes;

Table 3.A.2 Study eligibility criteria.

Criterion	Description
Field of study	Scientific literature; primary research
Study purpose	Studies are eligible if they involve universal, selective or indicated interventions to prevent or reduce the incidence of FASD
Study design	RCTs, CCTs and observational analytical studies (i.e., prospective and retrospective cohort studies with comparison groups). Interrupted time series and before-and-after studies with no comparison group were also included.
Population	Participants with a variety of risk-exposure levels (e.g., general population, pregnant women and their partners, women at reproductive age who use alcohol, or have previously abused alcohol while pregnant, or are at risk for conception, or who have had a child with FASD
Intervention	Any FASD-prevention approach that can be classified under the following: • Universal • Selective • Indicated
Comparator	Any comparator
Outcomes of interest	Incidence of FASD, maternal and child-related outcomes
Language of publication	English only
Study settings and geographic location	All settings and geographical locations, subject to language of publication and study design criteria

CCT = controlled clinical trial; FASD = fetal alcohol spectrum disorder; RCT = randomized controlled clinical trial.

risk-reduction measures; maternal outcomes (e.g., drinking behavior, relapse, number of subsequent deliveries); legal outcomes; family-related outcomes; and economic and healthcare-utilization outcomes. Outcomes were analyzed separate according to the follow-up period that was evaluated.

Secondary research (i.e., systematic reviews, health technology assessments, and evidence reports), editorials, letters, commentaries, position papers, and clinical practice guidelines were excluded from the review, and considered only as background information and to frame the analysis of the results. Studies were also excluded if the primary goal of the intervention was to prevent or terminate pregnancy.

Data Extraction

A pre-tested data-extraction form was used to extract information regarding the study design and methods (i.e., year, country of study, type of publication, duration of the study, number of participating centers, study design), characteristics of participants (i.e., demographic characteristics, inclusion/exclusion criteria), FASD-prevention strategy (i.e., setting, type of intervention) and comparators (i.e., control/comparison, waiting list, no intervention), and measures and outcomes of interest (i.e., type of change targeted, assessment instruments, assessment interval, effect size). Finally, information was collected on study conclusions, as reported by the authors of the primary studies. Data from the primary studies were extracted by one reviewer, and then independently verified for accuracy and completeness by a second reviewer. Any discrepancies in data extraction were resolved by consensus between the data extractor and the data verifier. Study selection, methodological quality assessment and data extraction were managed with Microsoft Excel™ (Microsoft Corporation, Redmond, WA, USA).

Methodological Quality Assessment

Due to the diversity of study designs that were included in the review, classic evidence classification systems, such as those recommended in the Cochrane Handbook [107], were not used for the review. A standard quality-rating tool developed by the PHRED and the EPHPP to evaluate studies on prevention strategies [98] was used to appraise the methodological quality of the studies (Table 3.A.3). The tool, which is based on guidelines set out by Mulrow *et al.* [108] and Jadad *et al.* [109], has been examined by experts in the field and received excellent ratings [99]. The tool consists of six criteria: selection bias; allocation bias; confounders; blinding of outcome assessors; data collection methods; and the handling of withdrawals and dropouts. Each criterion is rated as "strong," "moderate," or "weak," depending on characteristics of each criterion reported in the study. Once the ratings of characteristics are totaled, each study receives an overall assessment of strong, moderate, or weak quality. Two reviewers independently rated each relevant article for methodological quality. Discrepancies in quality assessment ratings were resolved by consensus.

Table 3.A.3 Methodological quality assessment tool.

EFFECTIVE PUBLIC HEALTH PRACTICE PROJECT (EPHPP)

```
Ref ID: _____
Author: _____
Year: _____
Reviewer: _____
```

QUALITY ASSESSMENT TOOL FOR QUANTITATIVE STUDIES

COMPONENT RATINGS

A) SELECTION BIAS

(Q1) Are the individuals selected to participate in the study likely to be representative of the target population?
1. Very likely
2. Somewhat likely
3. Not likely
4. Can't tell

(Q2) What percentage of selected individuals agreed to participate?
1. 80–100% agreement
2. 60–79% agreement
3. Less than 60% agreement
4. Not applicable
5. Can't tell

RATE THIS SECTION	STRONG	MODERATE	WEAK
See dictionary	1	2	3

B) STUDY DESIGN

1. Indicate the study design
2. Randomized controlled trial
3. Controlled clinical trial
4. Cohort analytic (two group pre + post)
5. Case-control
6. Interrupted time series
7. Cohort (one group pre + post (before–and-after))
8. Other specify _____
9. Can't tell

Was the study described as randomized? If NO, go to Component C.
No   Yes

If Yes, was the method of randomization described? (See dictionary)
No   Yes

If Yes, was the method appropriate? (See dictionary)
No   Yes

(Continued)

Table 3.A.3 (*Continued*)

RATE THIS SECTION See dictionary	STRONG 1	MODERATE 2	WEAK 3

C) CONFOUNDERS

(Q1) Were there important differences between groups prior to the intervention?
1. Yes
2. No
3. Can't tell

The following are examples of confounders:
1. Race
2. Sex
3. Marital status/family
4. Age
5. SES (income or class)
6. Education
7. Health status
8. Pre-intervention score on outcome measure

(Q2) If yes, indicate the percentage of relevant confounders that were controlled, either in the design (e.g. stratification, matching) or analysis.
1. 80–100%
2. 60–79%
3. Less than 60%
4. Can't Tell

RATE THIS SECTION See dictionary	STRONG 1	MODERATE 2	WEAK 3

D) BLINDING

(Q1) Was (were) the outcome assessor(s) aware of the intervention or exposure status of participants?
1. Yes
2. No
3. Can't tell

(Q2) Were the study participants aware of the research question?
1. Yes
2. No
3. Can't tell

RATE THIS SECTION See dictionary	STRONG 1	MODERATE 2	WEAK 3

Table 3.A.3 *(Continued)*

E) DATA COLLECTION METHODS

(Q1) Were data collection tools shown to be valid?
1. Yes
2. No
3. Can't tell

(Q2) Were data collection tools shown to be reliable?
1. Yes
2. No
3. Can't tell

RATE THIS SECTION See dictionary	STRONG 1	MODERATE 2	WEAK 3

F) WITHDRAWALS AND DROP-OUTS

(Q1) Were withdrawals and drop-outs reported in terms of numbers and/or reasons per group?
1. Yes
2. No
3. Can't tell

(Q2) Indicate the percentage of participants completing the study. (If the percentage differs by groups, record the lowest.)
1. 80–100%
2. 60–79%
3. Less than 60%
4. Can't tell

RATE THIS SECTION See dictionary	STRONG 1	MODERATE 2	WEAK 3

G) INTERVENTION INTEGRITY

(Q1) What percentage of participants received the allocated intervention or exposure of interest?
1. 80–100%
2. 60–79%
3. Less than 60%
4. Can't tell

(Q2) Was the consistency of the intervention measured?
1. Yes
2. No
3. Can't tell

(Q3) Is it likely that subjects received an unintended intervention (contamination or cointervention) that may influence the results?
1. Yes
2. No
3. Can't tell

(Continued)

Table 3.A.3 (*Continued*)

H) ANALYSES

(Q1) Indicate the unit of allocation (circle one)
community organization / institution practice / office individual

(Q2) Indicate the unit of analysis (circle one)
community organization / institution practice / office individual

(Q3) Are the statistical methods appropriate for the study design?
1. Yes
2. No
3. Can't tell

(Q4) Is the analysis performed by intervention allocation status (i.e., intention to treat) rather than the actual intervention received?
1. Yes
2. No
3. Can't tell

GLOBAL RATING

COMPONENT RATINGS

Please transcribe the information from the gray boxes on pages 1–4 onto this page.

A	**SELECTION BIAS**	RATE THIS SECTION See dictionary	STRONG 1	MODERATE 2	WEAK 3
B	**STUDY DESIGN**	RATE THIS SECTION See dictionary	STRONG 1	MODERATE 2	WEAK 3
C	**CONFOUNDERS**	RATE THIS SECTION See dictionary	STRONG 1	MODERATE 2	WEAK 3
D	**BLINDING**	RATE THIS SECTION See dictionary	STRONG 1	MODERATE 2	WEAK 3
E	**DATA COLLECTION METHODS**	RATE THIS SECTION See dictionary	STRONG 1	MODERATE 2	WEAK 3
F	**WITHDRAWALS AND DROPOUTS**	RATE THIS SECTION See dictionary	STRONG 1	MODERATE 2	WEAK 3

GLOBAL RATING FOR THIS PAPER (circle one):
1. STRONG   (four STRONG ratings with no WEAK ratings)
2. MODERATE   (less than four STRONG ratings and one WEAK rating)
3. WEAK   (two or more WEAK ratings)

Data Analysis and Synthesis of the Results

Each study that met the selection criteria for the review was classified into one of three main categories of universal, selective, and indicated FASD-prevention approaches. Characteristics of the included studies were summarized using descriptive statistics (i.e., proportions and percentages for categorical data; means with standard deviations (SD), or medians with interquartile ranges (IQR), for continuous data). A thematic analysis and synthesis of study results was undertaken. Evidence tables were constructed to describe study characteristics, quality and individual study results. The study outcomes were analyzed based on the report of statistically significant differences between the intervention and control.

Meta-analyses were planned as part of the data analysis to derive pooled estimates from individual RCTs or CCTs to support inferences regarding the efficacy and effectiveness of the FASD-prevention strategies. Individual study results would be pooled into a meta-analysis (weighted using the standard inverse variance method [107, 110]) when two or more studies assessed the same type of intervention, targeted similar populations, had similar study designs, and had usable data for outcomes of interest. The types of summary statistics to be considered in the meta-analyses were risk ratios or odds ratios (OR) with 95% confidence intervals (95% CI) for dichotomous outcomes and weighted or standardized mean differences (WMD and SMD, respectively) with 95% CI for continuous outcomes [107]. Meta-analyses would use a random-effect model. Statistical heterogeneity would be tested using the chi-square test [110] and quantified with the I^2 statistic [111]. If evidence of clinical or statistical heterogeneity among studies was identified, effect size estimates with corresponding 95% CI would be presented separately for each study [112, 113]. Heterogeneity would be characterized as small (I^2 <25%), moderate (I^2 26–74%) and high (≥75%) [111]. Sources of heterogeneity would be explored qualitatively. They may be due to methodological differences (differences in design or quality) or clinical differences (differences in key characteristics of participants, interventions or outcome measures) [107]. Where appropriate, subgroup analysis based on patient, intervention, follow-up period and study characteristics were to be conducted, if feasible. Statistical analyses would be conducted using Reviewer Manager 5 (Copenhagen: The Nordic Cochrane Center, The Cochrane Collaboration, 2008). Due to heterogeneity of populations, interventions, comparison groups, and outcomes of interest among the studies, meta-analyses were not conducted as part of the systematic review.

Appendix 3.B: Excluded Studies, Multiple Publications and Studies Pending Full Publication

Excluded Research Studies

The application of the selection criteria resulted in 128 studies being excluded from the systematic review. The primary reasons for exclusion were as follows:

- The study did not assess the efficacy/effectiveness of a prevention approach to FASD ($n = 60$).
- The study was not original research (e.g., narrative review, commentary, editorial) ($n = 37$).
- The study did not report measurable data for the outcomes of interest ($n = 14$).
- The study did not use any of the study designs considered in the review ($n = 8$).
- The study did not target the populations of interest ($n = 5$).
- The full text of the study was not retrieved ($n = 4$).

The excluded studies, and the reason(s) for their exclusion from the systematic review, are listed in Table 3.B.1.

Table 3.B.1 Excluded research studies.

Main reason for exclusion:
The study did not assess the efficacy/effectiveness of a prevention approach to FASD ($n = 60$)

Allen, C.D. and Ries, C.P. Smoking, alcohol, and dietary practices during pregnancy: comparison before and after prenatal education. *J. Am. Diet. Assoc.* 1985;85(5):605–606.

Astley, S.J., Bailey, D., Talbot, C., and Clarren, S.K. Fetal alcohol syndrome (FAS) primary prevention through FAS diagnosis: I. Identification of high-risk birth mothers through the diagnosis of their children. *Alcohol Alcohol.* 2000;35(5):499–508.

Astley, S.J., Bailey, D., Talbot, C., and Clarren, S.K. Fetal alcohol syndrome (FAS) primary prevention through FAS diagnosis: II. A comprehensive profile of 80 birth mothers of children with FAS. *Alcohol Alcohol.* 2000;35(5):509–519.

Autti-Ramo, I. Twelve-year follow-up of children exposed to alcohol in utero. *Dev. Med. Child. Neurol.* 2000;42(6):406–411.

Balachova, T., Bonner, B., Chaffin, M., Isurina, G., and Tsvetkova, L. Preventing fetal alcohol syndrome (FAS) and alcohol related neurodevelopmental disorders (ARND) in Russian children. *Alcohol. Clin. Exp. Res.* 2008;32(6):231A.

Berkowitz, G., Brindis, C., and Peterson, S. Substance use and social outcomes among participants in perinatal alcohol and drug treatment. *Women's Health* 1998;4(3):231–254.

Brindis, C. Options for recovery: Promoting perinatal drug and alcohol recovery, child health, and family stability. *J. Drug Issues* 1997;27(3):607–624.

Brindis, C.D., Clayson, Z., and Berkowitz, G. Options for recovery: California's perinatal projects. *J. Psychoactive Drugs* 1997;29(1):89–99.

Britt, G.C., Knisely, J.S., Dawson, K.S., and Schnoll, S.H. Attitude toward recovery and completion of a substance-abuse treatment program. *J. Subst. Abuse Treat.* 1995;12(5):349–353.

Burd, L., Klug, M.G., Martsolf, J.T., Martsolf, C., Deal, E., and Kerbeshian, J. A staged screening strategy for prenatal alcohol exposure and maternal risk stratification. *J. R. Soc. Health* 2006;126(2):86–94.

Centers for Disease Control and Prevention (CDC). Identification of children with fetal alcohol syndrome and opportunity for referral of their mothers for primary prevention–Washington, 1993–1997. *MMWR* 1998;47(40):861–864.

Table 3.B.1 (*Continued*)

Main reason for exclusion:
The study did not assess the efficacy/effectiveness of a prevention approach to FASD (*n* = 60)

Chang, G., Wilkins-Haug, L., Berman, S., and Goetz, M.A. Pregnant women with negative alcohol screens do drink less: a prospective study. *Am. J. Addict.* 1998;7(4):299–304.

Chang, G., Wilkins-Haug, L., Berman, S., Goetz, M.A., Behr, H., and Hiley, A. Alcohol use and pregnancy: improving identification. *Obstet. Gynecol.* 1998;91(6):892–898.

Chang, G., Wilkins-Haug, L., Berman, S., and Goetz, M.A. The TWEAK: application in a prenatal setting. *J. Stud. Alcohol* 1999;60(3):306–309.

Chang, G. Identifying prenatal alcohol use: Screening instruments versus clinical predictors. *Am. J. Addict.* 1999;8(2):87–93.

Clarren, S.K., Astley, S.J., Bailey, D., and Talbot, T. Prevention of fetal alcohol syndrome by direct outreach to mothers. *J. Intell. Disabil. Res.* 2000;44(3/4):239.

Coleman, M.A., Coleman, N.C., and Murray, J.P. Mutual support groups to reduce alcohol consumption by pregnant women: marketing implications. *Health Mark. Q.* 1990;7(3–4):47–63.

Connors, G.J. and Walitzer, K.S. Reducing alcohol consumption among heavy drinking women: evaluating the contributions of life-skills training and booster sessions. *J. Consult. Clin. Psychol.* 2001;69(3):447–456.

Czeizel, A.E. Ten years of experience in periconceptional care. *Eur. J. Obstet. Gynecol. Reprod. Biol.* 1999;84(1):43–49.

Dawson, D.A., Das, A., Faden, V.B., Bhaskar, B., Krulewitch, C.J., and Wesley, B. Screening for high- and moderate-risk drinking during pregnancy: a comparison of several TWEAK-based screeners. *Alcoholism* 2001;25(9):1342–1349.

Fleming, M.F., Barry, K.L., Manwell, L.B., Johnson, K., and London, R. Brief physician advice for problem alcohol drinkers. a randomized controlled trial in community-based primary care practices. *JAMA* 1997;277(13):1039–1045.

French, M.T., McCollister, K.E., Cacciola, J., Durell, J., and Stephens, R.L. Benefit-cost analysis of addiction treatment in Arkansas: specialty and standard residential programs for pregnant and parenting women. *Subst. Abuse* 2002;23(1):31–51.

Gifford, A., Farkas, K.J., Jackson, L.W., and Bearer, C.F. Cost benefit analysis of universal newborn screening for maternal alcohol use during pregnancy. *Pediatr. Res.* 2008;64(4):61.

Goransson, M., Magnusson, A., and Heilig, M. Identifying hazardous alcohol consumption during pregnancy: implementing a research-based model in real life. *Acta Obstet. Gynecol. Scand.* 2006;85(6):657–662.

Graves, K. An evaluation of the alcohol warning label: a comparison of the United States and Ontario, Canada in 1990 and 1991. *J. Public Policy Mark.* 1993;12(1):19–29.

Greenfield, T.K., Graves, K.L., and Kaskutas, L.A. Long-term effects of alcohol warning labels: findings from a comparison of the United States and Ontario, Canada. *Psychol. Mark.* 1999;16(3):261–282.

Grekin, E.R. and Ondersma, S.J. The relationship between prenatal care, personal alcohol abuse and alcohol abuse in the home environment. *Drugs Educ. Prev. Policy* 2009;16(5):463–470.

Hollstedt, C., Dahlgren, L., and Rydberg, U. Alcoholic women in fertile age treated at an alcohol clinic. *Acta Psychiatr. Scand.* 1983;67(3):195–204.

(*Continued*)

Table 3.B.1 (*Continued*)

Main reason for exclusion:
The study did not assess the efficacy/effectiveness of a prevention approach to FASD (*n* = 60)

Koniak-Griffin, D. Public health nursing care for adolescent mothers: impact on infant health and selected maternal outcomes at 1 year postbirth. *J. Adolesc. Health* 2002;30(1):44–54.

Kvigne, V.L., Bull, L.B., Welty, T.K., Leonardson, G.R., and Lacina, L. Relationship of prenatal alcohol use with maternal and prenatal factors in American Indian women. *Soc. Biol.* 1998;45(3–4):214–222.

Labs, S.M. Primary prevention of fetal alcohol syndrome: effects of target, threat noxiousness, and self-efficacy on the abstinence intentions of prospective mothers. The University of Alabama; Birmingham, 1993.

Laken, M.P. and Ager, J.W. Effects of case management on retention in prenatal substance abuse treatment. *Am. J. Drug Alcohol Abuse* 1996;22(3):439–448.

Larsson, G., Ottenblad, C., Hagenfeldt, L., Larsson, A., and Forsgren, M. Evaluation of serum gamma-glutamyl transferase as a screening method for excessive alcohol consumption during pregnancy. *Am. J. Obstet. Gynecol.* 1983;147(6):654–657.

Lee, S.H. and Grubbs, L.M. A comparison of self-reported self-care practices of pregnant adolescents. *Nurse Pract.* 1993;18(9):25–29.

Li, C., Olsen, Y., Kvigne, V., and Welty, T. Implementation of substance use screening in prenatal clinics. *SDJ Med.* 1999;52(2):59–64.

Little, B.B. Treatment of substance abuse during pregnancy and infant outcome. *Am. J. Perinatol.* 2003;20(5):255–262.

Little, R.E., Streissguth, A.P., Guzinski, G.M., Grathwohl, H.L., Blumhagen, J.M., and McIntyre, C.E. Change in obstetrician advice following a two-year community educational program on alcohol use and pregnancy. *Am. J. Obstet. Gynecol.* 1983;146(1):23–28.

Lumley, J. and Brown, S. Attenders and nonattenders at childbirth education classes in Australia: how do they and their births differ. *Birth-Iss. Perinat. Care* 1993;20(3):123–130.

Magnusson, A., Goransson, M., and Heilig, M. Unexpectedly high prevalence of alcohol use among pregnant Swedish women: failed detection by antenatal care and simple tools that improve detection. *J. Stud. Alcohol* 2005;66(2):157–164.

Manwell, L.B., Fleming, M.F., Mundt, M.P., Stauffacher, E.A., and Barry, K.L. Treatment of problem alcohol use in women of childbearing age: results of a brief intervention trial. *Alcoholism* 2000;24(10):1517–1524.

Marshall, S.K. and Stokl, M. Sheway's services for substance using pregnant and parenting women: evaluating the outcomes for infants. *Can. J. Commun. Mental Health* 2005;24(1):19–34.

Minor, M.J. and Van Dort, B. Prevention research on the teratogenic effects of alcohol. *Prev. Med.* 1982;11(3):346–359.

Mullins, S.M., Bard, D.E., and Ondersma, S.J. Comprehensive services for mothers of drug-exposed infants: relations between program participation and subsequent child protective services reports. *Child Maltreatment* 2005;10(1):72–81.

O'Connor, M.J. and Whaley, S.E. Health care provider advice and risk factors associated with alcohol consumption following pregnancy recognition. *J. Stud. Alcohol* 2006;67(1):22–31.

Perham-Hester, K.A. and Gessner, B.D. Correlates of drinking during the third trimester of pregnancy in Alaska. *Matern. Child Health J.* 1997;1(3):165–172.

Table 3.B.1 *(Continued)*

Main reason for exclusion:
The study did not assess the efficacy/effectiveness of a prevention approach to FASD (*n* = 60)

Perry, C., Williams, C.L., Veblen-Mortenson, S., Toomey, T.L., Komro, K., Anstine, P.S., *et al.* Project Northland: outcomes of a communitywide alcohol use prevention program during early adolescence. *Am. J. Pub. Health* 1996;86(7):956–965.

Project MATCH Research Group. Matching alcoholism treatments to client heterogeneity: Project MATCH three-year drinking outcomes. *Alcohol. Clin. Exp. Res.* 1998;22(6):1300–1311.

Russell, M., Martier, S.S., Sokol, R.J., Mudar, P., Bottoms, S., Jacobson, S., *et al.* Screening for pregnancy risk-drinking. *Alcoholism* 1994;18(5):1156–1161.

Russell, M., Martier, S.S., Sokol, R.J., Mudar, P., Jacobson, S., and Jacobson, J. Detecting risk drinking during pregnancy: a comparison of four screening questionnaires. *Am. J. Public Health* 1996;86(10):1435–1439.

Schinke, S., Schwinn, T., and Cole, K. Preventing alcohol abuse among early adolescents through family and computer-based interventions: four-year outcomes and mediating variables. *J. Dev. Phys. Disabil.* 2006;18(2):149–161.

Sokol, R.J., Janisse, J.J., Louis, J.M., Bailey, B.N., Ager, J., Jacobson, S.W., *et al.* Extreme prematurity: an alcohol-related birth effect. *Alccholism* 2007;31(6):1031–1037.

Spivak, K., Sanchez-Craig, M., and Davila, R. Assisting problem drinkers to change on their own: effect of specific and nonspecific advice. *Addiction* 1994;89:1135–1142.

St Pierre, A., Mark, P.M., Michelson, R., Condon, L.M., Nelson, A.F., and Rolnick, S.J. Alcohol and other drugs of abuse in pregnancy. *HMO Practice* 1996;10(3):114–118.

Stevens, S.J. and Arbiter, N. A therapeutic community for substance-abusing pregnant women and women with children: process and outcome. *J. Psychoact. Drugs* 1995;27(1):49–56.

Svikis, D.S. Brief interventions for alcohol, tobacco and other drugs 2000. Ongoing study. John Hopkins University. (Grant Number: 5R01AA11802–3).

Svikis, D.S., Golden, A.S., Huggins, G.R., Pickens, R.W., McCaul, M.E., Velez, M.L., *et al.* Cost-effectiveness of treatment for drug-abusing pregnant women. *Drug Alcohol Depend.* 1997;45:105–113.
Terza, J.V., Kenkel, D.S., Lin, T.F., and Sakata, S. Care-giver advice as a preventive measure for drinking during pregnancy: zeros, categorical outcome responses, and endogeneity. *Health Econ.* 2008;17(1):41–54.

Whaley, S.E. Increasing the report of alcohol use among low-income pregnant women. *Am. J. Health Promot.* 2003;17(6):369–372.

Wutzke, S.E., Conigrave, K.M., Saunders, J.B., and Hall, W.D. The long-term effectiveness of brief interventions for unsafe alcohol consumption: a 10-year follow-up. *Addiction* 2002;97:665–675.

Young, S. Fetal Alcohol Syndrome Disorder Training Project. *Nevada RNformation* 2009;18(4):6. Available at: http://www.nursingald.com/Uploaded/NewsletterFiles/NV11_09.pdf (accessed 2 December 2010).

Main reason for exclusion:
The study was not original research (e.g., narrative review, commentary, editorial) (*n* = 37)

Alpert, J.J. and Zuckerman, B.S. Prevention of fetal alcohol syndrome. *Pediatrics* 1993;92(5):739.

Altman, G.B. Educational strategies for a community program in preventing alcohol use during pregnancy. *Nurs. Adm. Q.* 1980;4(3):23–29.

(Continued)

Table 3.B.1 (Continued)

Main reason for exclusion:
The study was not original research (e.g., narrative review, commentary, editorial) (n = 37)

Anonymous. Program: Minnesota media campaign to promote alcohol-free pregnancy. *Health Educ. Q.* 1996;23(4):418–419.

Asante, K.O. and Robinson, G.C. Pregnancy outreach program in British Columbia: the prevention of alcohol-related birth defects. *Can. J. Publ. Health* 1990;81(1):76–77.

Babor, T.F. and Higgins-Biddle, J.C. Alcohol screening and brief intervention: dissemination strategies for medical practice and public health. *Addiction* 2000;95(5):677–686.

Best Start. Keys to a successful alcohol and pregnancy communication campaign. *Best Start* 2003. Available from: http://www.beststart.org/resources/alc_reduction/pdf/keys.pdf [cited 2009 Mar 30].

Bien, T.H., Miller, W.R., and Tonigan, J.S. Brief interventions of alcohol problems: a review. *Addiction* 1993;88:315–335.

Brindis, C.D., Berkowitz, G., Clayson, Z., and Lamb, B. California's approach to perinatal substance abuse: toward a model of comprehensive care. *J. Psychoact. Drugs* 1997;29(1):113–122.

Cockey, C.D. On the edge. Preventing fetal alcohol syndrome. *AWHONN Lifelines* 2001;5(4):23–24.

Colmorgen, G.H. Prevention of fetal alcohol syndrome. *Del. Med. J.* 1986;58(8):544–545.

Crome, I.B. Treatment of alcohol problems in pregnancy and prevention of fetal alcohol syndrome. *Eur. Psychiatr.* 2008;23:S57.

Dawson, D.A. Pre-pregnancy drinking: How drink size affects risk assessment. *Addiction* 2001;96(9):1361.

Fleming, M.F. Brief interventions and the treatment of alcohol use disorders: current evidence. *Recent Dev. Alcohol.* 2003;16:375–390.

Floyd, R.L., Ebrahim, S., Tsai, J., O'Connor, M., and Sokol, R. Strategies to reduce alcohol-exposed pregnancies. *Matern. Child Health J.* 2006;10(5 Suppl.):S149–S151.

Guarnera, D. Improving the response to FASD – fetal alcohol spectrum disorders. *Addiction Professional* 2009;7(5):30–33.

Gutzke, D.W. "The cry of the children": the Edwardian medical campaign against maternal drinking. *Br. J. Addict.* 1984;79(1):71–84.

Handmaker, N.S. and Wilbourne, P. Motivational interventions in prenatal clinics. *Alcohol Res. Health* 2001;25(3):219.

Hankin, J.R. Fetal alcohol syndrome prevention research. *Alcohol Res. Health* 2002;26:58–65.

Huntimer, C.M. The utilization of antenatal care in the prevention and intervention of the consequences of parental alcohol use. *SDJ Med.* 1987;40(7):25–30.

Jessup, M. and Green, J.R. Treatment of the pregnant alcohol-dependent woman. *J. Psychoact. Drugs* 1987;19(2):193–203.

Keough, V.A. and Jennrich, J.A. Including a screening and brief alcohol intervention program in the care of the obstetric patient. *J. Obstet. Gynecol. Neonatal. Nurs.* 2009;38(6):715–722.

Little, R.E., Streissguth, A.P., and Guzinski, G.M. Prevention of Fetal Alcohol Syndrome: a model program. *Alcoholism* 1980;4(2):185–189.

Table 3.B.1 *(Continued)*

Main reason for exclusion:
The study was not original research (e.g., narrative review, commentary, editorial) (*n* = 37)

Masotti, P., George, M.A., Szala-Meneok, K., Morton, A.M., Loock, C., Van Bibber, M., *et al*. Preventing fetal alcohol spectrum disorder in Aboriginal communities: a methods development project. *PLoS Med.* 2006;3(1):24–29.

Miller, W.R. and Rollnick, S. *Motivational interviewing: preparing people for change.* 2nd edn. New York: Guilford Press; 2009.

Miller, W.R. and Sanchez, V.C. Motivating young adults for treatment and lifestyle change, in: *Issues in Alcohol Use and Misuse in Young Adults* (ed. G. Howard), South Bend, IN: University of Notre Dame Press; 1994, pp.55–82.

Morse, B., Weiner, L., and Garrido, P. Focusing prevention of fetal alcohol syndrome on women at risk. *Ann. N. Y. Acad. Sci.* 1989;562:342–343.

Moyer, A., Finney, J.W., Swearingen, C.E., and Vergun, P. Brief interventions for alcohol problems: a meta-analytic review of controlled investigations in treatment seeking and non-treatment seeking populations. *Addiction* 2002;97:279–292.

Orgain, L.S. and Caporale, M.J. Using local media to educate young women about FAS and FAE. *Public Health Rep.* 1993;108(2):171.

Rosett, H.L. and Weiner, L. Identifying and treating pregnant patients at risk from alcohol. *Can. Med. Assoc. J.* 1981;125(2):149–154.

Senikas, V. Three national programs address fetal alcohol spectrum disorder. *J. Obstet. Gynaecol. Can.* 2009;31(2):172–186

Spong, C.Y., Toso, L., Roberson, R., Vink, J., and Abebe, D.T. Prevention of alcohol-induced damage in fetal alcohol syndrome with NAP and SAL. *Alcohol. Clin. Exp. Res.* 2008;32(6):314A.

Stockley, C.S. Effectiveness of strategies such as health warning labels to reduce alcohol-related harms – an Australian perspective. *Int. J. Drug Policy* 2001;12(2):153–166.

U.S. Preventive Service Task Force. Screening and behavioral counseling interventions in primary care to reduce alcohol misuse: recommendation statement. *Ann. Intern. Med.* 2004;140:554–556.

Velasquez, M.M., Mullen, P.D., and von Sternberg, K. Motivational interviewing for preventing alcohol-exposed pregnancies in women upon release from jail. *Alcohol. Clin. Exp. Res.* 2007;31(6):300A.

Velasquez, M.M. and von Sternberg, K. Project Choices: A Line of Research to Prevent Fetal Alcohol Spectrum Disorder. *Alcohol. Clin. Exp. Res.* 2009;33(6):345A.

Wallis, J. Intervention for alcohol use in pregnancy. *RCM Midwives* 2007;10(8):360.

Withlock, E.P., Polen, M.R., Green, C., Orleans, C.T., and Klein, J. Behavioral counseling interventions in primary care to reduce risky, harmful alcohol use by adults: a summary of the evidence for the U.S. Preventive Services Task Force. *Ann. Intern. Med.* 2004;140:558–569.

Main reason for exclusion:
The study did not report measurable data for the outcomes of interest (*n* = 14)

Corse, S.J. and Smith, M. Reducing substance abuse during pregnancy. Discriminating among levels of response in a prenatal setting. *J. Subst. Abuse Treat.* 1998;15(5):457–467.

(Continued)

Table 3.B.1 (*Continued*)

Main reason for exclusion:
The study did not report measurable data for the outcomes of interest (*n* = 14)

Dunnagan, T., Haynes, G., Christopher, S., and Leonardson, G. Formative evaluation of a multisite alcohol consumption intervention in pregnant women. *Neurotoxicol. Teratol.* 2003;25(6):745–755.

Escobar, G.J. How much does she really drink: HMO intervention. Kaiser Foundation Research Institute (Grant Number: 5R01AA12486-02); 2000.

Fleming, M.F. Brief alcohol intervention: Healthy Moms Project. University of Wisconsin Madison. (Grant Number: 3R01AA012522-01A2S1), 2000.

Glik, D., Prelip, M., Myerson, A., and Eilers, K. Fetal alcohol syndrome prevention using community-based narrowcasting campaigns. *Health Promot. Pract.* 2008;9(1):93–103.

Handmaker, N. Motivating pregnant problem drinkers to change. University of New Mexico Albuquerque. (Grant Number: 5R01AA12491-02), 2000.

Kenkel, D.S. Economic analysis of fetal alcohol syndrome preventive intervention. Cornell University (Grant Number: 1R01AA12487-01A1), 2000.

Kennedy, C., Finkelstein, N., Hutchins, E., and Mahoney, J. Improving screening for alcohol use during pregnancy: the Massachusetts ASAP program. *Matern. Child Health J.* 2004;8(3):137–147.

Kraemer, K.L. Brief intervention to prevent prenatal alcohol use. University of Pittsburgh (Grant Number: 5R01AA012485-04; 5R01AA12485-02), 2000.

Minnesota Department of Health. Program: Minnesota Media Campaign to promote alcohol-free pregnancy. *Health Educ. Q.* 1996;23(4):418.

Mullen, P.D. Preventing alcohol exposed pregnancy after a jail term. Ongoing study. University of Texas (Grant Number: 3R01AA012514-03S1; 5R01AA12514-02), 2000.

O'Connor, M.J. Preventing alcohol use in pregnant women utilizing WIC. Ongoing study. University of California Los Angeles (Grant Number: 3R01AA012480-03S1), 1999.

O'Connor, M.J. Preventing alcohol use in pregnant women utilizing WIC (Women, Infants, Children). University of California Los Angeles (Grant Number: 3R01AA012480-02), 2000.

Walsh Dotson, J.A., Henderson, D., and Magraw, M. A public health program for preventing fetal alcohol syndrome among women at risk in Montana. *Neurotoxicol. Teratol.* 2003;25(6):757–761.

Main reason for exclusion:
The study did not use any of the study designs considered in the review (*n* = 8)

Barrett, M.E., Wong, F.Y., and McKay, D.R. Self-reported alcohol use among women of childbearing age and their knowledge of alcohol warning labels and signs. *Arch. Fam. Med.* 1993;2(12):1260–1264.

Donnelly, F.M., Mowery, J.L., and McCarver, D.G. Knowledge and misconceptions among inner-city African American mothers regarding alcohol and drug use. *Am. J. Drug Alcohol Abuse* 1998;24(4):675–683.

Drinkard, C.R., Shatin, D., Luo, D., Heinen, M.J., Hawkins, M.M., and Harmon, R.G. Healthy pregnancy program in a national managed care organization: evaluation of satisfaction and health behavior outcomes. *Am. J. Manag. Care* 2001;7(4):377–386.

Glor, E.D. Impacts of a prenatal program. *Can. J. Publ. Health* 1987;78:249–254.

Table 3.B.1 *(Continued)*

Main reason for exclusion:
The study did not use any of the study designs considered in the review (*n* = 8)

Jones-Webb, R., McKiver, M., Pirie, P., and Miner, K. Relationships between physician advice and tobacco and alcohol use during pregnancy. *Am. J. Prev. Med.* 1999;16(3):244–247.

Kaskutas, L.A. Understanding drinking during pregnancy among urban American Indians and African Americans: health messages, risk beliefs, and how we measure consumption. *Alcohol. Clin. Exp. Res.* 2000;24(8):1241–1250.

Kaskutas, L.A. and Graves, K. Relationship between cumulative exposure to health messages and awareness and behavior-related drinking during pregnancy. *Am. J. Health Promotion* 1994;9(2):115–124.

Marin, G. Changes in reported awareness of product warning labels and messages in cohorts of California Hispanics and non-Hispanic whites. *Health Educ. Behav.* 1997;24(2):230–244.

Main reason for exclusion:
The study did not target the populations of interest (*n* = 5)

Grant, T., Huggins, J., Connor, P., Pedersen, J.Y., Whitney, N., and Streissguth, A. A pilot community intervention for young women with fetal alcohol spectrum disorders. *Community Ment. Health J.* 2004;40(6):499–511.

Greengield, T. and Kaskutas, L.A. Early impacts of alcoholic beverage warning labels: national study findings relevant to drinking and driving behavior. *Safety Sci.* 1993;16(5-6):689–707.

Handmaker, N.S., Hester, R.K., and Delaney, H.D. Videotaped training in alcohol counseling for obstetric care practitioners: a randomized controlled trial. *Obstet. Gynecol.* 1999;93(2):213–218.

Kaskutas, L. and Greenfield, T.K. First effects of warning labels on alcoholic beverage containers. *Drug Alcohol Depend.* 1992;31:1–14.

Weiner, L., Potter, D., McCarty, D., and Rosett, H.L. Fetal alcohol effects: prevention through training health-care professionals. *Alcohol. Clin. Exp. Res.* 1986;10(1):102.

Main reason for exclusion:
The full text of the study was not retrieved (*n* = 4)

Crosby, F.S. The effects of a fetal alcohol education intervention upon the knowledge, attitude and behavior of pregnant women in a health maintenance organization. *Dissertation Abstracts Int.* 1986;47(6-A).

Downer, G.A. Fetal alcohol syndrome: preventing birth defects through education. *HT: The Magazine for Healthcare Travel Professionals* 1997;4(6):18.

Holmes, L.B. Fetal Alcohol Damage Prevention Study. *Clinical Trials Gov.* 2008. Available from: http://clinicaltrials.gov/ct2/show/NCT00696085?term=fetal+alcohol&rank=2 [cited 2010 Apr 1].

Kirk, C., Lieberman, L., and Amaranth, K. The Multicultural Prenatal Drug and Alcohol Prevention Project of the Women's Action Alliance: final report of a 5 year CSAP demonstration project to the Center for Substance Abuse Prevention. New York: Women's Action Alliance; 1995.

Multiple Publications of Studies Included in the Review

Of the 70 included articles, 19 were identified as multiple publications; that is, cases in which the same study was published more than once or part of the data from an original report was republished. The multiple publications were not considered to be unique studies, and any information that they provided was included with the data reported in the main study.

Table 3.B.2 Multiple publications.

Multiple publications of studies included in the review (*n* = 19)

Chang, G., Goetz, M.A., Wilkins-Haug, L., and Berman, S. A brief intervention for prenatal alcohol use: an in-depth look. *J. Subst. Abuse Treat.* 2000;18(4):365–369. **Associated publication of Chang *et al.* (1999)**[33]

Chang, G., McNamara, T.K., Orav, E.J., and Wilkins-Haug, L. Brief intervention for prenatal alcohol use: the role of drinking goal selection. *J. Subst. Abuse Treat.* 2006;31(4):419–424. **Associated publication of Chang *et al.* (2005)**[34]

Centers for Disease Control and Prevention (CDC). Motivational intervention to reduce alcohol-exposed pregnancies: Florida, Texas, and Virginia, 1997–2001. *MMWR – Morbidity & Mortality Weekly Report* 2003;52(19):441–444. **Associated publication of Floyd *et al.* (2007)**[40]

Grant, T., Ernst, C.C., Pagalilauan, G., and Streissguth, A. Postprogram follow-up effects of paraprofessional intervention with high-risk women who abused alcohol and drugs during pregnancy. *J. Commun. Psychol.* 2003;31(3):211–222. **Associated publication of Grant *et al.* (2005)**[42]

Halmesmaki, E. Treatment program of pregnant alcoholics to prevent FAS. *Alcohol Alcohol.* 1988;23(3):A55. **Associated publication of Halmesmaki (1988)**[43]

Hankin, J.R. FAS prevention strategies: Passive and active measures. *Alcohol Health Res. World* 1994;18(1):62–66. **Associated publication of Hankin *et al.* (1996)**[46]

Hankin, J.R., Firestone, I.J., Sloan, J.J., Ager, J.W., Goodman, A.C., Sokol, R.J., *et al.* The impact of the alcohol warning label on drinking during pregnancy. *J. Public Policy Mark.* 1993;12(1):10–18. **Associated publication of Hankin *et al.* (1996)**[46]

Hankin, J.R., Sloan, J.J., Firestone, I.J., Ager, J.W., Sokol, R.J., and Martier, S.S. A time series analysis of the impact of the alcohol warning label on antenatal drinking. *Alcoholism* 1993;17(2):284–289. **Associated publication of Hankin *et al.* (1996)**[46]

Hankin, J.R., Sloan, J.J., Firestone, I.J., Ager, J.W., Sokol, R.J., Martier, S.S., *et al.* The alcohol beverage warning label: when did knowledge increase? *Alcoholism* 1993;17(2):428–430. **Associated publication of Hankin *et al.* (1996)**[46]

Hankin, J.R., Sloan, J.J., Firestone, I.J., Ager, J.W., Sokol, R.J., and Martier, S.S. Has awareness of the alcohol warning label reached its upper limit? *Alcoholism* 1996;20(3):440–444. **Associated publication of Hankin *et al.* (1996)**[46]

Hankin, J.R., Sloan, J.J., and Sokol, R.J. The modest impact of the alcohol beverage warning label on drinking during pregnancy among a sample of African American women. *J. Public Policy Mark.* 1998;17(1):61–69. **Associated publication of Hankin *et al.* (1996)**[46]

Table 3.B.2 *(Continued)*

Multiple publications of studies included in the review (*n* = 19)

Hankin, J. and Sokol, R. Brief postpartum intervention protects previously born children from alcohol-related developmental delay. *Am. J. Obstet. Gynecol.* 2003;189(6, Suppl. 1):S148. **Associated publication of Hankin (2003)[45]**

Ingersoll, K., Floyd, L., Sobell, M., and Velasquez, M.M., and the Project CHOICES Intervention Research Group. Reducing the risk of alcohol-exposed pregnancies: a study of a motivational intervention in community settings. *Pediatrics* 2003;111(5 Pt 2):1131–1135. **Associated publication of Floyd *et al.* (2007)[40]**

Little, R.E., Streissguth, A.P., Guzinski, G.M., Uhl, C.N., Paulozzi, L., Mann, S.L., *et al.* An evaluation of the pregnancy and health program. *Alcohol Health Res. World* 1985;10(1):44–53. **Associated publication of Little *et al.* (1984)[52]**

May, P.A., Miller, J.H., and Gossage, J.P. Enhanced case management to prevent fetal alcohol syndrome. *Alcohol. Clin. Exp. Res.* 2004;28(5):125A. **Associated publication of May *et al.* (2008)[57]**

Project Choices Intervention Research Group. Reducing the risk of alcohol-exposed pregnancies: a study of a motivational intervention in community settings. *Pediatrics* 2003;111:1131–1135. **Associated publication of Floyd *et al.* (2007)[40]**

Rosett, H.L., Ouellette, E.M., Weiner, L., and Owens, E. Therapy of heavy drinking during pregnancy. *Obstet. Gynecol.* 1978;51(1):41–46. **Associated publication of Rosett *et al.* (1983)[68]**

Rosett, H.L., Weiner, L., and Edelin, K.C. Strategies for prevention of fetal alcohol effects. *Obstet. Gynecol.* 1981;57(1):1–7. **Associated publication of Rosett *et al.* (1983)[68]**

Velasquez, M.M., Ingersoll, K.S., Sobell, M.B., Floyd, L., Sobell, L.C., and von Sternberg, K. A dual-focus motivational intervention to prevent alcohol-exposed pregnancy. *Alcohol. Clin. Exp. Res.* 2007;31(6):333A. **Associated publication of Floyd *et al.* (2007)[40]**

Studies Pending Full Publication

One study that was identified through gray literature searches and that met the selection criteria for the review was not included at this stage. After communication with the study authors, it was determined that results are being prepared for final publication. It was decided that the study would be referenced but not included in full in the systematic review as study results are being submitted to publication.

Studies pending full publication (*n* = 1)

Sobell, L.C. A Media-Based Motivational Intervention to Prevent Alcohol Exposed Pregnancies (AEPs) *Clinical Trials gov* 2009. Available at: http://clinicaltrials.gov/ct2/show/NCT00219336?term=fetal+alcohol&rank=9 [accessed 28 Mar 2010].

Appendix 3.C: Summary Tables of Overall Characteristics of Studies on Prevention Approaches to FASD

Table 3.C.1 Country of study.

Country	No. of studies	Reference List Number(s)
Canada	2	[31, 32]
Denmark	1	[65]
Finland	1	[43]
Latin America (Argentina, Brazil, Cuba, and Mexico)	1	[28]
Norway	1	[60]
Sweden	2	[51, 63]
UK	1	[73]
USA	41	[26, 27, 29, 30, 33–42, 44–50, 52–59, 61, 62, 64, 66–72, 74, 75]

UK = United Kingdom; USA = United States of America.

Table 3.C.2 Types of publication.

Type of publication	No. of studies	Reference List Numbers
Conference abstract/paper	2	[31, 45]
Journal article	46	[26–30, 32–35, 37, 39–44, 46–75]
Thesis/dissertation	2	[36, 38]

Table 3.C.3 Types of study design.

Study design	No. of studies	Reference List Number(s)
Before-and-after study	19	[27, 31, 35, 41–43, 48, 49, 51, 52, 54–58, 68, 71, 72, 75]
CCT	13	[28, 30, 38, 44, 45, 47, 50, 53, 64, 66, 67, 69, 73, 114]
Interrupted time series	1	[46]
Prospective analytical cohort study	5	[37, 60–62, 74]
RCT	6	[26, 33, 34, 36, 39, 40]
Retrospective analytical cohort study	6	[29, 32, 59, 63, 65, 70]

CCT = controlled clinical trial; RCT = Randomized controlled trial.

Table 3.C.4 Sources of funding.

Sources of funding	No. of studies	Reference List Numbers
Reported	37	[26–28, 32–34, 37, 39–44, 46–48, 50–52, 54–58, 60–66, 68–70, 73–75]
NR	13	[29–31, 35, 36, 38, 45, 49, 53, 59, 67, 71, 72]

NR = not reported.

Table 3.C.5 Study settings.

Study setting	No. of studies	Reference List Number(s)
Community	8	[27, 29, 31, 41, 48, 55, 59, 62]
Community and health facilities	1	[42]
Community, health facilities, and urban jail	1	[40]
Community, schools, and health facilities	2	[58, 66]
Health facilities	35	[26, 28, 30, 32–39, 43–46, 49, 51–53, 56, 57, 60, 61, 63–65, 67–75]
Schools	3	[47, 50, 54]

Table 3.C.6 Types of study population.

Study population	No. of studies	Reference List Number(s)
Broad public	7	[27, 31, 50, 54, 55, 58, 59]
Pregnant women	15	[28–30, 36, 38, 46, 49, 51, 52, 60, 61, 63, 65, 69, 73]
Pregnant women and women of childbearing age	1	[48]
Women of childbearing age	5	[32, 41, 53, 62, 72]
Women of childbearing age who consume alcohol	3	[40, 47, 66]
Women at risk of an alcohol-exposed pregnancy	19	[26, 33–35, 37, 39, 42–45, 56, 57, 64, 67, 68, 70, 71, 74, 75]

Table 3.C.7 Residential settings of study populations.

Residential setting	No. of studies	Reference List Numbers
Mix of urban and rural	9	[30–32, 39, 40, 52, 53, 61, 67]
Rural	5	[29, 49, 56–58]
Suburban/inner city	7	[35, 36, 46, 50, 68, 69, 71]
Urban	20	[27, 28, 33, 34, 38, 41, 42, 44, 47, 51 55, 60, 62, 64–66, 70, 73–75]
NR	9	[26, 37, 43, 45, 48, 54, 59, 63, 72, 114]

NR = not reported.

Table 3.C.8 Sex of target population.

Sex of target population	No. of studies	Reference List Numbers
Female only	42	[26, 28–30, 32, 33, 35–49, 51–53, 56, 57, 60–75]
Male and female	8	[27, 31, 34, 50, 54, 55, 58, 59]

Table 3.C.9 Age group of target population.

Age group	No. of studies	Reference List Numbers
Adult (≥18 years of age)	25	[31, 33, 34, 37–40, 42–45, 47, 55–57, 59–64, 70, 72, 74, 75]
Both youth and adults	11	[26, 27, 30, 32, 35, 36, 46, 51, 58, 67, 71]
Youth (<18 years of age)	6	[28, 41, 50, 54, 66, 69]
NR	8	[29, 48, 49, 52, 53, 65, 68, 73]

NR = not reported.

Table 3.C.10 Race of target population.

Race group	No. of studies	Reference List Numbers
Miscellaneous races	26	[26, 27, 30, 33–40, 42, 44, 45, 47, 50, 59, 64, 66–71, 74, 75]
Non-Caucasians only	11	[28, 29, 41, 46, 54–58, 61, 62]
NR	13	[31, 32, 43, 48, 49, 51–53, 60, 63, 65, 72, 73]

NR = not reported.

Table 3.C.11 Prevention approaches to FASD.

Prevention approach	No. of studies	Reference List Numbers
Universal	18	[27, 29–32, 41, 46, 48–50, 54, 55, 58, 59, 62, 65, 72, 73]
Selective	23	[26, 28, 33–40, 44, 47, 51, 52, 60, 61, 63, 64, 66, 67, 69, 71, 75]
Indicated	9	[42, 43, 45, 53, 56, 57, 68, 70, 74]

Table 3.C.12 General level of the intervention under study.

Level of the intervention	No. of studies	Reference List Number(s)
Community focused	10	[27, 31, 32, 41, 46, 52, 54, 58, 62, 65]
Community and system-level focused	3	[48, 55, 59]
Individual/family focused	36	[26, 28, 30, 33–40, 42–45, 47, 49–51, 53, 56, 57, 60, 61, 63, 64, 66–75]
System-level focused	1	[29]

Table 3.C.13 Types of public health preventive intervention implemented.

Type of intervention	No. of studies	Reference List Number(s)
Referral and follow-up	8	[35, 37, 42, 51–53, 56, 74]
Case management	8	[35, 37, 42, 53, 56, 57, 66, 68]
Delegated functions	0	NA
Screening	5	[35, 51, 52, 64, 71]
Case finding	3	[37, 51, 52]
Outreach	1	[35]
Disease and other health event investigation	0	NA
Surveillance	0	NA
Health teaching	18	[28, 33, 35, 36, 38, 49, 50, 52, 54, 58, 61, 64, 66, 67, 69, 71, 73, 74]
Counseling	25	[26, 33–35, 37, 39, 40, 43–45, 47, 51–53, 56, 57, 60, 63, 64, 66, 68, 70, 71, 74, 75]
Consultation	4	[53, 56, 60, 74]
Advocacy	1	[42]
Social marketing	11	[27, 31, 32, 41, 46, 48, 55, 59, 62, 65, 72]
Policy development and enforcement	4	[29, 48, 55, 59]
Community organizing	0	NA
Coalition building	0	NA
Collaboration	0	NA

NA = Not applicable.

Table 3.C.14 Theoretical frameworks underlying preventive approaches to FASD.

Theoretical framework	No. of studies	Reference List Number(s)
Activated health education model	1	[36]
Cognitive-behavioral approach	4	[39, 45, 66, 75]
Ecological model of social support	1	[28]
Health belief model	1	[53]
Health communication process model	1	[54]
Home visitation model	1	[42]
Miller's self-in-relation theory	1	[74]
Reasoned action and social learning theory	1	[49]
Social cognitive theory	3	[38, 64, 67]
Social marketing theory	4	[32, 41, 61, 62]
Transtheoretical model	1	[40]
NR	30	[26, 27, 29, 30, 33–35, 37, 43, 44, 46–48, 50–52, 55–60, 63, 65, 68–73]

NR = not reported.

Table 3.C.15 Types of intervention setting.

Type of intervention setting	No. of studies	Reference List Numbers
Community	14	[27, 29, 31, 32, 37, 41, 46, 48, 52, 55, 58, 59, 62, 65]
Health facility	27	[26, 30, 33, 34, 36, 38–40, 43, 45, 49, 51, 56, 57, 60, 61, 63, 64, 66, 68–75]
Health facility or home	3	[44, 53, 67]
Home	3	[28, 35, 42]
School	3	[47, 50, 54]

Table 3.C.16 Individual components implemented in the interventions.

Individual components implemented		No. of studies	Reference List Number(s)
Education	Mass media	6	[27, 31, 32, 48, 52, 62]
	Distribution of printed educational materials	11	[27, 28, 30, 41, 52, 54, 58, 62, 65, 72, 73]
	Educational sessions (workshops)	6	[36, 61, 66, 67, 69, 74]
	School curriculum	2	[54, 58]
	Alcohol-intake testing and counseling	1	[33]
	Motivational messages	7	[33, 36, 49, 61, 67, 69, 73]
	Computer-based education	2	[49, 50]
	Audio-visual materials	8	[29, 31, 49, 50, 54, 58, 62, 73]
Legal	Warning labels/Alcohol ban	5	[29, 46, 48, 55, 59]
Counseling activities	Alcohol-intake testing and counseling	1	[33]
	Counseling (individual or for couples)	23	[26, 33–35, 37, 39, 40, 43–45, 47, 51–53, 56, 57, 60, 63, 64, 68, 71, 74, 75]
	Case management	9	[35, 37, 42, 51, 53, 56, 57, 66, 68]
	Skills training	6	[36, 42, 53, 66, 70, 74]
	Support group	5	[37, 52, 53, 70, 74]
	Referral to available services	9	[35, 37, 42, 51–53, 56, 66, 74]

Table 3.C.17 Types of provider who delivered the preventive interventions.

Type of provider	No. of studies	Reference List Number(s)
Counselors	1	[40]
Physicians	3	[33, 43, 73]
Health educators	3	[36, 61, 67]
Self-applied (i.e., media or printed materials)	11	[27, 30–32, 38, 41, 48, 49, 62, 65, 69]
Midwives	2	[60, 63]
Multidisciplinary teams (two or more providers)	12	[26, 28, 35, 39, 51–53, 57, 66, 68, 74, 75]
Nurses	1	[34]
Nutritionists	1	[64]
Peers	2	[50, 58]
Public health nurses	2	[42, 71]
Social workers	1	[45]
Substance abuse counselors	1	[70]
NS	10	[29, 37, 44, 46, 47, 54–56, 59, 72]

NS = not specified.

Table 3.C.18 Types of outcome reported in the studies on the effectiveness of preventive approaches to FASD.

Type of outcome		No. of outcomes assessed at different follow-up periods				
		≤3 months	>3 months and ≤6 months	>6 months and ≤9 months	>9 months and ≤1 year	>1 year
Immediate	Knowledge about alcohol use during pregnancy/FASD	8 [30, 32, 38, 50, 54, 58, 72]	2 [36, 58]	3 [73]	2 [31, 41]	2 [62]
	Attitudes toward alcohol use during pregnancy	5 [30, 49, 50, 54]	1 [36]	–	2 [31, 52]	–
	Awareness of risk of alcohol use during pregnancy	–	1 [27]	–	1 [52]	1 [55]
	Perceptions about alcohol use during pregnancy	1 [50]	1 [53]	–	1 [59]	–
Intermediate	Alcohol intake	12 [37, 38, 44, 47, 66, 67]	12 [29, 33, 35–37, 39]	4 [28, 40, 61, 73]	20 [34, 43, 46, 48, 51, 57, 60, 63, 69–71, 74, 75]	2 [42, 65]
	Alcohol abstinence	2 [44, 67]	–	2 [64, 68]	2 [57, 60]	3 [42, 56, 65]
	Binge drinking	1 [47]	–	1 [40]	1 [40]	1 [65]
	Alcohol-exposed pregnancy	1 [47]	–	1 [40]	–	–
Ultimate	Neonatal and infant outcomes	–	–	1 [61]	21 [26, 33, 43, 47, 64, 69, 70, 74]	7 [42, 45, 59, 64]
	Maternal outcomes	–	–	2 [28, 61]	4 [74, 75, 115]	3 [42, 53]
	FASD outcomes	–	–	–	4 [36, 43, 51]	1 [57]
	Economic / Healthcare utilization outcomes	–	–	–	2 [47, 74]	–
	Family outcomes	–	–	–	–	1 [53]
	Legal outcomes	–	–	–	1 [35]	–

Table 3.C.19 Studies reporting on statistically significant results for any of the outcomes of interest in the review.

Reporting of statistically significant differences in the results	Study conclusions			
	No support of the superiority of the intervention	No conclusions regarding the superiority of the intervention	Partial support of the superiority of the intervention	Support of the superiority of the intervention
Studies that did not provide data on statistical testing of the differences	2 [62, 65]	11 [27, 31, 43, 48, 49, 53–56, 68, 75]	–	3 [35, 42, 71]
Studies that reported no statistically significant differences	8 [28, 33, 36, 41, 60, 63, 66, 69]	3 [46, 59, 73]	2 [51, 57]	3 [30, 34, 44]
Studies that reported statistically significant differences	–	1 [52]	3 [26, 38, 50]	14 [29, 32, 37, 39, 40, 45, 47, 58, 61, 64, 67, 70, 72, 74]

Table 3.C.20 Summary of individual components of the methodological quality assessment of studies included in the review.

Domains of Methodological Quality		No. of studies
Selection bias	Strong	4 [26, 39, 54, 65]
	Moderate	18 [28, 38, 42, 45, 46, 48–51, 55–57, 60, 62–64, 66, 67]
	Weak	28 [27, 29–37, 40, 41, 43, 44, 47, 52, 53, 58, 59, 61, 68–75]
Allocation bias	Strong	18 [26, 28, 30, 33, 34, 36, 38–40, 44, 45, 47, 50, 53, 64, 66, 67, 73]
	Moderate	32 [27, 29, 31, 32, 35, 37, 41–43, 46, 48, 49, 51, 52, 54–63, 65, 68–72, 74, 75]
	Weak	—
Confounders	Strong	19 [33, 34, 36, 38–40, 44, 45, 47, 53, 60, 61, 64, 66, 67, 69, 70, 73, 74]
	Moderate	2 [26, 28]
	Weak	29 [27, 29–32, 35, 37, 41–43, 46, 48–52, 54–59, 62, 63, 65, 68, 71, 72, 75]
Blinding	Strong	1 [39]
	Moderate	17 [27–30, 32, 33, 36, 37, 40, 42, 44, 46, 47, 53, 61, 65, 73]
	Weak	32 [26, 31, 34, 35, 38, 41, 43, 45, 48–52, 54–60, 62–64, 66–72, 74, 75]
Data collection methods	Strong	16 [30, 33–36, 38–40, 45–47, 50, 53, 63, 66, 74]
	Moderate	4 [51, 64, 69, 72]
	Weak	30 [26–29, 31, 32, 37, 41–44, 48, 49, 52, 54–62, 65, 67, 68, 70, 71, 73, 75]
Withdrawals and dropouts	Strong	15 [28, 30, 33–35, 39, 44, 50, 53, 54, 60, 61, 67, 69, 75]
	Moderate	10 [36, 38, 40, 42, 43, 47, 56, 63, 64, 66]
	Weak	25 [26, 27, 29, 31, 32, 37, 41, 45, 46, 48, 49, 51, 52, 55, 57–59, 62, 65, 68, 70–74]
Global rating	Strong	1 [39]
	Moderate	12 [28, 33, 36, 38, 40, 47, 50, 53, 61, 63, 64, 66]
	Weak	37 [26, 27, 29–32, 34, 35, 37, 41–46, 48, 49, 51, 52, 54–60, 62, 65, 67–75]

Table 3.C.21 Summary of other methodological aspects of the studies included in the review.

Domains		No. of studies
Report of starting and stopping accession dates	Yes	29 [26–32, 36, 37, 39–42, 45, 46, 48, 52, 55, 56, 58, 59, 62–65, 68–70, 73]
	No	18 [34, 35, 38, 43, 44, 47, 49, 50, 53, 54, 57, 60, 61, 66, 67, 72, 74, 75]
	Partial	3 [33, 51, 71]
Report of selection criteria	Inclusion and exclusion	5 [28, 33, 34, 67, 75]
	Inclusion only	36 [26, 29, 30, 32, 35–51, 54, 57, 59–62, 64–66, 68–73]
	NR	9 [27, 31, 52, 53, 55, 56, 58, 63, 74]
Report on patient eligibility	15 [26, 28, 33, 34, 36, 40, 42, 46, 56, 57, 59, 64, 65, 67, 68]	
Description of the frequency of the intervention	25 [8–26, 26–28, 28–32, 32, 33, 33, 34, 34, 35, 35, 36, 36–40, 43, 45, 47, 50, 60, 61, 63, 66, 68–70, 72–75]	
Description of the duration of the intervention	16 [26, 32–34, 38–40, 42, 49, 50, 62–64, 67, 68, 75]	

NR = not reported.

Appendix 3.D: Operational Definitions of Prevention Approaches to FASD

The following classification of prevention interventions for FASD was based on a conceptual framework proposed by the Institute of Medicine in the United States [4, 14] that describes three types of preventive approaches.

Table 3.D.1 Types of prevention approach.

Prevention approach	Description
Universal	Universal interventions attempt to educate the broad public about the risks of drinking during pregnancy. The aim of universal intervention is that the population be informed of, have knowledge of, and fully understand the relationship between the consumption of alcohol and its teratogenic effects. The purpose of this approach is to ensure that pregnant women, and possibly their male partners, do not engage in risky behaviors that are likely to harm their unborn child. Universal interventions may be designed specifically for women during pregnancy or the pre-conceptual period, and encourage abstinence as a responsible approach to motherhood. The alcohol beverage warning label is an example of a universal intervention that has been extensively studied. Public education through public service announcements, billboards, pamphlets in physicians' offices, and media advertisements serves to fulfill the universal model, but universal interventions also include changes in the social environment (e.g., changes in the law and regulation or changes in social and cultural norms related to the acceptability of alcohol consumption during pregnancy). Healthcare providers are ideally situated to use universal prevention models, given that the mother, and possibly also the father, will come into contact with a health professional at some stage in the pregnancy. These visits present opportunities to convey messages about the dangers of alcohol consumption during pregnancy.
Selective	Selective interventions target women (and their partners) who are at risk of having children with FASD; that is, all women of childbearing age who consume alcohol. An example of a selective prevention measure is the screening of pregnant women for use of alcohol, followed by the counseling of drinkers regarding risk to the fetus or, if warranted, referral to specialized treatment. Screening is focused on identifying alcohol dependence and a need for intervention in the addiction.
Indicated	Indicated interventions are directed at women who are at high risk of having a child with FASD, such as those who have previously abused alcohol while pregnant or while at risk for conception, or women who drink and have previously delivered an infant with FASD. This level of prevention includes treatment of alcoholism in women who are pregnant or likely to become pregnant. Women who are enrolled in alcohol-treatment programs might, for example, receive a psychosocial intervention that includes contingency management, motivational interviewing, psychotherapy, and behavioral therapy. The interventions are modified to target alcohol dependency in pregnant women as an appropriate preventive intervention for the developing fetus.

FASD = fetal alcohol spectrum disorder.

The following classification of preventive interventions for FASD is based on the Public Health Interventions (PHI) model [76] that describes three levels of public health practice.

The classification of prevention interventions for FASD shown in Figure 3.D.1 is based on an "Intervention Wheel" model [76] that includes 17 public health interventions: surveillance; disease and health threat investigation; outreach; screening; case-finding; referral and follow-up; case management; delegated functions; health teaching; counseling; consultation; collaboration; coalition-building; community-organizing; advocacy; social marketing; and policy development and enforcement.

1) **Referral and follow-up, case management, and delegated functions**
    1.1   **Referral and follow-up:** Referral and follow-up interventions assist individuals, families, groups, organizations and communities to make use of the resources needed to prevent or resolve problems or concerns. Referral and follow-up most often follow the implementation of another intervention, such as health teaching, counseling, delegated functions, consultation, screening, and case finding. They are also important components of case management. On occasion, they are implemented in conjunction with advocacy. Types: (a) early intervention services; (b) referral of mother to alcohol treatment programs; (c) counseling and support groups; (d) interdisciplinary teams or specialist in FASD; (e) follow-up care for developmental delay; and (f) respite care. Additional

Table 3.D.2   General level of intervention under study.

Level of intervention	Description
Community-focused	Community-focused interventions change community norms, community attitudes, community awareness, community practices and community behaviors, and are directed towards entire populations within the community, or occasionally towards target groups within those populations. They are also called "Social-focused" interventions.
Individual/ family-focused	Individual-focused interventions change knowledge, attitudes, beliefs, practices and behaviors of individuals. This practice level is directed at individuals alone.
Systems-focused	Systems-focused interventions change organizations, policies, laws and power structures. The focus is not directly on individuals and communities, but on the systems that impact health. They are also called "Policy-focused" interventions.
Unclear	It is not possible to categorize the general level of intervention based on the information provided by the authors.

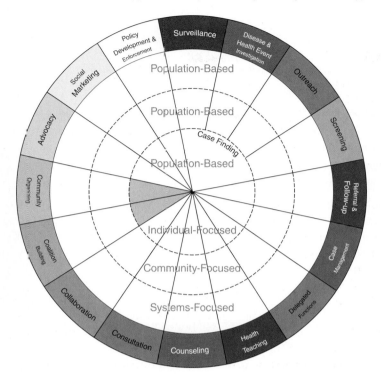

Figure 3.D.1 Classification of prevention interventions from a Public Health Perspective. Taken from Minnesota Department of Health Division of Community Health Services 2001 [76].

recommendations: referral to community services, crisis management, child welfare, public health nurses, therapeutic childcare, and agencies that monitor the home environment.

1.2 **Case management:** Case management interventions optimize self-care capabilities of individuals and families and the capacity of systems and communities to coordinate and provide services.

1.3 **Delegated functions:** Delegated functions are direct-care tasks that a registered professional nurse carries out under the authority of a health-care practitioner, as allowed by law. Delegated functions also include any direct-care tasks that a registered professional nurse entrusts to other appropriate personnel to perform.

2) **Screening, case finding, outreach, disease and health event investigation, and surveillance**
Screening, case finding, outreach, surveillance, and disease and other health event investigations often are implemented together. Case finding is closely

linked with screening of individuals and families, and the two terms are sometimes used interchangeably.

2.1 **Screening:** Screening interventions identify individuals with unrecognized health risk factors or asymptomatic disease conditions.

2.2 **Case finding:** Case-finding interventions locate individuals and families with identified risk factors and connect them to resources. This often leads to referral and follow-up.

2.3 **Outreach:** Outreach interventions locate populations of interest or populations at risk and provide information about the nature of the concern, what can be done about it, and how services can be obtained.

2.4 **Disease and other health event investigation:** Disease and other health event investigation interventions systematically gather and analyze data regarding threats to the health of populations, ascertain the source of the threats, identify cases and others at risk, and determine control measures.

2.5 **Surveillance:** Surveillance activities describe and monitor health events through ongoing and systematic collection, analysis and interpretation of health data for the purpose of planning, implementing and evaluating public health interventions.

3) **Health teaching, counseling, and consultation**

3.1 **Health teaching:** Health teaching interventions communicate facts, ideas and skills that change knowledge, attitudes, values, beliefs, behaviors, and practices and skills of individuals, families, systems and/or communities.

3.2 **Counseling:** Counseling interventions establish an interpersonal relationship with a community, system, family, or individual intended to increase or enhance their capacity for self-care and coping.

3.3 **Consultation:** Consultation seeks information and generates optional solutions to perceived problems or issues through interactive problem solving with a community, system, family or individual. The community, system, family or individual selects and acts on the option best meeting the circumstances.

4) **Advocacy, social marketing, and policy development and enforcement**

4.1 **Advocacy:** Advocacy interventions plead someone's cause or act on someone's behalf with a focus on developing the capacity of the community, system, individual, or family to plead their own cause or act on their own behalf. Advocacy is frequently used with other interventions, such as referral and follow-up, community organizing, and policy development and enforcement. Advocacy is often discussed in relation to case management.

4.2 **Social marketing:** Social marketing, a relatively new intervention first introduced in 1971, uses commercial marketing principles and technologies to design programs to influence the knowledge, attitudes, values, beliefs, behaviors, and practices of the population of interest.

4.3 **Policy development and enforcement:** Policy development and enforcement interventions help place health issues on decision makers' agendas, acquire a plan of resolution, and determine needed resources. Policy development results in laws, rules and regulations, ordinances, and policies. Policy enforcement compels others to comply with the laws, rules, regulations, ordinances, and policies created in conjunction with policy development.

5) **Collective actions (community organizing, coalition building, and collaboration)**
Collective action is the generic term for interventions characterized by groups of people or organizations coming together to address issues that matter to them jointly.

5.1 **Community organizing:** Community organizing helps community groups to identify common problems or goals, mobilize resources, and develop and implement strategies for reaching the goals they collectively have set.

5.2 **Coalition building:** Coalition building promotes and develops alliances among organizations or constituencies for a common purpose. It builds linkages, solves problems, and/or enhances local leadership to address health concerns.

5.3 **Collaboration:** Collaboration commits two or more persons or organizations to achieving a common goal through enhancing the capacity of one or more of them to promote and protect health.

Appendix 3.E: Study Evidence Tables

Table 3.E.1 Characteristics of studies on universal prevention approaches to FASD.

Study	Study design, objective and setting	Demographics and participant characteristics	Intervention	Outcomes/Results	Author conclusions
LaChausse [50] **Country:** USA **Source:** Journal article **Funding:** Society	CCT To evaluate the effectiveness of a multimedia program to prevent FAS **Study dates:** NR **Setting:** Suburban	**Study population:** Broad public **Selection criteria:** Youth from a suburban high school **No. of participants:** Enrolled = 114 Analyzed = 87 **Demographics:** – Females (%): 49 – Mean age: NR; SD = NR – Ethnicity: White = 14%; African American = 8%; Hispanic = 68%; Asian = 5%; Other = 5%	**Intervention:** FASTRAC Educational multimedia program No. enrolled = NR No. analyzed = 44 **Comparators:** No intervention No. enrolled = NR No. analyzed = 43	**Follow-up period:** ≤3 months **Outcomes and results:** 1. Fetal alcohol syndrome knowledge (mean score). TOA = 2 weeks |	Baseline	Endpoint
FASTRAC	6.7	7.6*
No intervention	7.1	7.4	 (p < 0.01) 2. Attitudes toward alcohol use during pregnancy (mean score). TOA = 2 weeks 		Baseline	Endpoint
FASTRAC	4.6	4.7
No intervention	4.5	4.4		The FASTRAC program significantly increased student knowledge regarding FAS, but had little impact on the participants' attitudes towards using alcohol during pregnancy, or their intention not to drink during pregnancy. The FASTRAC program did not make participants less likely to use alcohol during pregnancy. The program did not increase the perceived severity of using alcohol during pregnancy among program participants. **Statistically significant results:** Yes Partial support to the effectiveness of the intervention

Calabro *et al.* [30]

Country: USA

Source: Journal article

Funding: NR

CCT

To evaluate whether health education materials written at a lower rather than a higher reading level are more effective in producing changes in knowledge, attitude and behavioral intention to use alcohol

Study dates: Jul 1993 to Dec 1993

Setting: Mix

Study population: Pregnant women

Selection criteria: Women ≥15 years old who visited public health clinics for their first prenatal visit; English or Spanish language

No. of participants:
Enrolled = NR
Analyzed = 252

Demographics:
- Females (%): 100
- Mean age: NR; SD = NR
- Ethnicity:
  Hispanic = 65.5%; Asian American = 2.5%; African American = 19.4%; European American = 12.6%

Intervention: Health education materials (3rd grade reading level)

No. enrolled = NR

No. analyzed = NR

Comparators: Health education materials (10th grade reading level)

No. enrolled = NR

No. analyzed = NR

3. Perceived severity of alcohol use during pregnancy (mean score). TOA = 2 weeks

	Baseline	Endpoint
FASTRAC	3.5	3.8
No intervention	3.5	3.5

4. Intention to use alcohol during pregnancy (mean score). TOA = 2 weeks

	Baseline	Endpoint
FASTRAC	1.6	1.2
No intervention	1.6	1.4

Follow-up period: ≤3 months

Outcomes and results:

1. Change in knowledge, attitudes and intentions toward alcohol consumption while pregnant. TOA = Immediate

   1) Changes in statements from baseline reported as statistically significant ($p < 0.05$):

	3rd grade reading level	10th grade reading level
English-speaking women	6/9	4/9
Spanish-speaking women	2/9	1/9

Among English-speaking women, the material written at the lower reading level was shown to be more effective, whereas among Spanish-speaking participants, test scores were unchanged. Clinicians in public health clinics who have pregnant patients with low literacy levels should be cautioned not to rely on written materials to reinforce health messages about alcohol use during pregnancy, but rather keep them as supplemental.

Statistically significant results: No

Support to the effectiveness of the intervention

(Continued)

Table 3.E.1 *(Continued)*

Study	Study design, objective and setting	Demographics and participant characteristics	Intervention	Outcomes/Results	Author conclusions
				2. Change in behavioral intention to avoid alcohol consumption while pregnant (score; 1 = unlikely to 5 = very likely). TOA = Immediate	

– Among English-speaking women:

	Baseline	Endpoint
Health education – 3rd grade	4.7	4.9
Health education – 10th grade	4.6	4.7

– Among Spanish-speaking women:

	Baseline	Endpoint
Health education – 3rd grade	4.4	4.7
Health education – 10th grade	4.3	4.5

Waterson [73]	**Study population:**	**Intervention:**	**Follow-up period:** >6 mo and ≤9 mo
Country: UK	Pregnant women	*Trial #1:*	**Outcomes and results:**
Source: Journal article	**Selection criteria:** Pregnant women attending prenatal clinics	Prenatal educational information (written only)	1. Change in drinking behavior during pregnancy:
CCT	**No. of participants:**	No. enrolled = 477	– Among women who drank >7 units of alcohol/week before pregnancy (%). TOA = 28 weeks of pregnancy
To evaluate the effectiveness of two different methods of giving information in the antenatal clinic to prevent fetal alcohol exposure	Enrolled = 2100 Analyzed = 2100	No. analyzed = NR	
Funding: Government, society	**Demographics:** – Females (%): 100 – Mean age: NR; SD = NR – Ethnicity: NR	**Comparators:** Prenatal educational information (written + verbal reinforcement)	– Success
Study dates: May 1982 to Oct 1983		No. enrolled = 559	Written information (Trial 1)	63%
Setting: Urban		No. analyzed = NR	Written and verbal reinforcement (Trial 1)	68%
		Trial #2:	Written information (Trial 2)	69%
		Prenatal educational information (written only)	Written, verbal reinforcement and video (Trial 2)	66%
			– Partial success
		No. enrolled = 564	Written information (Trial 1)	22%
		No. analyzed = NR	Written and verbal reinforcement (Trial 1)	12%
		Comparators: Prenatal educational information (written + verbal reinforcement + video)	Written information (Trial 2)	14%
			Written, verbal reinforcement and video (Trial 2)	19%
			– No changes
		No. enrolled = 500	Written information (Trial 1)	9%
		No. analyzed = NR	Written and verbal reinforcement (Trial 1)	13%
			Written information (Trial 2)	12%
			Written, verbal reinforcement and video (Trial 2)	7%

Written information, personal advice and a video for alcohol prevention during pregnancy can be incorporated into the existing clinic routine.

Statistically significant results: No

No conclusions regarding the effectiveness of the intervention

(Continued)

Table 3.E.1 (Continued)

Study	Study design, objective and setting	Demographics and participant characteristics	Intervention	Outcomes/Results	Author conclusions
				2. Knowledge about "safe" daily alcohol intake when planning a pregnancy (%). TOA = 28 weeks of pregnancy	
				– Suggested "safe" daily intake ≤1 unit:	
				Written information (Trial 1) — 47%	
				Written and verbal reinforcement (Trial 1) — 50%	
				Written information (Trial 2) — 59%	
				Written, verbal reinforcement and video (Trial 2) — 64%	
				3. Knowledge about "safe" daily drinking when planning a pregnancy (%). TOA = 28 weeks of pregnancy	
				– Suggested "safe" daily intake ≤1 unit:	
				Written information (Trial 1) — 44%	
				Written and verbal reinforcement (Trial 1) — 45%	
				Written information (Trial 2) — 55%	
				Written, verbal reinforcement and video (Trial 2) — 60%	
				4. Knowledge about "safe" daily drinking when not pregnant or planning a pregnancy (≤4 units) (%). TOA = 28 weeks of pregnancy	
				Written information (Trial 1) — 67	
				Written and verbal reinforcement (Trial 1) — 74%	
				Written information (Trial 2) — 84%	
				Written, verbal reinforcement and video (Trial 2) — 83%	

Mengel *et al.* [62]

Country:
USA

Source:
Journal article

Funding:
Government, society

Prospective analytical cohort study

To evaluate the effectiveness of a targeted media campaign to increase knowledge of FASD

Study dates:
Oct 2002 to Mar 2004

Setting: Urban

Study population:
Women of childbearing age

Selection criteria:
African American women aged 18–35 years who were not pregnant

No. of participants:
Enrolled = 799 (pre)
Analyzed = 806 (post)

Demographics:
- Females (%): 100
- Mean age: NR; SD = NR
- Ethnicity: African American = 100%

Intervention:
Public education media campaign

No. enrolled = 418 (pre)

No. analyzed = 404 (post)

Comparators:
No public education media campaign community

No. enrolled = 381 (pre)

No. analyzed = 402 (post)

Follow-up period: >1 year

Outcomes and results:

1. Messages remembered (%). TOA = 18 months

	Media campaign	No media campaign
No safe level	29.7%	22.3%
No safe time	14.4%	10.3%

2. Knowledge about alcohol intake during pregnancy (% strongly agree) TOA = 18 months

   - Drinking a lot of alcohol during pregnancy is very harmful to babies:

	Before	After
Media campaign	94%	92.1%
No media campaign	87.9%	91.5%

   - It is safe for women to drink alcohol occasionally during pregnancy:

	Before	After
Media campaign	8.9%	7.9%
No media campaign	5.5%	5.2%

There was a small but statistically significant decline in knowledge scores comparing post-intervention results with pre-intervention. Knowledge scores increased in direct proportion to the number of times that respondents heard the message. The FAS intervention messages had to be heard 10 or more times in order to improve FAS-prevention knowledge. The targeted media campaign was ineffective in improving knowledge of FAS.

Statistically significant results: NR

Does not support the effectiveness of the intervention

(Continued)

Table 3.E.1 (Continued)

Study	Study design, objective and setting	Demographics and participant characteristics	Intervention	Outcomes/Results	Author conclusions
				– Pregnant women should not drink alcohol:	

	Before	After
Media campaign	95%	92.1%
No media campaign	89.2%	92.3%

– How much alcohol a woman drinks during pregnancy has little to do with how healthy her baby will be:

	Before	After
Media campaign	14.1%	18.3%
No media campaign	10.8%	11.2%

– A pregnant woman's drinking causes most of the damage to the baby during the first 3 months of pregnancy:

	Before	After
Media campaign	73%	68.1%
No media campaign	62.7%	72.6%

Mazis et al. [59]

Country: USA

Source: Journal article

Funding: NR

Retrospective analytical cohort study

To evaluate the impact of alcohol beverage warning labels

Study dates: May 1989 to May 1990

Setting: NR

Study population: Broad public

Selection criteria: >18 years of age

No. of participants:
Enrolled = 2324
Analyzed = 2028

Demographics:
- Females (%): 59
- Mean age: NR; SD = NR
- Ethnicity: NR

Intervention: Alcohol beverage warning label period (1990)

No. enrolled = 1220
No. analyzed = 1008

Comparators: No alcohol beverage warning label period (1989)

No. enrolled = 1104
No. analyzed = 1020

Follow-up period: >9 months and ≤1 year

Outcomes and results:

1. Perception of risk associated with consuming alcohol (%). TOA = 12 months

	No alcohol beverage warning period	Alcohol beverage warning period
	49.8%	54.1%

There was a slight increase from 1989 to 1990 in the public's perception of the risk associated with consuming alcohol beverages.

Statistically significant results: No

No conclusions regarding the effectiveness of the intervention

---

Casiro et al. [32]

Country: Canada

Source: Journal article

Funding: Society

Retrospective analytical cohort study (with historical control period)

To evaluate the effects of a television public awareness campaign on the public's knowledge of the risks of drinking alcohol during pregnancy

Study dates: Jun 1991 to Sep 1991

Setting: Mix

Study population: Women of childbearing age

Selection criteria: Women of childbearing age (15–45 years) attending physician practices, community health clinics, and nursing stations

No. of participants:
Enrolled = 3900
Analyzed = 2969

Demographics:
- Females (%): NR
- Mean age: NR; SD = NR
- Ethnicity: NR

Intervention: Television public awareness campaign

No. enrolled = 1900
No. analyzed = 1392

Comparators: No public awareness campaign period

No. enrolled = 2000
No. analyzed = 1577

Follow-up period: >3 months and ≤6 months

Outcomes and results:

1. Knowledge that drinking alcohol during pregnancy can cause abnormalities in the infant (%). TOA = 10 weeks

Knowledge of abnormalities due to alcohol effects	Campaign period	No campaign period
Mental	93%*	86.5%
Physical	91.8%*	86.9%
Behavioral	89.3%*	80.9%

*(p < 0.001)

A television campaign highlighting the potential risks of alcohol consumption during pregnancy may be an effective method of increasing public knowledge of alcohol-related birth defects.

Statistically significant results: Yes

Support to the effectiveness of the intervention

(*Continued*)

Table 3.E.1 (Continued)

Study	Study design, objective and setting	Demographics and participant characteristics	Intervention	Outcomes/Results	Author conclusions
				2. Knowledge that if a pregnant woman has an alcoholic drink, the alcohol will reach the baby (%). TOA = 10 weeks | Campaign period	No campaign period
97.4%	95.3%	 (p < 0.02)	
Bowerman [29] **Country:** USA **Source:** Journal article **Funding:** NR	Retrospective analytical cohort study To evaluate the effect of a community-initiated fetal alcohol syndrome intervention in arctic Alaska **Study dates:** Nov 1994 to Mar 1995 **Setting:** Rural	**Study population:** Pregnant women **Selection criteria:** Women with viable pregnancies **No. of participants:** Enrolled = NR, Analyzed = 348 **Demographics:** – Females (%): 100 – Mean age: NR; SD = NR – Ethnicity: Aboriginal = 100%	**Intervention:** Community-supported alcohol ban No. enrolled = NR No. analyzed = 73 **Comparators:** No alcohol ban community No. enrolled = NR No. analyzed = 275	**Follow-up period:** >3 months and ≤6 months **Outcomes and results:** 1. Change in regional self-reported alcohol abuse (%). TOA = 5 months | Before ban	After ban
42%	9%	 RR = 0.21; 95% CI = 0.08 to 0.55 2. First-trimester alcohol abuse (%). TOA = 5 months 	Before ban	After ban
43%	11%	 RR = 0.25; 95% CI = 0.07 to 0.94	There was a substantial reduction in regional prenatal alcohol consumption and fetal alcohol exposure during the initial period of the ban. Second- and third-trimester abuse fell, but not at significant levels. The alcohol ban appears to be a successful intervention in areas where FAS is high. **Statistically significant results:** Yes Support to the effectiveness of the intervention

Olsen *et al.* [65]

Country:
Denmark

Source:
Journal article

Funding:
Government,
society

Retrospective
analytical cohort
study

To evaluate the effect
of a comprehensive
health campaign to
influence pregnancy
outcomes by
reducing the intake
of alcohol and
tobacco during
pregnancy

Study dates:
Apr 1984 to Apr 1987

Setting: Urban

Study population:
Pregnant women

Selection criteria:
Pregnant women attending
midwife centers

No. of participants:
Enrolled = NR
Analyzed = 11 980

Demographics:
– Females (%): 100
– Mean age: NR; SD = NR
– Ethnicity: NR

Intervention:
Health education
campaign ("Healthy
Habits for Two," city
of Odense)

No. enrolled = 6268

No. analyzed = NR

Comparators:
No intervention (city
of Aalborg)

No. enrolled = 5712

No. analyzed = NR

Follow-up period: >1 year

Outcomes and results:

1. Teetotalers (%). TOA = 2 years

Cities	Before	After
Odense	16%	18%
Aalborg	19%	20%

2. Average number of drinks per week (mean).
TOA = 2 years

Cities	Before	After
Odense	1.8	1.8
Aalborg	1.5	1.5

3. Binge drinking (%). TOA = 2 years

Cities	Before	After
Odense	18%	19%
Aalborg	19%	18%

Alcohol consumption during
pregnancy remained unchanged.
There is need for more research
on what is important for the
success of a mass campaign
concerning changes in behavior.

Statistically significant results: NR

Does not support the effectiveness
of the intervention

(Continued)

Table 3.E.1 (*Continued*)

Study	Study design, objective and setting	Demographics and participant characteristics	Intervention	Outcomes/Results	Author conclusions
Hankin *et al.* [46] **Country:** USA **Source:** Journal article **Funding:** Government	Interrupted time series To evaluate the impact of an alcohol beverage warning label on drinking during pregnancy **Study dates:** Sept 1986 to May 1995 **Setting:** Inner city	**Study population:** Pregnant women **Selection criteria:** Pregnant African-American women attending perinatal clinics **No. of participants:** Enrolled = 17632 Analyzed = 17456 **Demographics:** – Females (%): 100 – Mean age: 23.7 years; SD = 6.1 – Ethnicity: African American = 100%	**Intervention:** Alcohol beverage warning label No. enrolled = 17632 No. analyzed = 17456 **Comparators:** NA	**Follow-up period:** >1 year **Outcomes and results:** 1. Periconceptional drinking (%). TOA = 9 months No numeric data. Report of statistically significant reduction among nulliparous (p < 0.04) but not for multiparous women	Multiparous women did not seem to be influenced by the warning label. The warning label had a significant, albeit small, impact on nulliparous women. **Statistically significant results:** No No conclusions regarding the effectiveness of the intervention
Awopetu *et al.* [27] **Country:** USA **Source:** Journal article **Funding:** Government	Before-and-after study To report the outcome of a pilot study on a FASD media intervention **Study dates:** July 2006 to Dec 2006 **Setting:** Urban	**Study population:** Broad public **Selection criteria:** NR **No. of participants:** Enrolled = NR Analyzed = 49 **Demographics:** – Females (%): 77.5 – Mean age: NR; SD = NR – Ethnicity: Black – 74.5%; White = 63.4%; Other = 6.1%	**Intervention:** Media public education campaign ("Be in the kNOw") No. enrolled = NR No. analyzed = 49 **Comparators:** NA	**Follow-up period:** >3 months and ≤6 months **Outcomes and results:** 1. Number of FAS-related telephone calls received through a hotline. TOA = 6 months **Baseline (prior to Jun 2006):** 5–6 **Endpoint (July to Dec 2006):** 49	The media intervention reached a wide geographic audience, provoking interest beyond the initial target area and expected age ranges. **Statistically significant results:** NR No conclusions regarding the effectiveness of the intervention

Carr and Brand [31]

Country
Canada

Source
Conference abstract

Funding
NR

Before-and-after study

To evaluate the impact of a multimedia FASD-prevention campaign on the public's knowledge of FASD

Study dates:
2005 to 2006

Setting: Mix

Study population:
Broad public

Selection criteria: NR

No. of participants:
Enrolled = NR
Analyzed = NR

Demographics
– Females (%): NR
– Mean age: NR; SD = NR
– Ethnicity: NR

Intervention:
Media public education campaign

No. enrolled
Pre-survey = 401;
Post-survey = 400

No. analyzed = NR

Follow-up period: >1 year

Outcomes and results

1. Proportion that perceived message effectiveness
   – TOA = 1 year
   – Results = 87%

2. Knowledge acquisition
   – TOA = 1 year
   – Results = 26%

A multimedia campaign can have an impact on the public's knowledge about FASD

Statistically significant results: NR

No conclusions regarding effectiveness of the intervention

Ma [54]

Country:
USA

Source:
Journal article

Funding:
Government

Before-and-after study

To evaluate a prevention strategy that targets Native American youth at highest risk of engaging in behaviors that lead to FAS births

Study dates: NR

Setting: NR

Study population:
Broad public

Selection criteria:
Native American youth (6th to 8th graders) at high risk of engaging in behaviors that lead to FAS births

No. of participants:
Enrolled = 90
Analyzed = 85

Demographics:
– Females (%): NR
– Mean age: NR; SD = NR
– Ethnicity: NR

Intervention:
Educational FAS prevention program

No. enrolled = 90
No. analyzed = 85

Comparators: NA

Follow-up period: ≤3 months

Outcomes and results:

1. Knowledge about FAS prevention (%).
   TOA = 2 weeks

	Before	After
Knowledge that alcohol affects body, emotions and behaviors	88.2%	95.2%
Knowledge that drinking alcohol in pregnancy hurts the baby	78.2%	97.2%
Knowledge that alcohol in breast milk affects the baby after birth	53%	81.2%
Knowledge that FAS causes mental retardation and other disorders	66.1%	89.3%
Native American 7th-generation concepts are clear	48.2%	96.4%

It is feasible to establish and implement FAS-prevention programs in schools that serve Native American youth, particularly those at highest risk of engaging in behaviors that result in FAS pregnancies.

Statistically significant results: NR

No conclusions regarding the effectiveness of the intervention

(Continued)

Table 3.E.1 (Continued)

Study	Study design, objective and setting	Demographics and participant characteristics	Intervention	Outcomes/Results	Author conclusions
Marin [55] **Country:** USA **Source:** Journal article **Funding:** Government	Before-and-after study To evaluate the impact of health-promotion messages on the levels of awareness among a Hispanic population **Study dates:** 1989 to 1992 **Setting:** Urban	**Study population:** Broad public **Selection criteria:** NR **No. of participants:** Enrolled = NR Analyzed = 4661 **Demographics:** – Females (%): 57.7 – Mean age: 37 years; SD = NR – Ethnicity: Hispanic = 100%	**Intervention:** Health-promotion messages No. enrolled = NR No. analyzed = 4661 **Comparators:** NA	**Follow-up period:** >1 year **Outcomes and results:** 1. Awareness of warning messages regarding alcohol and pregnancy (%). (Follow-up period = 3 years) 1989 93.8% · 1990 90.6% · 1991 95.8% · 1992 96.4% 2. Attitudes about FAS prevention (%). TOA = 2 weeks Both male and female are responsible for FAS prevention — Before 83.9%, After 89.3% FAS can be prevented — Before 66.1%, After 96.4% The person would not drink even if asked to do so by best friends — Before 76.8%, After 89.3% Making healthy choices is part of FAS prevention — Before 67%, After 75%	Continuous exposure to the warning messages seemed to increase the level of awareness of the message in the community. **Statistically significant results:** NR No conclusions regarding the effectiveness of the intervention

May and
Hymbaugh [58]

Country:
USA

Source:
Journal article

Funding:
Government

Before-and-after
study

To evaluate the
impact of a
comprehensive,
macro-level FASD
prevention program
on Native Americans
and Alaska Natives

Study dates:
Sept 1983 to Nov
1985

Setting: Rural

Study population:
Broad public

Selection criteria: NR

No. of participants:
Enrolled = NR
Analyzed = 215

Demographics:
– Females (%): NR
– Mean age: NR; SD = NR
– Ethnicity:
  Aboriginal = 100%

Intervention:
National Indian Fetal
Alcohol Syndrome
Prevention Program

No. enrolled = NR

No. analyzed = 215

Comparators: NA

Follow-up period: >3 months and ≤6 months

1. Knowledge gain–school children (mean
   score; max = 8). TOA = 3 to 3.5 months

Before	After
5.1	6.6

   (p < 0.05)

2. Knowledge gain–community (mean score;
   max = 110). TOA = 2 months

Before	After
55.1	86.1

   (p < 0.05)

A substantial amount of
knowledge is retained after
FAS-prevention program. A
macro-level health education
program can work.

Statistically significant results Yes

Support to the effectiveness of the
intervention

(Continued)

Table 3.E.1 (Continued)

Study	Study design, objective and setting	Demographics and participant characteristics	Intervention	Outcomes/Results	Author conclusions
Glik et al. [41] **Country:** USA **Source:** Journal article **Funding:** Private	Before-and-after study To evaluate the effectiveness of a social marketing intervention in raising awareness of FAS among Hispanic and African American youth **Study dates:** Apr 1998 to Jan 1999 **Setting:** Urban	**Study population:** Women of childbearing age **Selection criteria:** Female African American and Hispanic youth aged 13–19 years **No. of participants:** Enrolled = 971 Analyzed = 774 **Demographics:** – Females (%): 100 – Mean age: 15.1 years; SD = 2 – Ethnicity: African-American = 53.5%; Hispanic = 46.5%	**Intervention:** Social marketing campaign (Narrowcasting) No. enrolled = 971 No. analyzed = 774 **Comparators:** NA	**Follow-up period:** >6 months and ≤9 months **Outcomes and results:** 1. Knowledge about alcohol and pregnancy (%). TOA = 8 months – Hispanic group:	Exposure to the campaign was not correlated with knowledge increase. The authors concluded that a narrowcasting campaign is an effective means of filling in specific gaps in knowledge among well-defined groups, using methods and messages tailored to the audience. **Statistically significant results:** No Does not support the effectiveness of the intervention

	Before	After
It is OK for pregnant woman to drink alcohol without harming her baby	16.9%	12.8%
Baby can be harmed if pregnant woman drinks alcohol during the first few weeks of pregnancy	71.6%	78.4%
Baby can be harmed if pregnant woman drinks alcohol during the last few weeks of pregnancy	80.9%	85.4%
Baby can be harmed if pregnant woman drinks alcohol anytime during pregnancy	80.3%	86.5%

(Continued)

– African-American group:

	Before	After
It is OK for pregnant woman to drink alcohol without harming her baby	18.9%	10.4%
Baby can be harmed if pregnant woman drinks alcohol during the first few weeks of pregnancy	59.2%	75%
Baby can be harmed if pregnant woman drinks alcohol during the last few weeks of pregnancy	73.1%	84.3%
Baby can be harmed if pregnant woman drinks alcohol anytime during pregnancy	69%	85.4%

Table 3.E.1 (Continued)

Study	Study design, objective and setting	Demographics and participant characteristics	Intervention	Outcomes/Results	Author conclusions
Walker et al. [72] **Country:** USA **Source:** Journal article **Funding:** NR	Before-and-after study To evaluate the effectiveness of a brief intervention to increase knowledge about FASD among women requesting emergency contraception and/or a pregnancy test **Study dates:** Apr to Oct 2000 **Setting:** NR	**Study population:** Women of childbearing age **Selection criteria:** Women requesting a pregnancy test and/or emergency contraception; able to read and speak English **No. of participants:** Enrolled = 50 Analyzed = 50 **Demographics:** – Females (%): 100 – Mean age: 23.8 years; SD = 6.9 – Ethnicity: NR	**Intervention:** Brief intervention for prenatal alcohol use No. enrolled = 50 No. analyzed = 50 **Comparators:** NA	**Follow-up period:** ≤3 months **Outcomes and results:** 1. Knowledge about alcohol use during pregnancy (mean score; max = 8). TOA = Immediate | Before	After
---	---
5.8	6.7	 (p = 0.0001)	The brief intervention was effective in communicating knowledge about FASD to women of childbearing age. **Statistically significant results:** Yes Support to the effectiveness of the intervention
Kaskutas et al. [48] **Country:** USA **Source:** Journal article **Funding:** Government	Before-and-after study To evaluate the effects of health messages on drinking during pregnancy **Study dates:** 1989 to 1994 **Setting:** NR	**Study population:** Pregnant women and women of childbearing age **Selection criteria:** Pregnant women and women of childbearing age (<40 years) **No. of participants:** Enrolled = 365 Analyzed = 362 **Demographics:** – Females (%): 100 – Mean age: NR; SD = NR – Ethnicity: White = 77%; Black = 12%; Other = 11%	**Intervention:** Alcohol beverage warning label No. enrolled = 365 No. analyzed = 365 **Comparators:** NA	**Follow-up period:** >9 months and ≤1 year **Outcomes and results:** 1. Proportion of women that consumed a maximum number of drinks during pregnancy (%). TOA = 12 months | No. of drinks	Before	After
---	---	---
0	36.8%	74.8%
1–2	33.8%	21%
3–4	14.7%	3%
>5	14.7%	1.2%		Most drinking women reduced their drinking during pregnancy, and over half abstained completely. Pregnant women and women likely to become pregnant increasingly had been exposed to the container label that warns that pregnant women should not drink during pregnancy. However, there was a decrease in the proportion of pregnant women exposed to advertisements and to conversations about the risk of drinking during pregnancy. **Statistically significant results:** NR No conclusions regarding the effectiveness of the intervention

Kinzie *et al.* [49]	Before-and-after study	**Study population:** Pregnant women	**Intervention:** Prenatal alcohol educational multimedia program ("The Healthy Touch")	**Follow-up period:** ≤3 months	It is possible that the program had an impact on intentions to consume alcohol while pregnant.

Country: USA — To evaluate the impact of a computer-based multimedia prenatal alcohol education program

Selection criteria: Women presenting for prenatal care at a public clinic

No. enrolled = 59

Outcomes and results:

Statistically significant results: NR

Source: Journal article

Funding: NR

No. of participants:
Enrolled = 59
Analyzed = 59

No. analyzed = 59

Comparators: NA

1. Preference for alcoholic beverages in social situations (%). TOA = Immediate

No conclusions regarding the effectiveness of the intervention

Study dates: NR

Setting: Rural

Demographics:
– Females (%): 100
– Mean age: 23.5 years;
– SD = NR
– Ethnicity: NR

Before	After
39%	0%

CCT = controlled clinical trial; FAS = fetal alcohol syndrome; FASD = fetal alcohol spectrum disorder; FASTRAC = The Fetal Alcohol Spectrum Teaching and Research Awareness Campaign; max = maximum; IGR = intrauterine growth retardation; mo = month(s); NA = not applicable; NR = not reported; SD = standard deviation; TOA = time to outcome assessment; UK = United Kingdom; USA = United States of America.

Table 3.E.2 Characteristics of studies on selective prevention approaches to FASD.

Study	Study design, objective and setting	Demographics and Participant characteristics	Intervention	Outcomes/Results	Author conclusions

Floyd *et al.* [40]
 	
Country: USA
 	
Source: Journal article
 	
Funding: Government
	RCT
	
	To evaluate the impact of a brief motivational intervention to reduce the risk of an AEP
	
	Study dates: July 2002 to Jan 2004
	
	Setting: Mix
		Study population: Women of childbearing age who consume alcohol
		
		Selection criteria: Women of childbearing age (18–44 years); no condition causing infertility; not pregnant or planning to become pregnant in the next 9 months; had vaginal intercourse during the previous 3 months with a fertile man without using effective contraception; engaged in risky drinking
		
		No. of participants:
		Enrolled = 830
		Analyzed = 593
		
		Demographics:
		– Females (%): 100
		– Mean age: 29.6 years; SD = 7.5
		– Ethnicity: Black/not Hispanic = 47.2%
			Intervention: Project CHOICES
			
			No. enrolled = 416
			
			No. analyzed = 291
			
			Comparators: Information only
			
			No. enrolled = 414
			
			No. analyzed = 302
				Follow-up period: >6 months and ≤9 months
				
				Outcomes and results:
				1. Reduced AEP. TOA = 3, 6 and 9 months
				
				– Unadjusted ORs
				
				    OR 95% CI
				3 months 2.0 1.5 to 2.8
				6 months 1.9 1.4 to 2.6
				9 months 1.9 1.3 to 2.6
				
				– Adjusted ORs
				
				    OR 95% CI
				3 months 2.3 1.6 to 3.2
				6 months 2.1 1.5 to 3.0
				9 months 2.1 1.4 to 3.0
					A brief motivational intervention considerably decreased the risk of AEP, risky drinking and the use of ineffective contraception in high-risk women. The results were maintained at 9 months of follow-up. Project CHOICES intervention appears to be a good candidate for large-scale implementation in public health settings to reduce the risk of AEP in high-risk populations.
					
					Statistically significant results: Yes
					
					Support to the effectiveness of the intervention

(Continued)

2. Reduced risk drinking. TOA = 3, 6 and 9 months
   – Unadjusted ORs

	OR	95% CI
3 months	1.6	1.2 to 2.3
6 months	1.5	1.1 to 2.1
9 months	1.4	1.0 to 2.1

   – Adjusted ORs

	OR	95% CI
3 months	1.7	1.2 to 2.5
6 months	1.6	1.1 to 2.3
9 months	1.5	1.0 to 2.1

3. Number of binge-drinking episodes (mean). TOA = 9 months

	Baseline	Endpoint
CHOICES	30.1	7.1
Information only	29.1	9.8

Table 3.E.2 (*Continued*)

Study	Study design, objective and setting	Demographics and Participant characteristics	Intervention	Outcomes/Results	Author conclusions
				4. Median number of drinks/week. TOA = 9 months	

4. Median number of drinks/week. TOA = 9 months

	Baseline	Endpoint
CHOICES	36	2.3
Information only	38	3.1

5. Proportion of participants meeting risk reduction thresholds (%). TOA = 3, 6 and 9 mo:

– Alcohol use fewer than 8 drinks/week:

	CHOICES	Information only
3 months	46.4%	36.3%
6 months	46%	37.3%
9 months	54.9%	44%

– No binge drinking:

	CHOICES	Information only
3 months	52.1%	38.1%
6 months	52%	41.4%
9 months	57.9%	46.8%

Armstrong et al. [26]

Country: USA

Source: Journal article

Funding: Government

RCT

To evaluate the effects of two brief interventions in prenatal care clinics

Study dates: May 2000 to Jun 2004

Setting: Health facility

Study population: Women at risk of an AEP

Selection criteria: Women that were positive on a screening questionnaire for risk of alcohol use during pregnancy

No. of participants:
Enrolled = 1164
Analyzed = 908

Demographics:
- Females (%): 100
- Mean age: 15 to 44 years
- Ethnicity: White = 48%; Black = 9%; Hispanic = 21%; Asian = 6%; Other = 16%

Intervention: Brief intervention for prenatal alcohol use (Early Start Plus)

No. enrolled = 462
No. analyzed = 266

Comparators: Brief intervention for prenatal alcohol use (Early Start)

No. enrolled = 330
No. analyzed = 298
Standard prenatal care
No. enrolled = 372
No. analyzed = 344

- Reduced risk for drinking:

	CHOICES	Information only
3 months	42.2%	30.3%
6 months	42.4%	32.5%
9 months	48.8%	40.4%

- Reduced risk for AEP:

	CHOICES	Information only
3 months	63.6%	45.6%
6 months	63.9%	46.9%
9 months	69.1%	54.3%

Follow-up period
>9 months and ≤1 year

Outcomes and results

1. Assisted ventilation (%)
   - TOA = Postpartum period

ESP	ES	Control
2%	0.7%	2.2%

ESP vs. control OR = 0.80 (95% CI = 0.19, 3.35; p = 0.75);
ES vs. control OR = 0.05 (95% CI = 0.00, 2.34; p = 0.12);
ESP vs. ES OR = 5.58 (95% CI = 0.49, 64.72; p = 0.16)

Early Start Plus appears to be helpful in reducing the incidence of preterm events.

Statistically significant results: Yes

Partial support to the effectiveness of the intervention

(Continued)

Table 3.E.2 *(Continued)*

Study	Study design, objective and setting	Demographics and Participant characteristics	Intervention	Outcomes/Results	Author conclusions

2. Low birth weight (<2500 g)–
   TOA = Postpartum period

ESP	ES	Control
3.2%	3.7%	6.6%

ESP vs. control OR = 0.49 (95% CI = 0.20, 1.25; p = 0.12);ES vs. control OR = 0.28 (95% CI = 0.10, 0.80; p = 0.02);ESP vs. ES OR = 0.91 (95% CI = 0.29, 2.83; p = 0.86)3. Preterm delivery (<35 weeks gestational age)

– TOA = Postpartum period

ESP	ES	Control
0.4%	1.1%	2.2%

ESP vs. control OR = 0.08 (95% CI = 0.00, 1.99; p = 0.11); ES vs. control OR = 0.30 (95% CI = 0.05, 1.82; p = 0.17); ESP vs. ES OR = 0.37 (95% CI = 0.03, 5.25; p = 0.43)

4. NICU admission

– TOA = Postpartum period

ESP	ES	Control
10.8%	10.2%	10.4%

ESP vs. control OR = 0.78 (95% CI = 0.20, 2.97; p – 0.70); ES vs. control OR = 0.65 (95% CI – 0.16, 2.64; p = 0.52); ESP vs. ES OR = 1.24 (95% CI = 0.38, 4.01; p = 0.70)

(Continued)

5. Rehospitalization within 2 weeks of discharge
   - TOA = Postpartum period

ESP	ES	Control
1.6%	2.9%	4.1%

ESP vs. control OR = 0.27 (95% CI = 0.04, 1.77; p = 0.16);
ES vs. control OR = 0.62 (95% CI = 0.17, 2.29; p = 0.44);
ESP vs. ES OR = 1.95 (95% CI = 0.43, 8.94; p = 0.36)

6. Preterm labor
   - TOA = Postpartum period

ESP	ES	Control
6.4%	7.3%	9.1%

ESP vs. control OR = 0.44 (95% CI = 0.20, 0.97; p = 0.04);
ES vs. control OR = 0.55 (95% CI = 0.27, 1.14; p = 0.10);
ESP vs. ES OR = 0.91 (95% CI = 0.36, 2.31; p = 0.84)

Table 3.E.2 (*Continued*)

Study	Study design, objective and setting	Demographics and Participant characteristics	Intervention	Outcomes/Results	Author conclusions
				7. Pre-eclampsia – TOA = Postpartum period |	ESP	ES	Control
---	---	---	---
	5.2%	4.8%	4.1%	 ESP vs. control OR = 0.70 (95% CI = 0.27, 1.79; p = 0.42); ES vs. control OR = 0.54 (95% CI = 0.21, 1.40; p = 0.19); ESP vs. ES OR = 1.47 (95% CI = 0.58, 3.74; p = 0.39)	
Chang *et al.* [34] **Country:** USA **Source:** Journal article **Funding:** Government	RCT To evaluate the effectiveness of a brief intervention in the reduction of prenatal alcohol consumption **Study dates:** NR **Setting:** Urban	**Study population:** Women at risk of an AEP **Selection criteria:** Women with positive T-ACE results (total score >2); being at risk for prenatal alcohol use (any alcohol consumption in the 3 months before study enrollment, or consumption of at least one drink per day in the 6 months before study enrollment, or drinking during a previous pregnancy); gestation <28 weeks and intention to carry pregnancy to term **No. of participants:** Enrolled = 304 Analyzed = 304 **Demographics:** – Females (%): 100 – Mean age = 31.3 years; SD = NR – Ethnicity: NR	**Intervention:** Brief intervention for prenatal alcohol use including the partner No. enrolled = 152 No. analyzed = 152 **Comparators:** Assessment only No. enrolled = 152 No. analyzed = 152	**Follow-up period:** >9 months and ≤1 year **Outcomes and results:** 1. Mean % of drinking days at endpoint (%). TOA = Postpartum period | Brief intervention	Assessment only
---	---
1.9%	2%	 2. Proportion that had less than half a drink per episode until the time of delivery (%). TOA = Postpartum period 	Brief intervention	Assessment only
---	---
0.39%	0.4%		Both the brief intervention group and the assessment group demonstrated overall reduced alcohol consumption, but the brief intervention is more effective in reducing subsequent consumption in women who drink more often. **Statistically significant results:** No Support to the effectiveness of the intervention

Chang *et al.* [33]

Country: USA

Source: Journal article

Funding: Government

RCT

To evaluate the impact of a brief intervention on antepartum alcohol consumption

Study date: 1994

Setting: Urban

Study population: Women at risk of an AEP

Selection criteria: Pregnant women initiating prenatal care; alcohol consumption during the previous 6 months; positive alcohol screen (T-ACE >2 points); no seeking alcohol treatment

No. of participants:
Enrolled = 250
Analyzed = 247

Demographics:
– Females (%): 100
– Mean age: 30.7 years; SD = 5.4
– Ethnicity: Caucasian = 78%; African-American = 14%; Hispanic = 6%; Asian = 2%

Intervention: Brief intervention for prenatal alcohol use

No. enrolled = 123
No. analyzed = NR

Comparators: Assessment only

No. enrolled = 127
No. analyzed = NR

Follow-up period: >9 months and ≤1 year

Outcomes and results:

1. Net decrease of drinks per drinking day (mean). TOA = 22 weeks

Brief intervention	Assessment only
0.3	0.4

2. Number of drinking episodes in the antepartum (mean). TOA = 22 weeks

Brief intervention	Assessment only
0.7	1

3. Infant birth weight (mean g). TOA = Postpartum period

Brief intervention	Assessment only
3360	3406

4. Apgar scores (mean). TOA = Postpartum period
   – 1-min Apgar score:

	Brief intervention	Assessment only
1-min	8.1	7.8
5-min	8.9	8.7

Both groups reduced antepartum alcohol consumption, but differences between groups were not statistically significant. A comprehensive assessment of alcohol use helped to reduce antepartum alcohol consumption.

Statistically significant results: No

Does not support the effectiveness of the intervention

(Continued)

Table 3.E.2 (*Continued*)

Study	Study design, objective and setting	Demographics and Participant characteristics	Intervention	Outcomes/Results	Author conclusions

Fleming [39]
 	
Country:
USA
 	
Source:
Journal article
 	
Funding:
Government
	RCT
	
	To evaluate the efficacy of a brief alcohol intervention in postpartum women
	
	Study dates:
	2002 to 2005
	
	Setting:
	Health facility
		Study population:
		Women at risk of an AEP
		
		Selection criteria:
		Postpartum women 18 years and older, positive for high-risk drinking (>3 drinking days/week or ≥5 drinks/day or ≥7 drinks/ week prior to pregnancy). alcohol use once the woman knew she was pregnant, ≥7 drinks/week, ≥3 drinking days/week or ≥4 drinks on ≥2 days in the last 28 days, ≥2 positive responses on T-ACE at postpartum
		
		No. of participants:
		Enrolled = 235
		Analyzed = 235
		
		Demographics:
		– Females (%): 100
		– Mean age: 28 yr;
		  SD = NR
		– Ethnicity:
		  Caucasian = 81.7%;
		  African-
		  American = 6.8%; Native
		  American = 7.2%;
		  Asian = 0.9%;
		  Hispanic = 2.5%;
		  Other = 0.9%
			Intervention:
			Brief alcohol intervention
			
			No. enrolled = 122
			No. analyzed = 122
			
			Comparators:
			Usual care (health booklet)
			
			No. enrolled = 113
			No. analyzed = 113
				Follow-up period:
				>6 months and ≤9 months
				
				Outcomes and results:
				1. Total drinks in the previous 28 days (mean, SD)
				  – TOA = 6 months
				
				| BI
					Control

---	---
19.8 (19.2)	27.1 (22.1)	 ($p = 0.01$) 2. Number of drinking days – TOA = 6 months 	BI	Control
---	---
6.9 (6.3)	9.2 (22.1)	 ($p = 0.02$) 3. Number of heavy drinking days – TOA = 6 months 	BI	Control
---	---
1.7 (2.2)	2.6 (3.1)	 ($p = 0.01$)	A brief intervention can reduce alcohol use in postpartum women. **Statistically significant results: Yes** Support the effectiveness of the intervention

Crosby [36]

Country:
USA

Source:
Dissertation

Funding: NR

RCT

To evaluate the effects of an alcohol education intervention among pregnant women

Study dates:
Oct 1982 to Feb 1983

Setting:
Inner city

Study population:
Pregnant women

Selection criteria:
Women receiving prenatal care; early stage of pregnancy

No. of participants:
Enrolled = 80
Analyzed = 41

Demographics:
- Females (%): 100
- Mean age = 27.7 years; SD = NR
- Ethnicity: NR

Intervention:
Cognitive-based health education

No. enrolled = 29
No. analyzed = 20

Comparators:
Information only

No. enrolled = 31
No. analyzed = 21

Usual prenatal care

No. enrolled = 20
No. analyzed = 11

Follow-up period: >3 months and ≤6 months

Outcomes and results:

1. Attitudes toward alcohol use during pregnancy (mean subscore DDP questionnaire; 15 = low concern; 75 = high concern). TOA = 5 months

	Baseline	Endpoint
Cognitive-based education	66.7	69.6
Information only	69.5	69.8
Usual prenatal care	66.5	69.7

2. Knowledge about alcohol use during pregnancy (mean subscore DDP questionnaire; 17= low score; 29 = high score). TOA = 5 months

	Baseline	Endpoint
Cognitive-based education	22.5	23.6
Information only	22.7	23.9
Usual prenatal care	21.9	22.5

There were no differences among the groups in pre-to post-test changes in attitude toward and knowledge about alcohol use during pregnancy. Drinking and monthly alcohol intake before, early and late in the pregnancy were greatly reduced in all three groups from before to early in the pregnancy. The experimental groups reported higher pre-pregnant alcohol intake and showed a greater reduction in the amount of alcohol ingested from before to early pregnancy than the control group. The change in alcohol intake did not vary among groups from early to late pregnancy pre- to post-intervention. An elaborate instructional strategy is not needed for prenatal alcohol education. Prevention of fetal alcohol effects is an area in which self-instructional materials with a comprehensive self-test may be as effective as more expensive interventions.

Statistically significant results: No

Does not support the effectiveness of the intervention

(Continued)

Table 3.E.2 (*Continued*)

Study	Study design, objective and setting	Demographics and Participant characteristics	Intervention	Outcomes/Results	Author conclusions
				3. Alcohol use (%) before (1), early (2) and late (3) in pregnancy. TOA = 5 months	

3. Alcohol use (%) before (1), early (2) and late (3) in pregnancy. TOA = 5 months

	1	2	3
Cognitive-based education	79.3%	44.8%	61%
Information only	83.9%	38.7	44%
Usual prenatal care	85%	55%	54.5%

4. Monthly alcohol ingestion rate (mean) before (1), early (2) and late (3) in pregnancy. TOA = 5 months

	1	2	3
Cognitive-based education	11.7	1.8	2.4
Information only	8.1	1.9	1.4
Usual prenatal care	6.3	2.9	1.8

5. Risk for FAS. TOA = 5 months

Cognitive-based education	0
Information only	0
Usual prenatal care	0

Ingersoll et al. [47]
Country: USA
Source: Journal article
Funding: Government, society, internal

CCT
To evaluate the effects of a motivational interview-based intervention to reduce the risk of AEP
Study dates: NR
Setting: Urban

Study population: Women of childbearing age who consume alcohol

Selection criteria: Women of childbearing age (18–24 years) at risk for an AEP; having sexual intercourse with a man in the past 90 days while not using effective contraception; drinking at risky levels (engaging in at least one binge in the past 90 days or consuming an average of eight standard drinks/week)

No. of participants:
Enrolled = 228
Analyzed = 199

Demographics:
- Females (%): 100
- Mean age: 20.4 years; SD = 1.7
- Ethnicity:
  Caucasian = 69.8%;
  African-American = 16.6%;
  Asian = 5.8%;
  Hispanic = 2.3%;
  Other = 3.9%; Pacific Islander = 1.6%

Intervention: BALANCE Motivational interview

No. enrolled = 114
No. analyzed = 94

Comparators: Information only
No. enrolled = 114
No. analyzed = 105

Follow-up period: ≤3 mo

Outcomes and results:
1. Number of standard drinks/week (mean). TOA = 1 month

BALANCE	Information only
9.5	11.4

2. Binges in the past month (mean). TOA = 1 month
- Results = MI = 2.9; Control = 3.8

BALANCE	Information only
2.9	4.4

3. Highest number of standard drinks per day (mean). TOA = 1 month

BALANCE	Information only
5.9	7.1

($p < 0.003$)

The BALANCE intervention was efficacious in reducing the risk of AEP at 1 month follow-up.

Statistically significant results: Yes

Support to the effectiveness of the intervention

(Continued)

Table 3.E.2 (*Continued*)

Study	Study design, objective and setting	Demographics and Participant characteristics	Intervention	Outcomes/Results	Author conclusions
Palinkas *et al.* [66] **Country:** USA **Source:** Journal article **Funding:** Government	CCT To evaluate the effectiveness of social skills training and social network restructuring in the prevention of drug use among high-risk female youth **Study dates:** NR **Setting:** Urban	**Study population:** Women of childbearing age who consume alcohol **Selection criteria:** Women aged 14–19 years; English speakers; residing within San Diego city; not placed in a juvenile detention facility; at risk for drug use based on POSIT **No. of participants:** Enrolled = 296 Analyzed = 296 **Demographics:** – Females (%): 100 – Mean age: 16 years; SD = 1.4 – Ethnicity: African-American = 38%; Mexican Americans = 45%; non-Hispanic whites = 9%; Others = 8%	**Intervention:** Project PALS No. enrolled = 144 No. analyzed = NR **Comparators:** Education intervention only (Facts of Life) No. enrolled = 152 No. analyzed = NR	4. Drink risk (%), TOA = 1 month	The PALS skills training intervention may be ineffective, and is possibly counterproductive as a means of primary prevention in high-risk youth. Social skills training is no more effective as a means of secondary prevention than normative education alone. **Statistically significant results:** No Does not support the effectiveness of the intervention

Outcomes/Results (detail):

4. Drink risk (%), TOA = 1 month

BALANCE	Information only
70.7%	84.8%

5. AEP risk (%), TOA = 1 month

BALANCE	Information only
26.1%	45.7%

Effect size = 0.19; p < 0.005

Follow-up period: >9 months and ≤1 year

Outcomes and results:

1. Alcohol intake (%), TOA = 3 months

	Baseline	3 mo
PALS	42%	55.1%
Education	46.3%	57.4%

OR = 0.9 (95% CI = 0.5, 1.6)

2. Alcohol intake (no drug use at pre-intervention (%), TOA = 3 months

	Baseline	3 mo
PALS	0%	42.9%
Education	0%	37.7%

OR = 1.2 (95% CI = 0.5, 2.6)

O'Connor and Whaley [64]

Country: USA

Source: Journal article

Funding: Government

CCT

To evaluate the efficacy of a brief intervention for alcohol use by pregnant women

Study dates: Jun 2001 to Mar 2004

Setting: Urban

Study population: Women at risk of an AEP

Selection criteria: Pregnant drinkers screened at prenatal visits

No. of participants: Enrolled = 345 Analyzed = 255

Demographics:
- Females (%): 100
- Mean age: 28.1 years; SD = 5.9
- Ethnicity: White = 7%, Black = 17.3%; Hispanic = 70.6%; Other = 5.1%

Intervention: Brief intervention for prenatal alcohol use

No. enrolled = 162

No. analyzed = 117

Comparators: Assessment only

No. enrolled = 183

No. analyzed = 138

3. Alcohol intake (drug use at pre-intervention (%). TOA = 3 months

	Baseline	3 mo
PALS	100%	69.4%
Education	100%	75.9%

OR = 0.5 (95% CI = 0.3, 1.5)

Follow-up period: >6 months and ≤9 months

Outcomes and results:

1. Abstinence. TOA = Third trimester
 - Results: OR = 5.39; 95% CI = 1.59 to 18.25

2. Birth weight (g) among high-drinker mothers. TOA = Birth

Brief intervention	**Assessment only**
3486.1	3305.6

3. Birth weight (g) among low-drinker mothers. TOA = Birth

Brief intervention	**Assessment only**
3356.8	3421.9

4. Fetal mortality rate (%). TOA = NR

Brief intervention	**Assessment only**
0.9%	2.9%

Women receiving the brief intervention were five times more likely to report abstinence after intervention than women who received assessment only. Newborns whose mothers received brief intervention had higher birth weights and birth lengths. Fetal mortality rates were three times lower compared with newborns in the assessment-only condition. Brief intervention was more effective than assessment alone. More positive newborn outcomes were associated with brief intervention, particularly for newborns of heavier drinkers

Statistically significant results: Yes

Support to the effectiveness of the intervention

(Continued)

Table 3.E.2 (Continued)

Study	Study design, objective and setting	Demographics and Participant characteristics	Intervention	Outcomes/Results	Author conclusions
Reynolds *et al.* [67] **Country:** USA **Source:** Journal article **Funding:** NR	CCT To evaluate the effects of a cognitive-behavioral intervention for reducing alcohol consumption among economically disadvantaged pregnant women **Study dates:** NR **Setting:** Mix	**Study population:** Women at risk of an AEP **Selection criteria:** Pregnant women who reported drinking in the past month while screened at prenatal visits (T-ACE questionnaire) **No. of participants:** Enrolled = 78 Analyzed = 72 **Demographics:** – Females (%): 100 – Mean age: 22.4 years; SD = NR – Ethnicity: African-American = 67%; Caucasian = 33%	**Intervention:** Cognitive-behavioral self-help intervention No. enrolled = 42 No. analyzed = 39 **Comparators:** Usual prenatal care No. enrolled = 36 No. analyzed = 33	**Follow-up period:** ≤3 months **Outcomes and results:** 1. Alcohol quit rate (%). TOA = 2 months 2. Amount of alcohol consumed in the last month (%). TOA = 2 months	The self-help intervention produced greater alcohol cessation and greater reductions in the amount of alcohol consumed than the usual prenatal care. **Statistically significant results:** Yes Support to the effectiveness of the intervention

Outcome 1:

	Cognitive-behavioral	Usual prenatal care
	88%	69%

*(p < 0.05)

Outcome 2:

	Cognitive-behavioral	Usual prenatal care
<7 drinks	100%	71%*
≥7 drinks	73%	68%

*(p < 0.01)

Belizan et al. [28]	CCT	Study population: Pregnant women	Intervention: Health education (home visits)	Follow-up period: >9 months and ≤1 year

Follow-up period: >9 months and ≤1 year

Outcomes and results:

1. Change in daily alcohol drinking (%) TOA = 36 weeks

	Baseline	Endpoint
Health education	20.4%	19.1%
Usual prenatal care	17.6%	21.8%

2. Self-reported maternal morbidity (%)

- TOA = 36 weeks

	Health education	Usual prenatal care
Preterm labor	19.6%	18.5%
Premature rupture of membranes	2%	1.7%
IGR	1.4%	1.3%

An intervention of psychosocial support and health education during pregnancy failed to show any beneficial effects on perinatal outcome, health-related behavior, or utilization of health facilities. No differences in reduction of alcohol consumption were observed between the intervention and the control group.

Statistically significant results: No

Does not support the effectiveness of the intervention

Belizan et al. [28]

Country: Argentina, Brazil, Cuba, Mexico

Source: Journal article

Funding: Government

CCT

To evaluate the impact of health education during pregnancy on behavior and utilization of health resources

Study dates: Jan 1989 to Mar 1991

Setting: Urban

Study population: Pregnant women

Selection criteria: Women initiating prenatal care (15–20 weeks' gestation); singleton pregnancy; at least one of the following risk factors: low birth weight or preterm infants, previous fetal, neonatal or infant death; ≤17 years old; body weight ≤50 kg; height ≤1.50 m; low family income; ≤3 years schooling; smoking or heavy alcohol consumption; single, separated, divorced or widowed

No. of participants:
Enrolled = 2235
Analyzed = 2128

Demographics:
- Females (%): 100
- Mean age: 24.4 years;
- SD = 6.6
- Ethnicity: White = 60%; Other = 40%

Intervention: Health education (home visits)

No. enrolled = 1115
No. analyzed = 1009

Comparators: Usual prenatal care

No. enrolled = 1120
No. analyzed = 1019

(Continued)

Table 3.E.2 *(Continued)*

Study	Study design, objective and setting	Demographics and Participant characteristics	Intervention	Outcomes/Results	Author conclusions
Eustace [38] **Country:** USA **Source:** Dissertation **Funding:** NR	CCT To evaluate the effects of a nurse supportive-educative intervention on alcohol consumption behavior during pregnancy **Study dates:** NR **Setting:** Urban	**Study population:** Pregnant women **Selection criteria:** Pregnant women attending prenatal clinics; ≤30 weeks of gestation; English speakers **No. of participants:** Enrolled = 281 Analyzed = 281 **Demographics:** – Females (%): 100 – Mean age: 23 years; SD = 4.2 – Ethnicity: African-American = 80.7%; White = 14.6%; Hispanic = 2.5%; Other = 2.1%6	**Intervention:** Supportive-educative intervention (Positive teaching reinforcement–video) No. enrolled = 106 No. analyzed = NR **Comparators:** Supportive-educative intervention (Negative teaching reinforcement–video) No. enrolled = 84 No. analyzed = NR Information only (neutral video) No. enrolled = 91 No. analyzed = NR	**Follow-up period:** >3 months and ≤6 months **Outcomes and results:** 1. Knowledge about the effects of alcohol on fetus at baseline (1), 10-min (2), 6 weeks (3) and 12 weeks (4) (max score = 14). TOA = 12 weeks $*(p < 0.001)$ 2. Alcohol consumption behavior score (max = 4) at baseline (1), 6 weeks (2) and 12 weeks (3). TOA = 12 weeks 3. Mean amount of alcohol consumed in standard amounts (max = 5) at baseline (1), 6 weeks (2) and 12 weeks (3). TOA = 12 weeks	The two intervention groups showed significantly higher knowledge scores than baseline after the teaching intervention and remained stable over a 12-week period. The teaching interventions significantly increased knowledge of the danger of consuming alcohol during pregnancy. There was no statistically significant indication that education about the harmful effects of alcohol consumption during pregnancy decreased alcohol consumption during pregnancy. **Statistically significant results:** Yes Partial support to the effectiveness of the intervention

Table for outcome 1:

	1	2	3	4
Positive	11.7	12.7*	12.5*	12.5*
Negative	11.5	12.7*	12.5*	12.8*
Neutral	11.5	11.5	11.5	11.6

Table for outcome 2:

	1	2	3
Positive	0.3	0.4	0.2
Negative	0.4	0.7	0.07
Neutral	0.6	0.3	0.1

Table for outcome 3:

	1	2	3
Positive	0.09	0.1	0.06
Negative	0.08	0.3	0.00
Neutral	0.1	0.5	0.05

Sarvela and Ford [69]

Country:
USA

Source:
Journal article

Funding:
Government

CCT

To evaluate the effectiveness of a drug and alcohol abuse prenatal care health education program for pregnant youth

Study dates:
1989 to 1990

Setting:
Inner city

Study population:
Pregnant women

Selection criteria:
Pregnant youth attending two regional health centers; readability level equivalent to grades 5–9

No. of participants:
Enrolled = 212
Analyzed = 188

Demographics:
- Females (%): 100
- Mean age: NR; SD = NR
- Ethnicity: Black = 27.3%; White = 72.7%

Intervention:
ASPEN prenatal health education program

No. enrolled = 113

No. analyzed = 103

Comparators:
Usual prenatal care

No. enrolled = 99

No. analyzed = 85

Follow-up period: >9 months and ≤1 year

Outcomes and results:

1. Alcohol use in the last 5 months (%). TOA = Postpartum period

	Baseline	Endpoint
ASPEN	22.3%	3.6%
Usual prenatal care	15.1%	3.4%

2. Birth defects (%). TOA = Postpartum period

ASPEN	Usual prenatal care
10.5%	11%

3. Infant complications (%). TOA = Postpartum period

ASPEN	Usual prenatal care
78.1%	75.7%

RR = 0.96

Both the control and experimental groups decreased frequency of alcohol use from pre-test to post-test. The data appear to suggest that general prenatal care, as experienced by the control group, emphasizes the importance of reducing substance use during pregnancy.

Statistically significant results: No

Does not support the effectiveness of the intervention

(Continued)

Table 3.E.2 (*Continued*)

Study	Study design, objective and setting	Demographics and Participant characteristics	Intervention	Outcomes/Results	Author conclusions
				4. Meconium stool (%). TOA = Postpartum period	
				ASPEN **Usual prenatal care**	
				31.6% 31%	
				RR = 0.98	
				5. Birth weight (mean pounds). TOA = Postpartum period	
				ASPEN **Usual prenatal care**	
				7.1 7.3	
Handmaker *et al.* [44] **Country:** USA **Source:** Journal article **Funding:** Government	CCT To evaluate the efficacy of motivational interviewing in prenatal care clinics **Study dates:** NR **Setting:** Urban	**Study population:** Women at risk of an AEP **Selection criteria:** Pregnant women who reported consuming at least one drink in the past month **No. of participants:** Enrolled = 42 Analyzed = 34 **Demographics:** – Females (%): 100 – Mean age: 24 years; SD = 5.7 – Ethnicity: Hispanic = 53%; White = 38%; Black = 9%	**Intervention:** Motivational interview No. enrolled = 21 No. analyzed = 16 **Comparators:** Information only No. enrolled = 21 No. analyzed = 18	**Follow-up period:** ≤3 months **Outcomes and results:** 1. Reduction in total drinks consumed. TOA = 2 months – No data (p = 0.025) 2. Total abstinent days (%). TOA = 2 months **MI** **Information only** 44% 33%	Motivational interviewing shows promise as a specific intervention for initiating a reduction in drinking among pregnant women who are at greatest risk. **Statistically significant results:** No Support to superiority of the intervention compared to the provision of information only

Eisen et al. [37]

Country:
USA

Source:
Journal article

Funding:
Government

Prospective analytical cohort study

To evaluate the impact of a community-based drug prevention, education and treatment project for pregnant and postpartum women

Study dates:
Sept 1994 to Sept 1996

Setting: NR

Study population:
Women at risk of an AEP

Selection criteria:
Pregnant women that have used alcohol or other drugs during the pregnancy

No. of participants:
Enrolled = NR
Analyzed = 658

Demographics:
- Females (%): 100
- Mean age: NR; SD = NR
- Ethnicity: NR

Intervention:
PPWI treatment programs

No. enrolled = NR

No. analyzed = 370

Comparators:
No intervention

No. enrolled = NR

No. analyzed = 288

Follow-up period: >1 year

Outcomes and results:

1. Alcohol use in the last 30 days (%). TOA = 30 days

	Baseline	Endpoint
PPWI	33%	14%*
No intervention	23%	23%

*(p < 0.0001)

2. Alcohol use to intoxication in the last 30 days (%). TOA = from intake to delivery

	Baseline	Endpoint
PPWI	19%	4%*
No intervention	10%	6%

*(p < 0.0001)

3. Alcohol use in the last 30 days (%). TOA = 6 months postpartum

	Baseline	Endpoint
PPWI	32%	34%
No intervention	23%	35%

4. Alcohol use to intoxication in the last 30 days (%). TOA = 6 months postpartum

	Baseline	Endpoint
PPWI	14%	7%
No intervention	10%	8%

Participants in the intervention group had significantly lower 30-day rates of alcohol use from intake to delivery, but results were not maintained through 6 months postpartum.

Statistically significant results: Yes

Support to the effectiveness of the intervention

(Continued)

Table 3.E.2 (*Continued*)

Study	Study design, objective and setting	Demographics and Participant characteristics	Intervention	Outcomes/Results	Author conclusions
Meberg [60] **Country:** Norway **Source:** Journal article **Funding:** Society	Prospective analytical cohort study To evaluate the impact of an intervention program of supportive counseling focused on reduction of alcohol consumption in pregnant women **Study dates:** NR **Setting:** Urban	**Study population:** Pregnant women **Selection criteria:** Women registered for prenatal care **No. of participants:** Enrolled = 132 Analyzed = 132 **Demographics:** – Females (%): 100 – Mean age: 26.7 years; SD = NR – Ethnicity: NR	**Intervention:** Supportive counseling No. enrolled = 58 No. analyzed = 58 **Comparators:** Usual prenatal care No. enrolled = 74 No. analyzed = 74	**Follow-up period:** >9 months and ≤1 year **Outcomes and results:** 1. Teetotalers (%) before pregnancy (1) and after pregnancy (2). TOA = Postpartum period |	1	2 | Supportive counseling · 16% · 60% Usual prenatal care · 24% · 70% 2. Alcohol use (% g/day) before pregnancy (1) and during pregnancy (2). TOA = Postpartum period – <5 drinks |	1	2 | Supportive counseling · 62% · 34% Usual prenatal care · 64% · 27%	Drinking patterns changed during pregnancy in direction of abstinence and reduced alcohol consumption, independently of the intervention program introduced. **Statistically significant results:** No Does not support the effectiveness of the intervention

Mehl-Madrona [61]

Country: USA

Source: Journal article

Funding: Government

Prospective analytical cohort study

To evaluate the impact of a psychosocial prenatal intervention to reduce substance use among Native American women and other minority populations

Study dates: NR

Setting: Mix

Study population: Pregnant women

Selection criteria: Pregnant women >39 years attending prenatal clinics

No. of participants:
Enrolled = 640
Analyzed = 640

Demographics:
- Females (%): 100
- Mean age: 25 years; SD = 9
- Ethnicity: Black = 11%; Hispanic = 34%; Native American = 36%; White = 19%

Intervention: Psychosocial prenatal intervention

No. enrolled = 320
No. analyzed = 320

Comparators: Usual prenatal care

No. enrolled = 320
No. analyzed = 320

- ꝋ-10 drinks:

	1	2
Supportive counseling	12%	5%
Usual prenatal care	8%	3%

- 10–20 drinks:

	1	2
Supportive counseling	10%	0%
Usual prenatal care	4%	0%

Follow-up period: >6 months and ≤9 months

Outcomes and results:

1. Obstetric outcomes (%). TOA = 36–40 weeks of gestation

	Psychosocial intervention	Usual prenatal care
NSVD	79.6%	58.1%*
Cesarean	9.6%	21.8%*
Premature deliveries	5.3%	7.8%

*(p < 0.001)

The intervention was successful in increasing the number of normal spontaneous vaginal deliveries and decreasing the number of Cesarean births. It also had a significant impact in neonatal outcomes. Alcohol reductions were significant for heavy drinkers in the intervention group compared with the control group.

Statistically significant results: Yes

Support to the effectiveness of the intervention

(Continued)

Table 3.E.2 (*Continued*)

Study	Study design, objective and setting	Demographics and Participant characteristics	Intervention	Outcomes/Results	Author conclusions

2. Newborn outcomes. TOA = 36–40 weeks of gestation

	Psychosocial intervention	Usual prenatal care
Resuscitations	1.8%	2.5%
Special care nursery	7.5%	19%*
Apgar 1-min score < 7	21.5%	33.1%**
Apgar 5-min score < 7	9.3%	13.7%
Apgar 1-min score < 4	3.7%	11.5%**
Apgar 5-min score < 4	1.5%	5.9%***

*(p < 0.005); **(p < 0.001); ***(p < 0.01)

Nilsen *et al.* [63]

Country: Sweden

Source: Journal article

Funding: Government

Retrospective analytical cohort study

To compare current standard provision of alcohol advice during pregnancy with a more comprehensive counseling model

Study dates: Apr 2005 to Mar 2007

Setting: Health facility

Study population: Pregnant women

Selection criteria: NR

No. of participants: Enrolled = 2881
Analyzed = 1849

Demographics:
– Females (%): 100
– Mean age: NR
– Ethnicity: NR

Intervention: Questionnaire-based alcohol counseling

No. enrolled = 1348

No. analyzed = 931

Comparators: Standard counseling

No. enrolled = 1533

No. analyzed = 918

3. Alcohol use (%). TOA = 36–40 weeks of gestation

	Psychosocial intervention	Usual prenatal care
Alcohol use at conception	51.6%	50%
Alcohol use reduced	79.4%	73.8%
Heavy alcohol use at conception	9.7%	10.3%
Heavy alcohol use reduced	100%	36.4%

*(p < 0.02)

Follow-up period >9 months and ≤1 year

Outcomes and results

1. Frequency of drinking during pregnancy
   – TOA = Postpartum period

	Questionnaire-based counseling	Standard counseling
Ceased drinking	93.1%	93.2%

Questionnaire-based counseling was not more effective than standard counseling in its impact on the proportion of women who abstained from drinking during pregnancy.

Statistically significant results: No

Does not support the effectiveness of the intervention.

(Continued)

Table 3.E.2 (*Continued*)

Study	Study design, objective and setting	Demographics and Participant characteristics	Intervention	Outcomes/Results	Author conclusions

Corrarino *et al.* [35]
 	
Country:
USA
 	
Source:
Journal article
 	
Funding:
NR
	Before-and-after study
	
	To evaluate a pilot program that links substance-abusing pregnant women with treatment
	
	Study dates: NR
	
	Setting:
	Inner city
		Study population:
		Women at risk of an AEP
		
		Selection criteria:
		Pregnant substance-abusing women not in drug treatment upon entry into prenatal care
		
		No. of participants:
		Enrolled = 10
		Analyzed = 9
		
		Demographics:
		– Females (%): 100
		– Mean age: 22yr;
		  SD = NR
		– Ethnicity: White = 60%;
		  African-American = 30%;
		  Hispanic = 10%
			Intervention:
			Perinatal Outreach Project
			
			No. enrolled = 10
			
			No. analyzed = 9
			
			Comparators: NA
				Follow-up period: 3 months and ≤6 months
				
				Outcomes and results:
				
				1. Retention of custody of index child (%). TOA = Postpartum period
				
				    Custody retention 8/9
				
				2. Severity of addiction (% score). TOA = 6 months
				
				|
					Before	After

---	---	---
No problem (score 0–1)	0%	22.2%
Slight (score 2–3)	0%	22.2%
Moderate (score 4–5)	11.1%	22.2%
Considerable (score 6–7)	44.4%	22.2%
Extreme (score 8–9)	44.4%	11.1%		Further controlled studies are needed to determine more definitely the significance of the interventions provided in the study. The study supports the effectiveness of public health nurses and an interdisciplinary team in improving the health status of pregnant women. **Statistically significant results:** NR Support to the effectiveness of the intervention

Tavris [71]
Country: USA
Source: Journal article
Funding: NR

Before-and-after study

To evaluate the effectiveness of a prenatal care program in reducing self-reported risk factors for adverse pregnancy outcomes

Study dates: 1997

Setting: Inner city

Study population: Women at risk of an AEP

Selection criteria: Women with a risk of an adverse pregnancy outcome (State of Wisconsin Pregnancy Questionnaire score >40); on medical assistance from the state of Wisconsin

No. of participants: Enrolled = 166, Analyzed = 74

Demographics:
- Females (%): 100
- Mean age: 21.7 years; SD = NR
- Ethnicity: White = 84%; Hispanic = 12%; Other = 4%

Intervention: PNCC program
No. enrolled = 166
No. analyzed = 74
Comparators: NA

Follow-up period: >9 months and ≤1 year

Outcomes and results:

1. Alcohol intake (mean drinks per month). TOA = 38 weeks

3 months prior to pregnancy	After 38 weeks
9.6	0

2. Current alcohol intake (%). TOA = 38 weeks

3 months prior to pregnancy	After first prenatal visit
31.9%	2.5%

There were large and highly statistically significant improvements in several prenatal risk factors known to have large effects on pregnancy outcome in comparison with baseline values after participation in the PNCC program.

Statistically significant results: NR

Support to the effectiveness of the intervention

Yonkers [75]
Country: USA
Source: Journal article
Funding: Government

Before-and-after study

To evaluate the feasibility of delivering motivational interviewing and CBT in an obstetrical setting by non-behavioral health practitioners

Study dates: NR

Setting: Health facility

Study population: Women at risk of an AEP

Selection criteria: Pregnant women who self-reported alcohol or illicit drug use within the 28 days prior to study; English as primary language

No. of participants: Enrolled = 14, Analyzed = 14

Demographics:
- Females (%): 100
- Mean age: 27.4 years; SD = 6
- Ethnicity: African-American = 36%; Caucasian/white = 50%, Mixed = 14%

Intervention: Motivational interview + CBT
No. enrolled = 14
No. analyzed = 14
Comparators: NA

Follow-up period >9 months and ≤1 year

Outcomes and results

1. Depressive symptoms (mean IDS-SR score, SD)
   - TOA = Postpartum period

Before	After
23.9 (12.9)	17.1 (13.7)

2. Alcohol use (mean ASI score, SD)
   - TOA = Postpartum period

Before	After
0.16 (0.22)	0.06 (0.19)

Motivational interviewing and cognitive behavioral therapy delivered by non-behavioral health professionals has the potential to promote a reduction in hazardous substance use in pregnant women.

Statistically significant results: NR

No conclusions regarding the effectiveness of the intervention

(Continued)

Table 3.E.2 *(Continued)*

Study	Study design, objective and setting	Demographics and Participant characteristics	Intervention	Outcomes/Results	Author conclusions
Larsson [51] **Country:** Sweden **Source:** Journal article **Funding:** Government	Before-and-after study To evaluate the impact of an antenatal program for early detection of pregnancies at risk **Study dates:** 1979 **Setting:** Urban	**Study population:** Pregnant women **Selection criteria:** Pregnant women attending antenatal clinics **No. of participants:** Enrolled = 464 Analyzed = 464 **Demographics:** – Females (%): 100 – Mean age: NR; SD = NR – Ethnicity: NR	**Intervention:** Screening and treatment No. enrolled = 464 No. analyzed = 464 **Comparators:** NA	3. Average number of days of alcohol use in prior 28 days (mean, SD) – TOA = Postpartum period | Before	After
---	---
2.42 (5.7)	1.64 (4.7)	 **Follow-up period:** >9 months and ≤1 year **Outcomes and results:** 1. Reduction of alcohol intake or abstinence (%). TOA = Postpartum period For occasional drinkers 74% For excessive drinkers 100% For alcohol abusers 78% 2. FAS (n). TOA = Postpartum period For occasional drinkers 0 For excessive drinkers 1* For alcohol abusers 1 *partial FAS	Therapeutic assistance resulted in a substantial decline in alcohol intake among mothers who are heavy drinkers. **Statistically significant results:** No Partial support to the effectiveness of the intervention

Little *et al.* [52]

Country: USA

Source: Journal article

Funding: Government

Before-and-after study

To evaluate the impact of an educational program for maternal alcohol abuse during pregnancy

Study dates: 1979 to 1981

Setting: Mix

Study population: Pregnant women

Selection criteria: NR

No. of participants:
Enrolled = 688
Analyzed = 688

Demographics:
– Females (%): 100
– Mean age: NR; SD = NR
– Ethnicity: NR

Intervention:
Pregnancy and Health Program (PHP)

No. enrolled = 368 (pre)

No. analyzed = 320 (post)

Comparators: NA

Follow-up period: >9 months and ≤1 year

Outcomes and results:

1. Awareness of risk of alcohol use during pregnancy (%). TOA = 1 year

Before (1979)	After PHP program (1981)
98%	99%

2. Belief in alcohol abstinence as a beneficial behavior during pregnancy (%). TOA = 1 year

Before (1979)	After PHP program (1981)
48%*	56%

*(p < 0.05)

The PHP resulted in an increased belief in alcohol abstinence as a beneficial behavior during pregnancy. Education coupled with effective screening, and referral to treatment when needed, make the reduction of fetal alcohol effects a goal within reach for all communities.

Statistically significant results: Yes

No conclusions regarding the effectiveness of the intervention

---

95% CI = 95% confidence interval; AEP = alcohol-exposed pregnancy; AO = assessment only; ASI = Addictions Severity Index; ASPEN = Adolescent Substance Prevention Education Network; BALANCE = Birth Control and Alcohol Awareness: Negotiating Choices Effectively; BI = brief intervention; CCT = controlled clinical trial; DDP = Drinking During Pregnancy; ES = Early Start; ESP = Early Start Plus; FAS = fetal alcohol syndrome; g = gram(s); IDS-SR = Inventory of Depressive Symptomatology Self-Report; NA = not applicable; NR = not reported; NSVD = Normal spontaneous vaginal delivery; OR = odds ratio; PALS = Positive Adolescent Life Skills; PHP = Pregnancy and Health Program; PNCC = Prenatal Care Coordination Program; POSIT = Problem-Oriented Screening Instrument for Teenagers; PPWI = Pregnant and Postpartum Women and their Infant; RCT = randomized controlled trial; SD = standard deviation; TOA = time to outcome assessment; USA = United States of America.

Table 3.E.3 Characteristics of studies on indicated prevention approaches to FASD.

Study	Study design, objective and setting	Demographics and Participant characteristics	Intervention	Outcomes/Results	Author conclusions
Loudenburg [53] **Country:** USA **Source:** Journal article **Funding:** NR	CCT To evaluate the impact of a multifaceted intervention to reduce substance use in high-risk women of child-bearing age **Study dates:** NR **Setting:** Mix	**Study population:** Women of childbearing age **Selection criteria:** NR **No. of participants:** Enrolled = NR Analyzed = 302 **Demographics:** – Females (%): 100 – Mean age: NR; SD = NR – Ethnicity: NR	**Intervention:** Four-State FAS Consortium No. enrolled = NR No. analyzed = 156 **Comparators:** Usual prenatal care No. enrolled = NR No. analyzed = 146	**Follow-up period:** >3 months and ≤6 months **Outcomes and results:** 1. Perceptions of substance use. TOA = 6 months – Data for Four-State FAS only: Improvement in perception of controlling alcohol use — 20.6% Knowledge of harmful effects of alcohol and other drugs — 31.1% 2. Improvement in perceptions of family functioning. TOA = 6 months – Data for Four-State FAS only: Expression of affection for family members — 19.9% Parenting skills — 25.7% Overall functioning of family — 29.9%	The perceived improvements in each domain of intervention provide validation of the intervention design. The use of a multi-domain approach with high-risk populations is effective in maintaining abstinence or reducing substance use among high-risk women of childbearing age. **Statistically significant results:** NR No conclusions regarding the effectiveness of the intervention

Hankin [45]	**Study population:** Women at risk of an AEP
Country: USA	**Selection criteria:** Women consuming at least four drinks/week at the time they conceived an index pregnancy; women delivered an infant weighing more than 1500 g and were not sterilized at the time of delivery
Source: Journal article	
Funding: NR	

CCT

To evaluate the effect of a brief intervention designed to prevent drinking during the next pregnancy among women who drank heavily during an index pregnancy

Study dates: 1993 to 1995

Setting: NR

No. of participants:
Enrolled = NR
Analyzed = 96

Demographics:
– Females (%): 100
– Mean age: 25 years; SD = NR
– Ethnicity: Black = 84%; NR = 16%

Intervention:
Brief intervention for prenatal alcohol use

No. enrolled = NR
No. analyzed = 70

Comparators:
Assessment and information only

No. enrolled = NR
No. analyzed = 26

3. Improvement in perception of mental health status. TOA = 6 months

   – Data for Four-State FAS only

Dealing with stress	59.4%
General mental health	30%

4. Perception of general well-being. TOA = 6 months

   – Data for Four-State FAS only:

General physical health	20.4%

Follow-up period: >1 year

Outcomes and results:

1. Mental developmental delay (MDI Bailey scale) (%). TOA = 5 years

Brief intervention	Assessment only
11.4	11.5

2. Psychomotor developmental delay (PDI Bailey scale) (%). TOA = 5 years

Brief intervention	Assessment only
12.9	3.8

Index and subsequent infants born to the experimental group mothers were less likely to be delayed on the MDI, PDI and MDI-PDI Bailey scales. A brief intervention designed to reduce drinking among a group of at-risk drinkers protected their subsequent pregnancy as well as their index pregnancy. In the case of the index child who was exposed to alcohol *in utero*, the intervention may have improved the woman's mothering.

Statistically significant results: Yes

Support to the effectiveness of the intervention

(Continued)

Table 3.E.3 (*Continued*)

Study	Study design, objective and setting	Demographics and Participant characteristics	Intervention	Outcomes/Results	Author conclusions
				3. Developmental delay (MDI and PDI Bayley scales) (%). TOA = 5 years	
				Brief intervention	**Assessment only**	
				12.9	26.2	
				4. No developmental delays (Bailey MDI and PDI) (%). TOA = 5 years	
				Brief intervention	**Assessment only**	
				62.9%	57.8%	

Whiteside-Mansell [74]

Country:
USA

Source:
Journal article

Funding:
Government

Prospective analytical cohort study

To evaluate the impact of a comprehensive substance-use prevention and treatment program for low-income pregnant and parenting women

Study dates: NR

Setting: Urban

Study population:
Women at risk of an AEP

Selection criteria: NR

No. of participants:
Enrolled = 95
Analyzed = 37

Demographics:
- Females (%): 100
- Mean age: 28.2 years; SD = 5.2
- Ethnicity: African American = 73.6%; Other = 26.4%

Intervention:
AR-CARES

No. enrolled = 72

No. analyzed = 27

Comparators:
No intervention

No. enrolled = 23

No. analyzed = 10

Follow-up period:
Mother: >9 months and ≤1 year; Child: 6, 12, 18 months

Outcomes and results:

1. Alcohol use (%). TOA = Postpartum period

	Intake	Delivery
AR-CARES	83.6%	4.0%
No intervention	90.5%	33.3%

($p < 0.05$)

2. Obstetric complications (any) (%). TOA = Postpartum period

AR-CARES	No intervention
46%	40%

3. Fetal distress (%). TOA = Postpartum period

AR-CARES	No intervention
7%	0%

4. Meconium-stained amniotic fluid (%). TOA = Postpartum period

AR-CARES	No intervention
23%	10%

There was a significant reduction in the proportion of alcohol users among participants in the intervention group. Children from women in the participating group reached normal ranges of both growth and development. Program participation was associated with a significant reduction in alcohol use during the time before the birth of the target child. There are indications that the program may have had an impact on later child development.

Statistically significant results: Yes

Support to the effectiveness of the intervention

(Continued)

Table 3.E.3 (*Continued*)

Study	Study design, objective and setting	Demographics and Participant characteristics	Intervention	Outcomes/Results	Author conclusions
				5. Hospitalization outcomes. TOA = Postpartum period – Number of maternal hospital days (*n*):	

AR-CARES	No intervention
2.3	5

(p < 0.05)

– Number of infant hospital days (*n*):

AR-CARES	No intervention
3.1	4.3

– Number of days in NICU (*n*):

AR-CARES	No intervention
0.4	0.8

(Continued)

6. Neonatal and developmental outcomes.
   TOA = Postpartum period, 6, 12, 18 months
   - Infant weight at delivery (pounds):

AR-CARES	No intervention
6.5*	5.8

*(p < 0.05)
   - Infant length at delivery (inches):

AR-CARES	No intervention
18.7	19.8

   - Infant head circumference at delivery (cm):

AR-CARES	No intervention
35	33

(p < 0.10)
   - Mean Apgar scores:

	AR-CARES	No intervention
1-min	8	8
5-min	8	9

Table 3.E.3 (*Continued*)

Study	Study design, objective and setting	Demographics and Participant characteristics	Intervention	Outcomes/Results	Author conclusions
				– Bayley scales (score) (6 months):	

	AR-CARES	No intervention
MDI	99.4	100
PDI	98.4	102

– Weight percentile (6 months):

AR-CARES	No intervention
36.4	17.5

– Length percentile (6 months):

AR-CARES	No intervention
36.4	17.5

– Head circumference percentile (6 months):

AR-CARES	No intervention
47.1	17.5

(Continued)

- Bayley scales (score) (12 months):

	AR-CARES	No intervention
MDI	98.2	89.8
PDI	101.1	95

- Weight percentile (12 months):

AR-CARES	No intervention
50	11.67

- Length percentile (12 months):

AR-CARES	No intervention
55	10

- Head circumference percentile (12 months)

AR-CARES	No intervention
55	15

Table 3.E.3 *(Continued)*

Study	Study design, objective and setting	Demographics and Participant characteristics	Intervention	Outcomes/Results	Author conclusions
				– Bayley scales (score) (18 months):	

– Bayley scales (score) (18 months):

	AR-CARES	No intervention
MDI	91.7	79
PDI	97.5	79

– Weight percentile (18 months):

AR-CARES	No intervention
25	10

– Length percentile (18 months):

AR-CARES	No intervention
37.5	10

– Head circumference percentile (18 months):

AR-CARES	No intervention
37.5	5

Svikis *et al.* [70]	**Study population:** Women at risk of an AEP	**Intervention:** Counseling/support group	**Follow-up period:** >9 months and ≤1 year	No differences were found in the extent to which support group session and increased prenatal care separately contributed to improved outcomes. The authors endorse the use of support groups for pregnant, substance-abusing women in obstetric clinic settings.
Country: USA	**Selection criteria:**	No. enrolled = 54	**Outcomes and results:**	
Source: Journal article	Pregnant women attending prenatal care that screened positive for alcohol and/or drug use based on clinician interview (CAGE, ASI) or urinalysis drug toxicology at first prenatal visit; >28 weeks of gestation	No. analyzed = 54	1. Maternal alcohol use at delivery (self-report) (%). TOA = Postpartum period	
Funding: Internal		**Comparators.** No intervention		Support groups are inexpensive to implement and may serve as an attractive alternative for pregnant women who are unwilling to enter more formal treatment for their alcohol and drug problems.
Retrospective analytical cohort study		No. enrolled = 67		
To evaluate the clinical and economic efficacy of an on-site support group for drug-abusing pregnant women		No. analyzed = 67		

Retrospective analytical cohort study

To evaluate the clinical and economic efficacy of an on-site support group for drug-abusing pregnant women

Study dates: 1989 to 1990

Setting: Urban

No. of participants: Enrolled = 121 Analyzed = 121

Demographics:
– Females (%): 100
– Mean age: 25.1 years; SD = 4.5
– Ethnicity: African American = 87.6%; Other = 12.4%

1. Maternal alcohol use at delivery (self-report) (%). TOA = Postpartum period

Counseling	No intervention
38%	54%

2. Positive urinalysis drug toxicology at delivery (%). TOA = Postpartum period

Counseling	No intervention
48%	54%

Statistically significant results: Yes

Support to the effectiveness of the intervention

(Continued)

Table 3.E.3 (*Continued*)

Study	Study design, objective and setting	Demographics and Participant characteristics	Intervention	Outcomes/Results	Author conclusions
				3. Meconium staining (%). TOA = Postpartum period	

Counseling	No intervention
35%	48%

4. Infant birth weight (mean g). TOA = Postpartum period

Counseling	No intervention
3137	2805

(p < 0.002)

5. Low infant birth weight (<2500 g) (%). TOA = Postpartum period

Counseling	No intervention
15%	25%

(*Continued*)

6. Apgar scores. TOA = Postpartum period

   – 1-min Apgar score:

Counseling	No intervention
7.9*	7.2

   *(p < 0.02)

   2) 5-min Apgar score:

Counseling	No intervention
8.8	8.5

7. Medical care costs (mean in US$). TOA = 3 weeks after delivery

   – Maternal:

Counseling	No intervention
4095*	5016

   *(p < 0.01)

   – Infant:

Counseling	No intervention
1604*	3250

   *(p < 0.01)

Table 3.E.3 *(Continued)*

Study	Study design, objective and setting	Demographics and Participant characteristics	Intervention	Outcomes/Results	Author conclusions
Grant *et al.* [42] **Country:** USA **Source:** Journal article **Funding:** Government, society, internal	Before-and-after study To evaluate the impact of a paraprofessional intervention with high-risk women who abused alcohol and drugs during pregnancy **Study dates:** July 1991 to Dec 1992 and July 1994 to Dec 1995 **Setting:** Urban	**Study population:** Women at risk of an AEP **Selection criteria:** Pregnant or postpartum women; self-report of heavy alcohol or illicit drug use during pregnancy (≥5 alcoholic drinks/occasion ≥ once/month and/or use of any illicit substance ≥ once/week during pregnancy; ineffective or non-engagement with community social services **No. of participants:** Enrolled = 249 Analyzed = 216 **Demographics:** – Females (%): 100 – Mean age: 28.4 years; SD = NR – Ethnicity: White = 42.5%; African-American = 38.8%; Native American = 11.2%; Other (Hispanic, Asian) = 7.5%	**Intervention:** PCAP No. enrolled = 249 No. analyzed = 216 **Comparators:** NA	**Follow-up period:** >1 year **Outcomes and results:** 1. Addiction Severity Index (ASI) summary score. TOA = 3 years |	Baseline	Endpoint
---	---	---
Original site	−20.7	17
Replication site	−11	26	 2. Abstinence from alcohol/drugs at program exit (%). TOA = 3 years – Results = ≥6 months at program exit: 		Original	Replication
---	---	---
≥6 months at program exit	28%	41%
≥1 year at program exit	17%	33%
≥1 year during program	37%	53%		The PCAP community-based intervention offers hope to high-risk families and has proven to be a cost-effective strategy. **Statistically significant results:** NR Support to the effectiveness of the intervention

Halmesmaki [43]

Country:
Finland

Source:
Journal article

Funding:
Government

Before-and-after study

To evaluate the impact of a treatment program for pregnant alcoholics to prevent FAS

Study dates: NR

Setting:
Health facility

Study population:
Women at risk of an AEP

Selection criteria:
Pregnant alcohol abusers in their 8th to 12th gestational week

No. of participants:
Enrolled = NR
Analyzed = 85

Demographics:
– Females (%): 100
– Mean age: 28.1 years; SD = 6.1
– Ethnicity: NR

Intervention:
Counseling, psychological support and prenatal care

No. enrolled = NR

No. analyzed = 85

Comparators: NA

3. Subsequent pregnancy unexposed to alcohol/drugs (%) TOA – 3 years

Original site	Replication site
18%	36%

4. Index children in custody of their mothers (%). TOA = 3 years

Original site	Replication site
71%	73.5%

Follow-up period: >9 months and ≤1 year

Outcomes and results:

1. Alcohol use reduction (%). TOA = Postpartum period

All	64.5%
Alcoholics	55.1%
Heavy drinkers	56.6%
Moderate drinkers	84.6%

2. Fetal damage (%). TOA = Postpartum period

All	49%
Among those that reduced drinking	32.7%
Heavy drinkers	56.6%
Among those that continued drinking	80%

Two out of three drinkers reduced their alcohol consumption in the treatment program, and this decreased the risk of fetal damage.

Statistically significant results: NR

No conclusions regarding the effectiveness of the intervention

(Continued)

Table 3.E.3 *(Continued)*

Study	Study design, objective and setting	Demographics and Participant characteristics	Intervention	Outcomes/Results	Author conclusions
				3. Perinatal and neonatal mortality rates (%). TOA = Postpartum period	
				Perinatal mortality 2.4% Neonatal mortality 4.7%	
				4. FAS (%) TOA = Postpartum period	

				All 27.7%
				    Among those that reduced drinking 16%
				    Among those that continued drinking 48%	

				5. FAE (%) TOA = Postpartum period	

				All 30.5%
				    Among those that reduced drinking 24%
				    Among those that continued drinking 41%	

				6. Healthy infants (%) TOA = Postpartum period	

				All 41.6%
				    Among those that reduced drinking 60%
				    Among those that continued drinking 11%	

Masis *et al.* [56] **Country:** USA **Source:** Journal article **Funding:** Government	Before-and-after study To evaluate the impact of a hospital-based, comprehensive approach to the prevention of FAS **Study dates:** Jan 1988 to July 1989 **Setting:** Rural	**Study population:** Women at risk of an AEP **Selection criteria:** NR **No. of participants:** Enrolled = 39 Analyzed = 31 **Demographics:** – Females (%): 100 – Mean age: 27.2 years; SD = NR – Ethnicity: Aboriginal = 100%	**Intervention:** FAS Prevention Project No. enrolled = 39 No. analyzed = 31 **Comparison groups:** NA	**Follow-up period:** >1 year **Outcomes and results:** 1. Alcohol abstinence (%). TOA = 18 months Alcohol abstinence 56.3% The effectiveness of the prevention program depends not only on knowledge, case finding and treatment efforts, but also on the involvement of multiple constituencies in the community. **Statistically significant results:** NR No conclusions regarding effectiveness of the intervention
May *et al.* [57] **Country:** USA **Source:** Journal article **Funding:** Government	Before-and-after study To evaluate the impact of a case-management approach to preventing FAS in Northern Plains communities **Study dates:** NR **Setting:** Rural	**Study population:** Women at risk of an AEP **Selection criteria:** Women identified for second level screening for risk of alcohol abuse during pregnancy **No. of participants:** Enrolled = 137 Analyzed = 137 **Demographics:** – Females (%): 100 – Mean age: 24.1 years; SD = 6.5 – Ethnicity: Aboriginal = 100%	**Intervention:** Case management No. enrolled = 137 No. analyzed = NR **Comparators:** NA	**Follow-up period:** >1 year **Outcomes and results:** 1. Stopped drinking completely in the past 6 months (%). TOA = 6, 12 months Case management can be an efficacious intervention for women at high risk for births of children with FASD. **Statistically significant results:** No Partial support to the effectiveness of the intervention

Outcome 1 (May et al.):

Baseline	6 months	12 months
67.9%	60.5%	56.8%

2. Drinks consumed in the past 30 days (*n*). TOA = 6, 12 months

	Baseline	6 months	12 months
All women	24.2	23.5	36.2
Drinkers	55.3	45.8	54.3

(Continued)

Table 3.E.3 *(Continued)*

Study	Study design, objective and setting	Demographics and Participant characteristics	Intervention	Outcomes/Results	Author conclusions
				3. Times "high" or drunk in the past 6 months (%). TOA = 6, 12 months	

	Baseline	6 months	12 months
All women	15%	4.3%	7.2%
Drinkers	17.3%	8.6%	12%

4. Peak BAC (g of alcohol per 100 ml of blood) in past 6 months. TOA = 6, 12 months

	Baseline	6 months	12 months
Drinkers	0.27	0.23	0.26

5. FASD (*n* per child births). TOA = NR

FASD   2/150

Rosett *et al.* [68] **Country:** USA **Source:** Journal article **Funding:** Government, society	Before-and-after study To evaluate the effect of integrating therapy for heavy drinking with routine prenatal care **Study dates:** May 1974 to Sept 1979 **Setting:** Inner city	**Study population:** Women at risk of an AEP **Selection criteria:** Pregnant women identified as heavy drinkers (a minimum of 45 drinks/ months, with at least five drinks on some occasions) **No. of participants:** Enrolled = 162 Analyzed = 49 **Demographics:** – Females (%): 100 – Mean age: 25.2 years; SD = NR – Ethnicity: African- American = 59%; Other = 41%	**Intervention:** Screening and supportive counseling No. enrolled = 162 No. analyzed = 49 **Comparators:** NA

Follow-up period: >6 months and ≤9 months

Outcomes and results:

1. Alcohol abstinence or reduced alcohol consumption (%). TOA = 3rd trimester

Statistically significant results: NR

Marked reduction before the 3rd trimester	67%
Total abstinence for the reminder of pregnancy	38.7%
No longer met criteria for heavy drinking	28.6%

Women who drink heavily will respond to individual supportive counseling provided by their healthcare professionals.

No conclusions regarding the effectiveness of the intervention

AR-CARES = Arkansas Center for Addictions Research, Education, and Services; ASI = Addiction Severity Index; BAC = Blood alcohol content; CCT = controlled clinical trial; FAS = fetal alcohol syndrome; FASD = fetal alcohol spectrum disorder; MDI = mental development index; MI = motivational interview; NA = not applicable; NICI = neonatal intensive care unit; NR = not reported; PCAP = Parent-Child Assistance Program; PDI = psychomotor development index; SD = standard deviation; T-ACE = Tolerance, Annoyed, Cut down, Eye-opener; TOA = time to outcome assessment.

Appendix 3.F: Characteristics of the Interventions

Table 3.F.1 Characteristics of universal prevention interventions.

Study	Type of intervention	Classification of the Intervention (Public Health Perspective)	Individual Components of the Intervention	Characteristics of the Intervention
LaChausse [50]	FASTRAC educational multimedia program Multimedia, peer-delivered educational PowerPoint presentation that includes information on the history of FASD, information on FAS and the effects of alcohol on the fetus	**Intervention setting:** School **General level of the intervention:** Individual/ family-focused Health teaching	**Education:** Computer-based education Audio-visual materials	**Theoretical framework:** Can't tell **Frequency:** One session **Duration:** 45 min/ session **Type of provider:** Peers **Availability of a manual:** NR **Training of providers:** NR
Calabro et al. [30]	Health education materials Health education materials (3rd grade reading level) delivered at the first prenatal visit aimed to influence knowledge, attitude and behavioral intention to avoid alcohol consumption while pregnant	**Intervention setting:** Health facility **General level of the intervention:** Individual/ family-focused Health teaching	**Education:** Distribution of printed educational materials (e.g., fact sheets, posters)	**Theoretical framework:** Can't tell **Frequency:** NR **Duration:** NR **Type of provider:** Media/Printed materials **Availability of a manual:** NR **Training of providers:** NR
Waterson [73]	Education prenatal information Written information about the risks of alcohol in pregnancy; personal advice and reinforcement given by a doctor; educational video	**Intervention setting:** Health facility **General level of the intervention:** Individual/ family-focused Health teaching	**Education:** Distribution of printed educational materials (e.g., fact sheets, posters) Motivational messages Audio-visual materials	**Theoretical framework:** Can't tell **Frequency:** One session **Duration:** NR **Type of provider:** Doctor (Multimedia + doctor) **Availability of a manual:** NR **Training of providers:** NR

Table 3.F.1 (Continued)

Study	Type of intervention	Classification of the Intervention (Public Health Perspective)	Individual Components of the Intervention	Characteristics of the Intervention
Mengel et al. [62]	Media public education campaign Media campaign built around four FASD prevention messages. Visual, audio and print advertisements, direct marketing to the community, public relations/media interviews, displays at community events, educational videos for high school students	**Intervention setting:** Community **General level of the intervention:** Community-focused Social marketing	**Education:** Mass media Distribution of printed educational materials (e.g., fact sheets, posters) Audio-visual materials	**Theoretical framework:** Social marketing theory **Frequency:** NR **Duration:** 18 months **Type of provider:** Media **Availability of a manual:** NR **Training of providers:** NR
Mazis et al. [59]	Alcohol beverage warning label Warning label on alcohol beverages about drinking during pregnancy	**Intervention setting:** Community **General level of the intervention:** Community-focused, system-level-focused Social marketing and policy development	**Legal:** Warning labels	**Theoretical framework:** Can't tell **Frequency:** NR **Duration:** NR **Type of provider:** NR **Availability of a manual:** NR **Training of providers:** NR
Casiro et al. [32]	Television public awareness campaign Television public awareness campaign (30-s television public service announcement) with a message on alcohol and pregnancy. Announcement broadcast in both prime time and non-prime time viewing hours	**Intervention setting:** Community **General level of the intervention:** Community-focused Social marketing	**Education:** Mass media	**Theoretical framework:** Social marketing theory **Frequency:** 585 times **Duration:** 30 s **Type of provider:** Media **Availability of a manual:** NR **Training of providers:** NR
Bowerman [29]	Community-supported alcohol ban Prohibition of alcohol possession in the community	**Intervention setting:** Community **General level of the intervention:** System-level-focused Policy development and enforcement	**Legal:** Ban	**Theoretical framework:** Can't tell **Frequency:** NR **Duration:** NR **Type of provider:** NR **Availability of a manual:** NR **Training of providers:** NR

(Continued)

Table 3.F.1 (*Continued*)

Study	Type of intervention	Classification of the Intervention (Public Health Perspective)	Individual Components of the Intervention	Characteristics of the Intervention
Olsen *et al.* [65]	Health education campaign ("Healthy Habits for Two") Health campaign (Brochure about smoking and drinking during pregnancy, and stickers)	**Intervention setting:** Community **General level of the intervention:** Community-focused Social marketing	**Education:** Distribution of printed educational materials (e.g., fact sheets, posters)	**Theoretical framework:** Can't tell **Frequency:** NR **Duration:** NR **Type of provider:** Media **Availability of a manual:** NR **Training of providers:** NR
Hankin *et al.* [46]	Alcohol beverage warning label Federal alcoholic beverage warning label urging women not to drink during pregnancy because of the risk of birth defects	**Intervention setting:** Community **General level of the intervention:** Community-focused Social marketing and policy development	**Legal:** Warning labels	**Theoretical framework:** Can't tell **Frequency:** NR **Duration:** NR **Type of provider:** NR **Availability of a manual:** NR **Training of providers:** NR
Awopetu *et al.* [27]	Media public education campaign ("Be in the kNOw") Public education through mass media advertisement. Billboard and transit route posters, local newspapers, radio public service announcements, website. Content on negative consequences of alcohol consumption in pregnancy. Provision of resources for women who have alcohol dependency.	**Intervention setting:** Community **General level of the intervention:** Community-focused Social marketing	**Education:** Mass media Distribution of printed educational materials (e.g., fact sheets, posters)	**Theoretical framework:** Can't tell **Frequency:** NR **Duration:** NR **Type of provider:** Media **Availability of a manual:** NR **Training of providers:** NR

Table 3.F.1   *(Continued)*

Study	Type of intervention	Classification of the Intervention (Public Health Perspective)	Individual Components of the Intervention	Characteristics of the Intervention
Carr and Brand [31]	Media public education campaign Multimedia FASD campaign	**Intervention setting:** Community **General level of the intervention:** Community-focused Social marketing	**Education:** Mass media Multimedia materials	**Theoretical framework:** Health Promotion, Social Marketing, Communications and Instructional Design theory **Frequency:** NR **Duration:** NR **Type of provider:** Media **Availability of a manual:** NR **Training of providers:** NR
Ma [54]	Educational FAS-prevention program Community-based prevention program targeting 6th through 8th grade students (Multimedia FAS-prevention package, videos, computer-assisted technology, videotape to accompany a curriculum guide featuring 19 lessons with specific goals, project flyers, program brochure, World Wide Web page)	**Intervention setting:** School **General level of the intervention:** Community-focused Health teaching	**Education:** Distribution of printed educational materials (e.g., fact sheets, posters) School curriculum Audio-visual materials	**Theoretical framework:** Health communication process model **Frequency:** NR **Duration:** NR **Type of provider:** NR **Availability of a manual:** NR **Training of providers:** NR
Marin [55]	Health promotion messages Warning label on alcohol beverages about drinking during pregnancy	**Intervention setting:** Community **General level of the intervention:** Community-focused, system-level-focused Social marketing and policy development	**Legal:** Warning labels	**Theoretical framework:** Can't tell **Frequency:** NR **Duration:** NR **Type of provider:** NR **Availability of a manual:** NR **Training of providers:** NR

(Continued)

Table 3.F.1 (*Continued*)

Study	Type of intervention	Classification of the Intervention (Public Health Perspective)	Individual Components of the Intervention	Characteristics of the Intervention
May and Hymbaugh [58]	National Indian Fetal Alcohol Syndrome Prevention Program Macro-level FAS prevention program aimed at providing local people and communities with comprehensive knowledge, skills and materials to carry out prevention and intervention on their own.	**Intervention setting:** Community **General level of the intervention:** Community-focused Health teaching	**Education:** Distribution of printed educational materials (e.g. fact sheets, posters) School curriculum Audio-visual materials	**Theoretical framework:** Can't tell **Frequency:** NR **Duration:** 30–60 min/session **Type of provider:** Peers **Availability of a manual:** NR **Training of providers:** NR
Glik *et al.* [41]	Social marketing campaign (Narrowcasting) Social marketing intervention using a "narrowcasting" approach to raise awareness of the risks of drinking during pregnancy. Small posters and tear-off cards put in places youth frequent.	**Intervention setting:** Community **General level of the intervention:** Community-focused Social marketing	**Education:** Distribution of printed educational materials (e.g., fact sheets, posters)	**Theoretical framework:** Social marketing theory **Frequency:** NR **Duration:** NR **Type of provider:** Media/Printed materials **Availability of a manual:** NR **Training of providers:** NR
Walker *et al.* [72]	Brief intervention for prenatal alcohol use Education brochure (Facts About Fetal Alcohol Syndrome)	**Intervention setting:** Health facility **General level of the intervention:** Individual/family-focused Social marketing	**Education:** Distribution of printed educational materials (e.g., fact sheets, posters)	**Theoretical framework:** Can't tell **Frequency:** NA **Duration:** NR **Type of provider:** NR **Availability of a manual:** NR **Training of providers:** NR
Kaskutas *et al.* [48]	Alcohol beverage warning label Health messages on drinking during pregnancy (alcohol beverage container labels, point of sale signs, advertisements)	**Intervention setting:** Community **General level of the intervention:** Community-focused, system-level-focused Social marketing and policy development	**Education:** Mass media **Legal:** Warning labels	**Theoretical framework:** Can't tell **Frequency:** NR **Duration:** NR **Type of provider:** Media **Availability of a manual:** NR **Training of providers:** NR

Table 3.F.1 (*Continued*)

Study	Type of intervention	Classification of the Intervention (Public Health Perspective)	Individual Components of the Intervention	Characteristics of the Intervention
Kinzie et al. [49]	Prenatal alcohol educational multimedia program ("The Healthy Touch") Computer-based multimedia educational program that addresses alcohol use in pregnancy	**Intervention setting:** Health facility **General level of the intervention:** Individual/ family-focused Health teaching	**Education:** Motivational messages Computer-based education Audio-visual materials	**Theoretical framework:** Reasoned action and social learning theory **Frequency:** NR **Duration:** 20 min/ session **Type of provider:** Media **Availability of a manual:** NR **Training of providers:** NR

FAS = fetal alcohol syndrome; FASD = fetal alcohol spectrum disorder; FASTRAC = The Fetal Alcohol Spectrum Teaching and Research Awareness Campaign; NR = not reported.

Table 3.F.2 Characteristics of selective prevention interventions.

Study	Type of intervention	Classification of the Intervention (Public Health Perspective)	Individual Components of the Intervention	Characteristics of the Intervention
Floyd et al [40]	Project CHOICES Motivational interviewing brief intervention; counseling sessions, contraception consultation and services visit and information	**Intervention setting:** Health facility **General level of the intervention:** Individual/ family-focused Counseling	**Counseling and brief interventions:** Individual counseling	**Theoretical framework:** Transtheoretical model **Frequency:** Four sessions **Duration:** 45–60 min **Type of provider:** Counselors **Availability of a manual:** NR **Training of providers:** Yes
Armstrong et al. [26]	Brief intervention for prenatal alcohol use (Early Start Plus) Alcohol counseling, psychological support and prenatal care	**Intervention setting:** Health facility **General level of the intervention:** Individual/ family-focused Counseling	**Counseling and brief interventions:** Individual counseling	**Theoretical framework:** Can't tell **Frequency:** One **Duration:** 20–25 min **Type of provider:** Social worker, substance-abuse treatment providers **Availability of a manual:** NR **Training of providers:** NR

(*Continued*)

Table 3.F.2 *(Continued)*

Study	Type of intervention	Classification of the Intervention (Public Health Perspective)	Individual Components of the Intervention	Characteristics of the Intervention
Chang *et al.* [34]	Brief intervention for prenatal alcohol use, including the partner Single-session brief intervention enhanced by including a partner chosen by a pregnant women. Structure of the session: (1) knowledge assessment with feedback; (2) contracting and goal setting; (3) behavioral modification; (4) summary	**Intervention setting:** Health facility **General level of the intervention:** Individual/ family-focused Counseling	**Counseling and brief interventions:** Individual counseling	**Theoretical framework:** Can't tell **Frequency:** One session **Duration:** 25 min **Type of provider:** Nurse **Availability of a manual:** NR **Training of providers:** Yes
Chang *et al.* [33]	Brief intervention for prenatal alcohol use Comprehensive assessment of alcohol use and brief intervention; patient education and a self-help manual	**Intervention setting:** Health facility **General level of the intervention:** Individual/ family-focused Health teaching Counseling	**Education:** Alcohol-intake testing and counseling Motivational messages **Counseling and brief interventions:** Individual counseling	**Theoretical framework:** Can't tell **Frequency:** One session **Duration:** 45 min **Type of provider:** Doctor (Health provider) **Availability of a manual:** Yes **Training of providers:** NR
Fleming [39]	Brief alcohol intervention Alcohol counseling, psychological support	**Intervention setting:** Health facility **General level of the intervention:** Individual/ family-focused Counseling	**Counseling and brief interventions:** Individual counseling	**Theoretical framework:** Cognitive behavioral approach **Frequency:** Four sessions **Duration:** 15 min **Type of provider:** Obstetric nurses, research staff **Availability of a manual:** Yes **Training of providers:** Yes
Sobell [114]	Promoting Self Change (brief motivational intervention) Project CHOICES – Promoting Self Change (motivational materials targeting a number of health behaviors besides alcohol and contraception)	**Intervention setting:** Home **General level of the intervention:** Individual/ family-focused Health teaching	**Education:** Motivational messages No	**Theoretical framework:** Can't tell **Frequency:** NR **Duration:** NR **Type of provider:** Media/ Printed materials **Availability of a manual:** NR **Training of providers:** NR

Table 3.F.2 *(Continued)*

Study	Type of intervention	Classification of the Intervention (Public Health Perspective)	Individual Components of the Intervention	Characteristics of the Intervention
Crosby [36]	Cognitive-based health education Activated health education. Behavioral-based instructional model focused upon participants' involvement in defining awareness concepts and responsibility implementation.	**Intervention setting:** Health facility **General level of the intervention:** Individual/family-focused Health teaching	**Education:** Educational sessions (workshops) Motivational messages **Counseling and brief interventions:** Skills training	**Theoretical framework:** Activated Health Education Model **Frequency:** One session **Duration:** 50 min **Type of provider:** Health educator **Availability of a manual:** Yes **Training of providers:** Yes
Ingersoll et al. [47]	BALANCE program Motivational interviewing brief intervention. Personalized feedback and counseling on drinking and contraception	**Intervention setting:** School **General level of the intervention:** Individual/family-focused Counseling	**Counseling and brief interventions:** Individual counseling	**Theoretical framework:** Can't tell **Frequency:** One session **Duration:** 60–75 min **Type of provider:** NR **Availability of a manual:** Yes **Training of providers:** Yes
Palinkas et al. [66]	Project PALS Cognitive and behavioral skills training and education intervention (Facts of Life) Cognitive and behavioral techniques to improve social skills and to restructure social networks, and a normative education program that includes information on the hazards of drug use. Teaching sessions (group format) plus individual case sessions	**Intervention setting:** Health facility **General level of the intervention:** Individual/family-focused Case management Health teaching Counseling	**Education:** Educational sessions (workshops) **Counseling and brief interventions:** Case management Skills training Referral to available services	**Theoretical framework:** Cognitive behavioral approach **Frequency:** One weekly session for 16 weeks **Duration:** 90 min **Type of provider:** Multidisciplinary (Social workers and health educators) **Availability of a manual:** NR **Training of providers:** Yes
O'Connor and Whaley [64]	Brief intervention for prenatal alcohol use Counseling aimed at increasing awareness of the negative consequences of drinking, advice focused on identifying risky situations, actions aimed at reducing alcohol consumption and assistance with formulating drinking-reduction goals. Education, feedback, cognitive behavioral procedures, goal setting and contracting	**Intervention setting:** Health facility **General level of the intervention:** Individual/family-focused Screening Health teaching Counseling	**Counseling and brief interventions:** Individual counseling	**Theoretical framework:** Social cognitive theory **Frequency:** NR **Duration:** 10–15 min **Type of provider:** Nutritionist **Availability of a manual:** Yes **Training of providers:** Yes

(Continued)

Table 3.F.2 (Continued)

Study	Type of intervention	Classification of the Intervention (Public Health Perspective)	Individual Components of the Intervention	Characteristics of the Intervention
Reynolds *et al.* [67]	Cognitive-behavioral self-help intervention Self-help program to reduce alcohol consumption among pregnant women (10 min educational session and a nine-step self-help manual)	**Intervention setting:** Health facility and Home **General level of the intervention:** Individual/family-focused Health teaching	**Education:** Educational sessions (workshops) Motivational messages	**Theoretical framework:** Social cognitive theory **Frequency:** One session **Duration:** 10 min **Type of provider:** Health educator **Availability of a manual:** Yes **Training of providers:** Yes
Belizan *et al.* [28]	Health education (home visits) Health education consisting of: (1) reinforcement of social support network; (2) knowledge about pregnancy and delivery; (3) reinforcement of adequate health services utilization	**Intervention setting:** Home **General level of the intervention:** Individual/family-focused Health teaching	**Education:** Distribution of printed educational materials (e.g., fact sheets, posters)	**Theoretical framework:** Ecological model of social support **Frequency:** Four visits (22, 26, 30 and 34 weeks of gestation) **Duration:** NR **Type of provider:** Multidisciplinary (Social workers and obstetric nurses) **Availability of a manual:** Yes **Training of providers:** Yes
Eustace [38]	Supportive educative intervention Positive-teaching reinforcement education intervention about the dangers of alcohol consumption during pregnancy	**Intervention setting:** Health facility **General level of the intervention:** Individual/family-focused Health teaching	**Education:** Audio-visual materials	**Theoretical framework:** Social cognitive theory **Frequency:** One session **Duration:** 10 min **Type of provider:** Media **Availability of a manual:** NR **Training of providers:** NR
Sarvela and Ford [69]	ASPEN prenatal health education program Self-administered series of eight educational modules (one per each prenatal visit) completed by patients at the participating clinics while they waited to see a physician.	**Intervention setting:** Health facility **General level of the intervention:** Individual/family-focused Health teaching	**Education:** Educational sessions (workshops) Motivational messages	**Theoretical framework:** Can't tell **Frequency:** Eight sessions **Duration:** NR **Type of provider:** Media/Printed materials **Availability of a manual:** NR **Training of providers:** NR
Handmaker *et al.* [44]	Motivational interview **Description:** Motivational interviewing; brief intervention.	**Intervention setting:** Health facility or home **General level of the intervention:** Individual/family-focused Counseling	**Counseling and brief interventions:** Individual counseling	**Theoretical framework:** Can't tell **Frequency:** NR **Duration:** NR **Type of provider:** NR **Availability of a manual:** NR **Training of providers:** NR

Table 3.F.2   (*Continued*)

Study	Type of intervention	Classification of the Intervention (Public Health Perspective)	Individual Components of the Intervention	Characteristics of the Intervention
Eisen *et al.* [37]	PPWI treatment programs (a) Case management with provision or referral to individual and group counseling; or b) day treatment with direct provision of individual and group counseling services)	**Intervention setting:** Community **General level of the intervention:** Individual/ family-focused Referral and follow-up Case management Case finding Counseling	**Counseling and brief interventions:** Individual counseling Case management Support group Referral to available services	**Theoretical framework:** Can't tell **Frequency:** NR **Duration:** NR **Type of provider:** NR **Availability of a manual:** NR **Training of providers:** NR
Meberg [60]	Supportive counseling Structured interviews during pregnancy, including counseling focused on reduction of alcohol consumption and potential benefits to the fetus, and interview after delivery	**Intervention setting:** Health facility **General level of the intervention:** Individual/ family-focused Counseling Consultation	**Counseling and brief interventions:** Individual counseling	**Theoretical framework:** Can't tell **Frequency:** Two sessions **Duration:** 60 min **Type of provider:** Midwife **Availability of a manual:** NR **Training of providers:** NR
Mehl-Madrona [61]	Psychosocial prenatal intervention with endorsement and support by health care providers plus intrapartum labor support Psychosocial prenatal intervention for reducing substance use and perceived life stress: seven sessions dedicated to addressing fears, getting support, stress reduction, attachment to unborn child, preparation for birth and environmental awareness	**Intervention setting:** Health facility **General level of the intervention:** Individual/ family-focused Health teaching	**Education:** Educational sessions (workshops) Motivational messages	**Theoretical framework:** Social marketing theory **Frequency:** Seven sessions. One session every 2–3 weeks until week 36–40 of gestation **Duration:** NR **Type of provider:** Health educator **Availability of a manual:** NR **Training of providers:** Yes
Nilsen *et al.* [63]	Questionnaire-based alcohol counseling	**Intervention setting:** Health facility **General level of the intervention:** Individual/ family-focused Counseling	**Counseling and brief interventions:** Individual counseling	**Theoretical framework:** Can't tell **Frequency:** Two sessions **Duration:** 60–90 min **Type of provider:** Midwife **Availability of a manual:** NR **Training of providers:** NR

(*Continued*)

Table 3.F.2 (*Continued*)

Study	Type of intervention	Classification of the Intervention (Public Health Perspective)	Individual Components of the Intervention	Characteristics of the Intervention
Corrarino *et al.* [35]	Perinatal Outreach Project (home visits, counseling) Identification of women having an untreated alcohol or illicit drug problem; home visits, health education regarding pregnancy-related preventive health care, services of a substance abuse counselor, follow-up of needs; referral to community and social services as needed, referral to substance abuse treatment when the woman was ready; interdisciplinary-team case follow-up and evaluation	**Intervention setting:** Home **General level of the intervention:** Individual/family-focused Referral and follow-up Case management Screening Outreach Health teaching Counseling	**Education:** Alcohol-intake testing and counseling **Counseling and brief interventions:** Individual counseling Case management Referral to available services	**Theoretical framework:** Can't tell **Frequency:** Five to nine sessions (mean = 7) **Duration:** NR **Type of provider:** Multidisciplinary (Public health nurses + substance abuse counselor + interdisciplinary team) **Availability of a manual:** NR **Training of providers:** NR
Tavris [71]	PNCC Prenatal Care Coordination Program Assessment, preventive counseling and follow-up	**Intervention setting:** Health facility **General level of the intervention:** Individual/family-focused Screening Health teaching Counseling	**Counseling and brief interventions:** Individual counseling	**Theoretical framework:** Can't tell **Frequency:** NR **Duration:** NR **Type of provider:** Public health nurses **Availability of a manual:** NR **Training of providers:** NR
Yonkers [75]	Motivational interview + CBT Motivational interview and cognitive behavioral therapy delivered by non-behavioral health professionals	**Intervention setting:** Health facility **General level of the intervention:** Individual/family-focused Counseling	**Counseling and brief interventions:** Individual counseling	**Theoretical framework:** Cognitive behavioral approach **Frequency:** Six sessions **Duration:** 30 min **Type of provider:** Nurses, medical students **Availability of a manual:** NR **Training of providers:** Yes

Table 3.F.2 (*Continued*)

Study	Type of intervention	Classification of the Intervention (Public Health Perspective)	Individual Components of the Intervention	Characteristics of the Intervention
Larsson [51]	Screening and treatment of alcoholic pregnant women Structured interview for early detection of maternal alcohol abuse and referral to treatment for women with excessive alcohol consumption	**Intervention setting:** Health facility **General level of the intervention:** Individual/family-focused Referral and follow-up Screening Case finding Counseling	**Counseling and brief interventions:** Individual counseling Case management Referral to available services	**Theoretical framework:** Can't tell **Frequency:** NR **Duration:** NR **Type of provider:** Multidisciplinary (midwives, social workers) **Availability of a manual:** NR **Training of providers:** NR
Little *et al.* [52]	PHP education, screening and intervention program Public education, professional training, telephone information service, screening and counseling services, pregnancy outcome assessment	**Intervention setting:** Community **General level of the intervention:** Community-focused Referral and follow-up Screening Case finding Health teaching Counseling	**Education:** Mass media Distribution of printed educational materials (e.g., fact sheets, posters) **Counseling and brief interventions:** Individual counseling Support group Referral to available services	**Theoretical framework:** Can't tell **Frequency:** NR **Duration:** NR **Type of provider:** Multidisciplinary (nurse, certified alcoholism therapists) **Availability of a manual:** NR **Training of providers:** NR

ASPEN = Adolescent Substance Prevention Education Network; BALANCE = Birth Control and Alcohol Awareness: Negotiating Choices Effectively; NR = not reported; PALS = Positive Adolescent Life Skills; PHP = Pregnancy and Health Program; PNCC = prenatal counseling and supervision; PPWI = Pregnant and Postpartum Women and their Infant.

Table 3.F.3 Characteristics of indicated prevention interventions.

Study	Type of intervention	Classification of the Intervention (Public Health Perspective)	Individual Components of the Intervention	Characteristics of the Intervention
Loudenburg *et al.* [53]	Four-State FAS Consortium **Description:** Case management and home visit programs. Multifaceted intervention (intensive home visit/case management, motivational interviewing)	**Intervention setting:** Health facility + Home **General level of the intervention:** Individual/family-focused Referral and follow-up Case management Counseling Consultation	**Counseling and brief interventions:** Individual counseling Case management Skills training Support group Referral to available services	**Theoretical framework:** Health beliefs model **Frequency:** NR **Duration:** NR **Type of provider:** Multidisciplinary (NS) **Availability of a manual:** NR **Training of providers:** Yes
Hankin [45]	Brief intervention for prenatal alcohol use **Description:** Intensive brief intervention; counseling sessions that included reviewing the definition of a standard drink, helping the women set the goal of abstention or reduction of alcohol use, establishing limits on consumption, and teaching ways to slow down drinking	**Intervention setting:** Health facility **General level of the intervention:** Individual/family-focused Counseling	**Counseling and brief interventions:** Individual counseling	**Theoretical framework:** Cognitive behavioral approach **Frequency:** From 1 month postpartum to 13 months postpartum (four sessions) and booster sessions over a 5-year period **Duration:** NR **Type of provider:** Social worker **Availability of a manual:** NR **Training of providers:** NR

Table 3.F.3 (*Continued*)

Study	Type of intervention	Classification of the Intervention (Public Health Perspective)	Individual Components of the Intervention	Characteristics of the Intervention
Whiteside-Mansell *et al.* [74]	AR-CARES **Description:** Intensive outpatient program; treatment day, assistance in locating child care in the community, alcohol and drug use assessment, education and treatment, mental health assessment and referral, life skills assessment and development, group and individual counseling, parenting education and support, health services, health education, service coordination	**Intervention setting:** Health facility **General level of the intervention:** Individual/family-focused Referral and follow-up Health teaching Counseling Consultation	**Education:** Educational sessions (workshops) **Counseling and brief interventions:** Individual counseling Skills training Support group Referral to available services	**Theoretical framework:** Miller's self-in-relation theory **Frequency:** 4 1/2 h per day, 5 days per week **Duration:** NR **Type of provider:** Multidisciplinary (social worker, nurse practitioner, case managers, consultants in medicine, addictions, psychology and law/ethics) **Availability of a manual:** NR **Training of providers:** NR
Svikis *et al.* [70]	Counseling and support group **Description:** On-site support group for drug-abusing pregnant women. Sessions included discussions on how to avoid relapse, dangers of drugs to the fetus, mother's health needs, establishment of social support networks to avoid drug use, behavioral contracting for attendance to the sessions	**Intervention setting:** Health facility **General level of the intervention:** Individual/family-focused Counseling	**Counseling and brief interventions:** Skills training Support group	**Theoretical framework:** Can't tell **Frequency:** Once a week **Duration:** 60 min **Type of provider:** Substance abuse counselor **Availability of a manual:** NR **Training of providers:** NR

(*Continued*)

Table 3.F.3 (*Continued*)

Study	Type of intervention	Classification of the Intervention (Public Health Perspective)	Individual Components of the Intervention	Characteristics of the Intervention
Grant *et al.* [42]	PCAP **Description:**Home visitation; advocacy and case management to obtain alcohol and drug treatment and to stay in recovery; linking with comprehensive community resources	**Intervention setting:** Home **General level of the intervention:** Individual/family-focused Referral and follow-up Case management Advocacy	**Counseling and brief interventions:** Case management Skills training Referral to available services	**Theoretical framework:** Home visitation model **Frequency:** NR **Duration:** 1 h **Type of provider:** Public health nurses **Availability of a manual:** NR **Training of providers:** Yes
Halmesmaki [43]	Counseling, psychological support and prenatal care **Description:** Alcohol counseling, psychological support and prenatal care	**Intervention setting:** Health facility **General level of the intervention:** Individual/family-focused Counseling	**Counseling and brief interventions:** Individual counseling	**Theoretical framework:** Can't tell **Frequency:** First visit at 8–12 gestational week and then every 1–4 weeks **Duration:** NR **Type of provider:** Doctor (Obstetrician) **Availability of a manual:** NR **Training of providers:** NR
Masis and May [56]	FAS Prevention Project **Description:** Clinical assessment, community outreach and case management. Case management and support of women at risk of having a FASD-FAE child. Counseling, detoxification, individual and group alcohol treatment, follow-up, voluntary birth control	**Intervention setting:** Health facility **General level of the intervention:** Individual/family-focused Referral and follow-up Case management Counseling Consultation	**Counseling and brief interventions:** Individual counseling Case management Referral to available services	**Theoretical framework:** Can't tell **Frequency:** NR **Duration:** NR **Type of provider:** NR **Availability of a manual:** NR **Training of providers:** NR

Table 3.F.3   *(Continued)*

Study	Type of intervention	Classification of the Intervention (Public Health Perspective)	Individual Components of the Intervention	Characteristics of the Intervention
May *et al.* [57]	Case management **Description:** Case management and motivational interviewing	**Intervention setting:** Health facility **General level of the intervention:** Individual/ family-focused Case management Counseling	**Counseling and brief interventions:** Individual counseling Case management	**Theoretical framework:** Can't tell **Frequency:** NR **Duration:** NR **Type of provider:** Multidisciplinary (prevention and case managers) **Availability of a manual:** NR **Training of providers:** Yes
Rosett *et al.* [68]	Screening and supportive counseling **Description:** Counseling and treatment for pregnant problem drinkers: assess drinking patterns, evaluate psychopathology and strengths, explain effects of alcohol on the fetus, recognize pregnancy as a normal crisis, use mother's concern for unborn child to engage her in supportive psychotherapy, assist with real social problems, avoid use of disulfiram and other potential teratogens, withdraw alcohol gradually if tolerance was developed, plan aftercare before delivery	**Intervention setting:** Health facility **General level of the intervention:** Individual/ family-focused Case management Counseling	**Counseling and brief interventions:** Individual counseling Case management	**Theoretical framework:** Can't tell **Frequency:** Three or more sessions **Duration:** 30 min **Type of provider:** Multidisciplinary (psychiatrist, counselor) **Availability of a manual:** NR **Training of providers:** NR

AR-CARES = Arkansas Center for Addictions Research, Education, and Services; FAE = fetal alcohol effects; FAS = fetal alcohol syndrome; FASD = fetal alcohol spectrum disorder; NR = not reported; PCAP = Parent-Child Assistance Program.

Appendix 3.G: Methodological Quality of the Studies Included in the Review

Table 3.G.1 Methodological quality assessment of studies on universal prevention approaches to FASD.

Study	Intervention/Target population	Study results	Selection bias	Allocation bias	Confounders	Blinding	Data Collection Methods	Withdrawals/ Dropouts	Global Rating
LaChausse [50] CCT	FASTRAC Educational multimedia program / Broad public	Statistically significant results: Yes / Partial support of effectiveness of the intervention	Moderate	Strong	Weak	Moderate	Weak	Weak	Moderate
Calabro et al. [30] CCT	Health education materials / Pregnant women	Statistically significant results: No / Support effectiveness of the intervention	Weak	Strong	Weak	Weak	Weak	Weak	Weak
Waterson [73] CCT	Education prenatal information / Pregnant women	Statistically significant results: No / No conclusions regarding effectiveness of the intervention	Weak	Strong	Weak	Weak	Weak	Weak	Weak
Mengel et al. [62] Prospective analytical cohort study	Media public education campaign / Women of childbearing age	Statistically significant results: NR / Do not support effectiveness of the intervention	Moderate	Moderate	Weak	Weak	Weak	Weak	Weak
Mazis et al. [59] Retrospective analytical cohort study	Alcohol beverage warning label / Broad public	Statistically significant results: No / No conclusions regarding effectiveness of the intervention	Weak	Moderate	Weak	Weak	Weak	Weak	Weak

Study	Intervention	Population	Statistically significant results	Conclusion							
Casiro et al. [32] Retrospective analytical cohort study	Television public awareness campaign	Women of childbearing age	Statistically significant results: Yes	Support effectiveness of the intervention	Weak	Moderate	Weak	Moderate	Strong	Weak	Weak
Bowerman et al. [29] Retrospective analytical cohort study	Community-supported alcohol ban	Pregnant women	Statistically significant results: Yes	Support effectiveness of the intervention	Weak	Moderate	Weak	Moderate	Weak	Weak	Weak
Olsen et al. [65] Retrospective analytical cohort study	Health education campaign	Pregnant women	Statistically significant results: NR	Do not support effectiveness of the intervention	Strong	Moderate	Strong	Moderate	Weak	Weak	Weak
Hankin et al. [46] Interrupted time series	Alcohol beverage warning label	Pregnant women	Statistically significant results: No	No conclusions regarding effectiveness of the intervention	Moderate	Moderate	Weak	Weak	Weak	Weak	Weak
Awopetu et al. [27] Before-and-after study	Media public education campaign	Broad public	Statistically significant results: NR	No conclusions regarding the effectiveness of the intervention	Weak	Moderate	Weak	Weak	Weak	Weak	Weak
Carr and Brand [31] Before-and-after study	Multimedia FASD campaign	Broad public	Statistically significant results: NR	No conclusions regarding effectiveness of the intervention	Weak	Moderate	Weak	Weak	Weak	Weak	Weak

(Continued)

Table 3.G.1 *(Continued)*

Study	Intervention/Target population	Study results	Selection bias	Allocation bias	Confounders	Blinding	Data Collection Methods	Withdrawals/ Dropouts	Global Rating
Ma [54] Before-and-after study	Educational FAS prevention program	Statistically significant results: NR	Strong	Moderate	Weak	Weak	Weak	Strong	Weak
	Broad public	No conclusions regarding effectiveness of the intervention							
Marin [55] Before-and-after study	Health promotion messages	Statistically significant results: NR	Moderate	Moderate	Moderate	Moderate	Weak	Strong	Moderate
	Broad public	No conclusions regarding effectiveness of the intervention							
May and Hymbaugh [58] Before-and-after study	National Indian Fetal Alcohol Syndrome Prevention Program	Statistically significant results: Yes	Weak	Moderate	Weak	Weak	Strong	Strong	Weak
	Broad public	Support effectiveness of the intervention							
Glik et al. [41] Before-and-after study	Social marketing campaign	Statistically significant results: No	Weak	Moderate	Weak	Moderate	Weak	Weak	Weak
	Women of childbearing age	Do not support effectiveness of the intervention							

Study / design	Intervention	Population	Results							
Walker *et al.* [72] Before-and-after study	Brief intervention for prenatal alcohol use	Women of childbearing age	Statistically significant results: Yes; Support effectiveness of the intervention	Weak	Weak	Moderate	Moderate Strong	Strong	Weak	Weak
Kaskutas *et al.* [48] Before-and-after study	Alcohol beverage warning label	Pregnant women and women of childbearing age	Statistically significant results: NR; No conclusions regarding effectiveness of the intervention	Moderate	Moderate	Moderate	Moderate Weak	Weak	Weak	Weak
Kinzie *et al.* [49] Before-and-after study	Prenatal alcohol educational multimedia program	Pregnant women	Statistically significant results: NR; No conclusions regarding effectiveness of the intervention	Moderate	Moderate	Weak	Weak	Weak	Weak	Weak

CCT = controlled clinical trial; FAS = fetal alcohol syndrome; NR = not reported; FASTRAC = The Fetal Alcohol Spectrum Teaching and Research Awareness Campaign; RCT = randomized controlled trial.

Table 3.G.2 Methodological quality assessment of studies on selective prevention approaches to FASD.

Study	Intervention/Target population	Study results	Selection bias	Allocation bias	Confounders	Blinding	Data Collection Methods	Withdrawals/ Dropouts	Global Rating
Floyd et al. [40] RCT	Project CHOICES Women of childbearing age who consume alcohol	Statistically significant results: Yes Support effectiveness of the intervention	Weak	Strong	Strong	Moderate	Strong	Moderate	Moderate
Armstrong et al. [26] RCT	Brief intervention for prenatal alcohol use (Early Start Plus) Women at risk of an AEP	Statistically significant results: Yes Partial support to effectiveness of the intervention	Strong	Strong	Moderate	Weak	Weak	Weak	weak
Chang et al. [33] RCT	Brief intervention for prenatal alcohol use Women at risk of an AEP	Statistically significant results: No Do not support effectiveness of the intervention	Weak	Strong	Strong	Moderate	Strong	Strong	Moderate
Chang et al. [34] RCT	Brief intervention for prenatal alcohol use including the partner Women at risk of an AEP	Statistically significant results: No Support effectiveness of the intervention	Weak	Strong	Strong	Weak	Strong	Strong	Moderate
Fleming [39] RCT	Brief alcohol intervention Women at risk of an AEP	Statistically significant results: Yes Support effectiveness of the intervention	Strong	Strong	Strong	Strong	Strong	Strong	Strong

Study / Design	Intervention / Population	Results							
Sobel [114] RCT	Brief motivational intervention	NA (pending full publication by study authors. Sobel, M. 2010, pers. comm.)	NA (pending full publication by study authors. Sobel, M. 2010, pers. comm.)	NA (pending full publication by study authors. Sobel, M. 2010, pers. comm.)	NA (pending full publication by study authors. Sobel, M. 2010, pers. comm.)	NA (pending full publication by study authors. Sobel, M. 2010, pers. comm.)	NA (pending full publication by study authors. Sobel, M. 2010, pers. comm.)	NA (pending full publication by study authors. Sobel, M. 2010, pers. comm.)	NA (pending full publication by study authors. Sobel, M. 2010, pers. comm.)
Crosby [36] RCT	Cognitive-based health education; Pregnant women	Statistically significant results: No; Do not support effectiveness of the intervention	Weak	Strong	Strong	Moderate	Strong	Moderate	Moderate
Ingersoll *et al.* [47] CCT	Motivational interview (BALANCE); Women of childbearing age who consume alcohol	Statistically significant results: Yes; Support effectiveness of the intervention	Weak	Strong	Strong	Moderate	Strong	Moderate	Moderate
Palinkas *et al.* [66] CCT	Project PALS; Women of childbearing age who consume alcohol	Statistically significant results: No; Do not support effectiveness of the intervention	Moderate	Strong	Strong	Weak	Strong	Moderate	Moderate
O'Connor and Whaley [64] CCT	Brief intervention for prenatal alcohol use; Women at risk of an AEP	Statistically significant results: Yes; Support effectiveness of the intervention	Moderate	Strong	Strong	Weak	Moderate	Moderate	Moderate
Reynolds *et al.* [67] CCT	Cognitive-behavioral self-help intervention; Women at risk of an AEP	Statistically significant results: Yes; Support effectiveness of the intervention	Moderate	Strong	Strong	Weak	Weak	Strong	Moderate

(Continued)

Table 3.G.2 (*Continued*)

Study	Intervention/Target population	Study results	Selection bias	Allocation bias	Confounders	Blinding	Data Collection Methods	Withdrawals/Dropouts	Global Rating
Belizan et al. [28] CCT	Health education Pregnant women	Statistically significant results: No Do not support effectiveness of the intervention	Moderate	Strong	Weak	Weak	Moderate	Weak	Weak
Eustace [38] CCT	Supportive-educative intervention Pregnant women	Statistically significant results: Yes Partial support of effectiveness of the intervention	Moderate	Strong	Strong	Weak	Strong	Moderate	Moderate
Sarvela and Ford [69] CCT	ASPEN prenatal health education program Pregnant women	Statistically significant results: No Do not support effectiveness of the intervention	Weak	Moderate	Strong	Weak	Moderate	Strong	Weak
Handmaker et al. [44] CCT	Motivational interview Women at risk of an AEP	Statistically significant results: No Support effectiveness of the intervention	Weak	Strong	Strong	Moderate	Weak	Strong	Weak
Eisen et al. [37] Prospective analytical cohort study	PPWI treatment programs Women at risk of an AEP	Statistically significant results: Yes Support effectiveness of the intervention	Weak	Moderate	Weak	Moderate	Weak	Weak	Weak
Meberg [60] Prospective analytical cohort study	Supportive counseling Pregnant women	Statistically significant results: No Do not support effectiveness of the intervention	Moderate	Moderate	Strong	Weak	Weak	Strong	Weak

Study	Intervention	Participants	Statistically significant results		Support effectiveness						
Mehl-Madrona [61] Prospective analytical cohort study	Psychosocial prenatal intervention	Pregnant women	Statistically significant results: Yes	Weak	Support effectiveness of the intervention	Moderate	Strong	Moderate	Weak	Strong	Moderate
Nilsen et al. [63] Retrospective analytical cohort study	Questionnaire-based alcohol counseling	Pregnant women	Statistically significant results: No	Moderate	Do not support effectiveness of the intervention	Moderate	Weak	Weak	Strong	Moderate	Moderate
Corrarino et al. [35] Before-and-after study	Perinatal Outreach Project	Women at risk of an AEP	Statistically significant results: NR	Weak	Support effectiveness of the intervention	Moderate	Weak	Weak	Strong	Strong	Weak
Tavris [71] Before-and-after study	PNCC	Women at risk of an AEP	Statistically significant results: NR	Weak	Support effectiveness of the intervention	Moderate	Weak	Weak	Weak	Weak	Weak
Yonkers [75] Before-and-after study	Motivational interview + CBT	Women at risk of an AEP	Statistically significant results: NR	Weak	No conclusions regarding effectiveness of the intervention	Moderate	Weak	Weak	Weak	Strong	Weak
Larsson [51] Before-and-after study	Screening and treatment of alcoholic pregnant women	Pregnant women	Statistically significant results: No	Moderate	Partial support of effectiveness of the intervention	Moderate	Weak	Weak	Moderate	Weak	Weak
Little et al. [52] Before-and-after study	PHP	Pregnant women	Statistically significant results: Yes	Weak	No conclusions regarding effectiveness of the intervention	Moderate	Weak	Weak	Weak	Weak	Weak

ASPEN = Adolescent Substance Prevention Education Network; BALANCE = Birth Control and Alcohol Awareness: Negotiating Choices Effectively; CBT = cognitive behavioral therapy; CCT = controlled clinical trial; FAS = fetal alcohol syndrome; NR = not reported; PALS = Positive Adolescent Life Skills; PHP = Pregnancy and Health Program; PNCC = Prenatal Care Coordination Program; PPWI = Pregnant and Postpartum Women and their Infant; RCT = randomized controlled trial.

Table 3.G.3 Methodological quality assessment of studies on indicated prevention approaches to FASD.

Study	Intervention/Target population	Study Results	Selection Bias	Allocation Bias	Confounders	Blinding	Data Collection Methods	Withdrawals/ Dropouts	Global Rating
Loudenburg [53] CCT	Four-State FAS Consortium Women of childbearing age	Statistically significant results: NR No conclusions regarding effectiveness of the intervention	Weak	Strong	Strong	Moderate	Strong	Strong	Moderate
Hankin [45] CCT	Brief intervention for prenatal alcohol use Women at risk of an AEP	Statistically significant results: Yes Support effectiveness of the intervention	Moderate	Strong	Strong	Weak	Strong	Weak	Weak
Whiteside-Mansell et al. [74] Prospective analytical cohort study	AR-CARES Women at risk of an AEP	Statistically significant results: Yes Support effectiveness of the intervention	Weak	Moderate	Strong	Weak	Strong	Weak	Weak
Svikis et al. [70] Retrospective analytical cohort study	Counseling, support group Women at risk of an AEP	Statistically significant results: No Support effectiveness of the intervention	Weak	Moderate	Strong	Weak	Weak	Weak	Weak
Grant et al. [42] Before-and after study	PCAP Women at risk of an AEP	Statistically significant results: NR Support effectiveness of the intervention	Moderate	Moderate	Weak	Moderate	Weak	Moderate	Weak

Study	Intervention	Results							
Halmesmaki [43] Before-and-after study	Counseling, psychological support and prenatal care / Women at risk of an alcohol-exposed pregnancy	Statistically significant results: NR / No conclusions regarding effectiveness of the intervention	Weak	Moderate	Weak	Weak	Weak	Moderate	Weak
Masis and May [56] Before-and-after study	FAS Prevention Project / Women at risk of an AEP	Statistically significant results: NR / No conclusions regarding effectiveness of the intervention	Moderate	Moderate	Weak	Weak	Weak	Moderate	Weak
May et al. [57] Before-and-after study	Case management / Women at risk of an AEP	Statistically significant results: No / Partial support of effectiveness of the intervention	Moderate	Moderate	Weak	Weak	Weak	Weak	Weak
Rosett et al. [68] Before-and-after study	Screening and supportive counseling / Women at risk of an AEP	Statistically significant results: NR / No conclusions regarding effectiveness of the intervention	Weak	Moderate	Weak	Weak	Weak	Weak	Weak

AR-CARES = Arkansas Center for Addictions Research, Education and Services; CCT = controlled clinical trial; FAS = fetal alcohol syndrome; NR = not reported; PCAP = Parent-Child Assistance Program.

References

1 Sokol, R.J., Delaney-Black, V., and Nordstrom, B. (2003) Fetal alcohol spectrum disorder. *JAMA*, **290**, 2996–2999.

2 Astley, S.J. and Clarren, S.K. (2000) Diagnosing the full spectrum of fetal alcohol-exposed individuals: introducing the 4-digit diagnostic code. *Alcohol Alcohol.*, **35**, 400–410.

3 May, P.A. and Gossage, J.P. (2001) Estimating the prevalence of Fetal Alcohol Syndrome: a summary. *Alcohol Res. Health*, **25**, 159–167.

4 Institute of Medicine (1996) *Fetal Alcohol Syndrome: Diagnosis, Epidemiology, Prevention, and Treatment*, National Academy Press, Washington, DC.

5 Robinson, G.C., Conry, J.L., and Conry, R.F. (1987) Clinical profile and prevalence of fetal alcohol syndrome in an isolated community in British Columbia. *Can. Med. Assoc. J.*, **137** (3), 203–207.

6 Williams, R.J., Odaibo, F.S., and McGee, J.M. (1999) Incidence of fetal alcohol syndrome in northeastern Manitoba. *Can. J. Public Health*, **90** (3), 192–194.

7 Square, D. (1997) Fetal alcohol syndrome epidemic on Manitoba reserve. *Can. Med. Assoc. J.*, **157** (1), 59–60.

8 Asante, K.O. and Nelms-Maztke, J. (1985) *Report on the Survey of Children with Chronic Handicaps and Fetal Alcohol Syndrome in the Yukon and Northwest British Columbia*, Council for Yukon Indians, Whitehorse.

9 Alberta Children and Youth Services (2009) Fetal alcohol spectrum disorders. Government of Alberta. Available at: http://www.child.gov.ab.ca/home/594.cfm (accessed 2 April 2009).

10 Abel, E.L. and Sokol, R.J. (1987) Incidence of fetal alcohol syndrome and economic impact of FAS-related anomalies. *Drug Alcohol Depend.*, **19**, 51–70.

11 Abel, E.L. and Hannigan, J.H. (1995) Maternal risk factors in fetal alcohol syndrome: provocative and permissive influences. *Neurotoxicol. Teratol.*, **17**, 445–462.

12 Elliott, L., Coleman, K., Suebwongpat, A., and Norris, S. (2008) Fetal Alcohol Spectrum Disorders (FASD): systematic reviews of prevention, diagnosis and management. *HSAC Rep.*, **1** (9), i-535.

13 Toward Optimized Practice (TOP) (2007) *Physicians for Fetal Alcohol Spectrum Disorder Prevention*, Alberta Health and Wellness, Edmonton.

14 Institute of Medicine (1994) *Reducing Risks for Mental Disorders: Frontiers for Preventive Intervention Research*, National Academy Press, Washington, DC.

15 May, P.A., Gossage, J.P., Marais, A.S., Hendricks, L.S., Snell, C.L., Tabacnnick, B.G., *et al.* (2008) Maternal risk factors for fetal alcohol syndrome and partial fetal alcohol syndrome in South Africa: a third study. *Alcohol. Clin. Exp. Res.*, **32** (5), 738–753.

16 FASD Service networks (2007) Fetal Alcohol Spectrum Disorder Cross-Ministry Committee. Available from: http://www.fasd-cmc.alberta.ca/home/serviceNetworks.cfm (accessed 2 Apr 2009).

17 Hankin, J.R. (2002) Fetal alcohol syndrome prevention research. *Alcohol Res. Health*, **26**, 58–65.

18 National Institute on Alcohol Abuse and Alcoholism (2000) *Tenth Special Report to the U.S. Congress on Alcohol and Health*, Department of Health and Human Services, Washington, DC.

19 Waterson, E.J. and Murray-Lyon, I.M. (1990) Preventing alcohol related birth damage: a review. *Soc. Sci. Med.*, **30** (3), 349–364.

20 Schorling, J.B. (1993) The prevention of prenatal alcohol use: a critical analysis of intervention studies. *J. Stud. Alcohol*, **54** (3), 261–267.

21 Anonymous (2001) The problem of multiple publication. *Bancolier*, **91**, 91–96.

22 Bailey, B.J. (2002) Duplicate publication in the field of otolaryngology-head and neck surgery. *Arch. Otolaryngol.*, **126**, 211–216.

23 Tramer, M.R., Reynolds, D.J.M., Moore, R.A., and McQuay, H.J. (1997) Impact of covert duplicate publication on meta-analysis; a case study. *Br. Med. J.*, **315**, 635–640.

24 Huston, P. and Moher, D. (1996) Redundancy, disaggregation, and the integrity of medical research. *Lancet*, **347**, 1024–1026.

25 The Cochrane Collaboration (2008) *The Cochrane Handbook for Systematic Reviews of Interventions Version 5.0.0* (updated February 2008). The Cochrane Collaboration.

26 Armstrong, M.A., Kaskutas, L.A., Witbrodt, J., Taillac, C.J., Hung, Y.Y., Osejo, V.M., *et al.* (2009) Using drink size to talk about drinking during pregnancy: a randomized clinical trial of Early Start Plus. *Soc. Work Health Care*, **48** (1), 90–103.

27 Awopetu, O., Brimacombe, M., and Cohen, D. (2008) Fetal alcohol syndrome disorder pilot media intervention in New Jersey. *Can. J. Clin. Pharmacol.*, **15** (1), e124–e131.

28 Belizan, J.M., Barros, F., Langer, A., Farnot, U., and Victora, C., and Villar, J., on behalf of the Latin American Network for Perinatal and Reproductive Research (1995) Impact of health education during pregnancy on behavior and utilization of health resources. *Am. J. Obstet. Gynecol.*, **173** (3 Pt 1), 894–899.

29 Bowerman, R.J. (1997) The effect of a community-supported alcohol ban on prenatal alcohol and other substance abuse. *Am. J. Public Health*, **87** (8), 1378–1379.

30 Calabro, K., Taylor, W.C., and Kapadia, A. (1996) Pregnancy, alcohol use and the effectiveness of written health education materials. *Patient Educ. Couns.*, **29** (3), 301–309.

31 Carr, T. and Brand, L.E. (2007) Assessing the public's knowledge of FASD: the impact of a multimedia campaign. *Can. J. Clin. Pharmacol.*, **14** (3), e317.

32 Casiro, O.G., Stanwick, R.S., Pelech, A., and Taylor, V. (1994) Public awareness of the risks of drinking alcohol during pregnancy: the effects of a television campaign. Child Health Committee, Manitoba Medical Association. *Can. J. Public Health*, **85** (1), 23–27.

33 Chang, G., Wilkins-Haug, L., Berman, S., and Goetz, M.A. (1999) Brief intervention for alcohol use in pregnancy: a randomized trial. *Addiction*, **94** (10), 1499–1508.

34 Chang, G., McNamara, T.K., Orav, E.J., Koby, D., Lavigne, A., Ludman, B., *et al.* (2005) Brief intervention for prenatal alcohol use: a randomized trial. *Obstet. Gynecol.*, **105** (5 Pt 1), 991–998.

35 Corrarino, J.E., Williams, C., Campbell, W.S., III, Amrhein, E., LoPiano, L., and Kalachick, D. (2000) Linking substance-abusing pregnant women to drug treatment services: a pilot program. *J. Obstet. Gynecol. Neonatal Nurs.*, **29** (4), 369–376.

36 Crosby, F.S. (1986) The effects of a fetal alcohol education intervention upon the knowledge, attitude and behavior of pregnant women in a health maintenance organization. Dissertation, State University of New York, Buffalo, New York.

37 Eisen, M., Keyser-Smith, J., Dampeer, J., and Sambrano, S. (2000) Evaluation of substance use outcomes in demonstration projects for pregnant and postpartum women and their infants: findings from a quasi-experiment. *Addict. Behav.*, **25** (1), 123–129.

38 Eustace, L.W. (2000) *Fetal Alcohol Syndrome Prevention: Affecting Maternal Alcohol Consumption Behavior through Nurse Supportive-Educative Intervention*, University of Alabama, Birmingham, AL.

39 Fleming, M. (2007) Healthy Moms alcohol intervention. Available at: www.ClinicalTrials.gov (accessed 2 April 2010).

40 Floyd, R.L., Sobell, M., Velasquez, M.M., Ingersoll, K., Nettleman, M., Sobell, L., *et al.* (2007) Preventing alcohol-exposed pregnancies: a randomized controlled trial. *Am. J. Prev. Med.*, **32** (1), 1–10.

41 Glik, D., Halpert-Schilt, E., and Zhang, W. (2001) Narrowcasting risks of drinking during pregnancy among African American and Latina adolescent

girls. *Health Promot. Pract.*, **2** (3), 222–232.

42 Grant, T.M., Ernst, C.C., Streissguth, A., and Stark, K. (2005) Preventing alcohol and drug exposed births in Washington state: intervention findings from three parent-child assistance program sites. *Am. J. Drug Alcohol Abuse*, **31** (3), 471–490.

43 Halmesmaki, E. (1988) Alcohol counselling of 85 pregnant problem drinkers: effect on drinking and fetal outcome. *Br. J. Obstet. Gynaecol.*, **95** (3), 243–247.

44 Handmaker, N.S., Miller, W.R., and Manicke, M. (1999) Findings of a pilot study of motivational interviewing with pregnant drinkers. *J. Stud. Alcohol*, **60** (2), 285–287.

45 Hankin, J.R. (2003) *Protecting the Next Pregnancy: Maternal Drinking and Infant Developmental Outcomes*, American Sociological Association, pp. 1–14.

46 Hankin, J.R., Firestone, I.J., Sloan, J.J., Ager, J.W., Sokol, R.J., and Martier, S.S. (1996) Heeding the alcoholic beverage warning label during pregnancy: multiparae versus nulliparae. *J. Stud. Alcohol*, **57** (2), 171–177.

47 Ingersoll, K.S., Ceperich, S.D., Nettleman, M.D., Karanda, K., Brocksen, S., and Johnson, B.A. (2005) Reducing alcohol-exposed pregnancy risk in college women: initial outcomes of a clinical trial of a motivational intervention. *J. Subst. Abuse Treat.*, **29** (3), 173–180.

48 Kaskutas, L.A., Greenfield, T., Lee, M.E., and Cote, J. (1998) Reach and effects of health messages on drinking during pregnancy. *J. Health Educ.*, **29** (1), 11–20.

49 Kinzie, M.B., Schorling, J.B., and Siegel, M. (1993) Prenatal alcohol education for low-income women with interactive multimedia. *Patient Educ. Couns.*, **21** (1-2), 51–60.

50 Lachausse, R.G. (2008) The effectiveness of a multimedia program to prevent fetal alcohol syndrome. *Health Promot. Pract.*, **9** (3), 289–293.

51 Larsson, G. (1983) Prevention of fetal alcohol effects. An antenatal program for early detection of pregnancies at risk. *Acta Obstet. Gynecol. Scand.*, **62** (2), 171–178.

52 Little, R.E., Young, A., Streissguth, A.P., and Uhl, C.N. (1984) Preventing fetal alcohol effects: effectiveness of a demonstration project. *Ciba Found. Symp.*, **105**, 254–274.

53 Loudenburg, R. (2003) A multifaceted intervention strategy for reducing substance use in high-risk women. *Neurotoxicol. Teratol.*, **25** (6), 737–744.

54 Ma, G.X. (1998) Fetal Alcohol Syndrome among Native American adolescents: a model prevention program. *J. Prim. Prev.*, **19** (1), 43–55.

55 Marin, G. (1997) Changes across 3 years in self-reported awareness of product warning messages in a Hispanic community. *Health Educ. Res.*, **12** (1), 103–116.

56 Masis, K.B. and May, P.A. (1991) A comprehensive local program for the prevention of fetal alcohol syndrome. *Public Health Rep.*, **106** (5), 484–489.

57 May, P.A., Miller, J.H., Goodhart, K.A., Maestas, O.R., Buckley, D., Trujillo, P.M., *et al.* (2008) Enhanced case management to prevent fetal alcohol spectrum disorders in Northern Plains communities. *Matern. Child Health J.*, **12** (6), 747–759.

58 May, P.A. and Hymbaugh, K.J. (1989) A macro-level fetal alcohol syndrome prevention program for Native Americans and Alaska Natives: description and evaluation. *J. Stud. Alcohol*, **50** (6), 508–518.

59 Mazis, M.B., Morris, L.A., and Swasy, J.L. (1991) An evaluation of the alcohol warning label – initial survey results. *J. Public Policy Mark.*, **10** (1), 229–241.

60 Meberg, A. (1986) Moderate alcohol consumption – Need for intervention programs in pregnancy? *Acta Obstet. Gynecol. Scand.*, **65** (8), 861–864.

61 Mehl-Madrona, L.E. (2000) Psychosocial prenatal intervention to reduce alcohol, smoking and stress and improve birth outcome among minority women. *J. Prenat. Perinat. Psychol. Health*, **14** (3-4), 257–278.

62 Mengel, M.B., Ulione, M., Wedding, D., Jones, E.T., and Shum, D. (2005)

Increasing FASD knowledge by a targeted media campaign: outcome determined by message frequency. *J. FAS Int.*, **3**, e13.

63 Nilsen, P., Holmqvist, M., Bendtsen, P., Hultgren, E., and Cedergren, M. (2010) Is questionnaire-based alcohol counseling more effective for pregnant women than standard maternity care? *J. Women's Health*, **19** (1), 161–167.

64 O'Connor, M.J. and Whaley, S.E. (2007) Brief intervention for alcohol use by pregnant women. *Am. J. Public Health*, **97** (2), 252–258.

65 Olsen, J., Frische, G., Poulsen, A.O., and Kirchheiner, H. (1989) Changing smoking, drinking, and eating behaviour among pregnant women in Denmark. Evaluation of a health campaign in a local region. *Scand. J. Soc. Med.*, **17** (4), 277–280.

66 Palinkas, L.A., Atkins, C.J., Miller, C., and Ferreira, D. (1996) Social skills training for drug prevention in high-risk female adolescents. *Prev. Med.*, **25** (6), 692–701.

67 Reynolds, K.D., Coombs, D.W., Lowe, J.B., Peterson, P.L., and Gayoso, E. (1995) Evaluation of a self-help program to reduce alcohol consumption among pregnant women. *Int. J. Addict.*, **30** (4), 427–443.

68 Rosett, H.L., Weiner, L., and Edelin, K.C. (1983) Treatment experience with pregnant problem drinkers. *JAMA*, **249** (15), 2029–2033.

69 Sarvela, P.D. and Ford, T.D. (1993) An evaluation of a substance abuse education program for Mississippi delta pregnant adolescents. *J. Sch. Health*, **63** (3), 147–152.

70 Svikis, D., McCaul, M., Feng, T., Stuart, M., Fox, M., and Stokes, E. (1998) Drug dependence during pregnancy: effect of an on-site support group. *J. Reprod. Infant Psychol.*, **43** (9), 799–805.

71 Tavris, D. (2000) Evaluation of a pregnancy outcome risk reduction program in a local health department. *Wis. Med. J.*, **99** (2), 47–57.

72 Walker, D.S., Fisher, C.S., Sherman, A., Wybrecht, B., and Kyndely, K. (2005) Fetal alcohol spectrum disorders prevention: an exploratory study of women's use of, attitudes toward, and knowledge about alcohol. *J. Am. Acad. Nurse Pract.*, **17** (5), 187–193.

73 Waterson, E.J. (1990) Preventing fetal alcohol effects; A trial of three methods of giving information in the antenatal clinic. *Health Educ. Res.*, **5** (1), 53–61.

74 Whiteside-Mansell, L., Crone, C.C., and Conners, N.A. (1999) The development and evaluation of an alcohol and drug prevention and treatment program for women and children. The AR-CARES program. *J. Subst. Abuse Treat.*, **16** (3), 265–275.

75 Yonkers, K.A. (2009) A treatment for substance abusing pregnant women. *Arch. Women's Ment. Health*, **12** (4), 221–227.

76 Public Health Nursing Section (2001) *Public Health Interventions: Applications for Public Health Nursing Practice.* Minnesota Department of Health, St Paul, MN. Available at: http://www.health.state.mn.us/divs/cfh/ophp/resources/docs/phinterventions_manual2001.pdf (accessed 2 December 2010).

77 Bull, L.B., Kvigne, V.L., Leonardson, G.R., Lacina, L., and Welty, T.K. (1999) Validation of a self-administered questionnaire to screen for prenatal alcohol use in Northern Plains Indian women. *Am. J. Prev. Med.*, **16** (3), 240–243.

78 Floyd, R.L., Ebrahim, S.H., Boyle, C.A., and Gould, D.W. (1999) Observations from the CDC. Preventing alcohol-exposed pregnancies among women of childbearing age: the necessity of a preconceptional approach. *J. Women's Health Gender-Based Med.*, **8** (6), 733–736.

79 Parkes, T., Poole, N., Salmon, A., Greaves, L., and Urquhart, C. (2008) *Double Exposure: A Better Practices Review on Alcohol Interventions during Pregnancy*, Centre of Excellence for Women's Health, Vancouver, BC.

80 Masotti, P., George, M.A., Szala-Meneok, K., Morton, A.M., Loock, C., Van Bibber, M., *et al.* (2006) Preventing fetal alcohol spectrum disorder in aboriginal communities: a methods

development project. *PLoS Med.*,
3 (1), e8.

81 Macmillan, H.L., Walsh, C.A.,
Jamieson, E., Faries, E.J., McCue, H.,
MacMillan, A.B., *et al.* (2003) The
health of Ontario First Nations people:
results from the Ontario First Nations
Regional Health Survey. *Can. J. Public
Health*, **94** (3), 168–172.

82 Segal, B. (1998) Drinking and
drinking-related problems among
Alaska natives. *Alcohol Health Res.
World*, **22** (4), 276–280.

83 MacMillan, H.L., and MacMillan, A.B.
(1996) Aboriginal health. *Can. Med.
Assoc. J.*, **155** (11), 1569–1578.

84 Burd, L. (1994) Epidemiology of fetal
alcohol syndrome in American Indians,
Alaskan Natives, and Canadian
aboriginal peoples: a review of the
literature. *Public Health Rep.*, **109** (5),
688–693.

85 May, P.A. (1995) Prevention of alcohol
misuse: a review of health promotion
efforts among American Indians. *Am. J.
Health Promot.*, **9** (4), 288–299.

86 Tait, C. (2004) *Fetal Alcohol Syndrome
and Fetal Alcohol Effects: The "Making" of
A Canadian Aboriginal Health and Social
Problem*, McGill University, Montreal.

87 Smylie, J. (2001) A guide for health
professionals working with Aboriginal
peoples: health issues affecting
Aboriginal peoples. *J. Soc. Obstet.
Gynaecol. Can.*, **100**, 54–68.

88 Leff, S.S., Hoffman, J.A., and Lakin
Gullan, R. (2009) Intervention integrity:
new paradigms and applications. *Sch.
Ment. Health*, **1**, 103–106.

89 Dane, A.V. and Schneider, B.H. (1998)
Program integrity in primary and early
secondary prevention: are
implementation effects out of control?
Clin. Psychol. Rev., **18**, 23–45.

90 Bellg, A.J., Borrelli, B., Resnick, B.,
Hecht, J., Minicucci, D.S., Ory, M., *et
al.* (2004) Treatment Fidelity
Workgroup of the NIH Behavior
Change Consortium. Enhancing
treatment fidelity in health behavior
change studies: best practices and
recommendations from the NIH
Behavior Change Consortium. *Health
Psychol.*, **23** (5), 443–451.

91 Chudley, A.E., Conry, J., Cook, J.L., and
Loock, C. (2005) Fetal alcohol spectrum
disorder: Canadian guidelines for
diagnosis. *Can. Med. Assoc. J.*, **172**, S1.

92 Piantadosi, S. (2005) *Clinical Trials: A
Methodological Perspective*, 2nd edn,
John Wiley & Sons, Inc., Hoboken,
New Jersey.

93 Murphy-Brennan, M.G. and Oei, T.P.
(1999) Is there evidence to show that
fetal alcohol syndrome can be
prevented? *J. Drug Educ.*, **29** (1), 5–24.

94 Juni, P., Altman, D.G., and Mathhias,
E. (2001) Assessing the quality of
randomised controlled trials, in
*Systematic Reviews in Health Care:
Meta-Analysis in Context*, 2nd edn (eds
M. Egger, G. Davey Smith, and D.G.
Altman), British Medical Journal,
London.

95 Moher, D., Jadad, A.R., Nichol, G.,
Penman, M., Tugwell, P., and Walsh, S.
(1995) Assessing the quality of
randomized controlled trials: an
annotated bibliography of scales and
checklists. *Control. Clin. Trials*, **16**,
62–73.

96 West, S., King, V., Carey, T.S., Lohr,
K.N., McKoy, N., Sutton, S.F., *et al.*
(2002) Systems to Rate the Strength of
Scientific Evidence. Evidence Report/
Technology Assessment No. 47. AHRQ
Publication no. 02-E016. Agency for
Healthcare Research and Quality,
Rockville, MD.

97 Juni, P., Witschi, A., Bloch, R., and
Egger, M. (1999) The hazards of scoring
the quality of clinical trials for
meta-analysis. *JAMA*, **282**, 1054–1060.

98 Thomas, H., Ciliska, D., Dobbins, M.,
and Micucci, S. (2004) A process for
systematically reviewing the literature:
providing the research evidence for
public health nursing interventions.
Worldviews Evid.-Based Nurs., **2**, 91–99.

99 Deeks, J.J., Dinnes, J., D'Amico, R.,
Sowden, A.J., Sakarovitch, C., Song, F.,
et al. (2003) Evaluating non-randomised
intervention studies. *Health Technol.
Assess.*, **7** (1), iii–x and 1–173.

100 Easterbrook, P.J., Berlin, J.A., Gopalan,
R., and Matthews, D.R. (1991)
Publication bias in clinical research.
Lancet, **337**, 867–872.

101 Moher, D., Pham, B., and Klassen, T.P. (2000) What contributions do languages other than English make on the results of meta-analyses? *J. Clin. Epidemiol.*, **53**, 964–972.

102 Juni, P., Holenstein, F., Sterne, J., Barlett, C., and Egger, M. (2002) Direction and impact of language bias in meta-analyses of controlled trials: empirical study. *Int. J. Epidemiol.*, **31**, 115–123.

103 Society for Prevention Research (2003) *Standards of Evidence: Criteria for Efficacy, Effectiveness and Dissemination*, Society for Prevention Research, Falls Church, VA.

104 Flay, B., Biglan, A., Boruch, R.F., Gonzalez Castro, F., Gottfredson, D., Kellam, S., *et al.* (2005) Standards of evidence: criteria for efficacy, effectiveness and dissemination. *Prev. Sci.*, **6** (3), 151–175.

105 Boutron, I., Moher, D., Altman, D.G., Schulz, K., and Ravaud, P., for the CONSORT group (2008) Methods and processes of the CONSORT Group: example of an extension for trials assessing nonpharmacologic treatments. *Ann. Intern. Med.*, **148** (4), W60–W67.

106 Von Elm, E., Altman, D.G., Egger, M., Pocock, S.J., Gøtzsche, P.C., Vanderbroucke, J.P., *et al.* (2008) Strengthening the Reporting of OBservational studies in Epidemiology (STROBE) statement: guidelines for reporting observational studies. *J. Clin. Epidemiol.*, **61** (4), 344–349.

107 Higgins, J.P.T. and Green, S. (2008) *Cochrane Handbook for Systematic Reviews of Interventions*, John Wiley & Sons, Ltd, Chichester, UK.

108 Mulrow, C.D., Cook, D.J., and Davidoff, F. (1997) Systematic reviews: critical links in the great chain of evidence. *Ann. Intern. Med.*, **126**, 389–391.

109 Jadad, A.R., Moore, R.A., Carroll, D., Jenckinson, C., Reynolds, D.J., Gavaghan, D.J., *et al.* (1996) Assessing the quality of reports of randomized clinical trials: is blinding necessary? *Control. Clin. Trials*, **17** (1), 1–12.

110 Deeks, J., Altman, D.G., and Bradburn, M.J. (2001) Statistical methods for examining heterogeneity and combining results from several studies in meta-analysis, in *Systematic Reviews in Health Care: Meta-analysis in Context*, 3rd edn (eds M. Egger, G.D. Smith, and D.G. Altman), BMJ Publishing Group, London, pp. 285–312.

111 Higgins, J.P.T., Thompson, S.G., Deeks, J., and Altman, D.G. (2003) Measuring inconsistency in meta-analyses. *Br. Med. J.*, **327**, 557–560.

112 Greenland, S. (1994) A critical look at some popular meta-analysis methods. *Am. J. Epidemiol.*, **140**, 290–296.

113 Dwyer, T., Couper, D., and Walter, S.D. (2001) Sources of heterogeneity in the meta-analysis of observational studies: the example of SUDS and sleeping position. *J. Clin. Epidemiol.*, **54**, 440–447.

114 Sobell, L.C. (2009) A Media-based motivational intervention to prevent alcohol-exposed pregnancies (AEPs). Nova Southeastern University. Available at: www.ClinicalTrials.gov (accessed 2 December 2010).

115 Glik, D., Prelip, M., Myerson, A., and Eilers, K. (2008) Fetal alcohol syndrome prevention using community-based narrowcasting campaigns. *Health Promot. Pract.*, **9** (1), 93–103.

4

Five Perspectives on Prevention of FASD

Lola Baydala, Robin Thurmeier, June Bergman, Nancy Whitney, and Amy Salmon

This chapter contains speeches delivered at the IHE 2009 Consensus Development Conference on "Fetal Alcohol Spectrum Disorder FASD–Across the life span" (available at: www.ihe.ca). They are reprinted from the Proceedings of that conference, with the permission of the authors and the IHE.

4.1
Pre-Conception Initiatives

Lola Baydala, *Associate Professor of Pediatrics, University of Alberta*
   The questions I have been asked to address are: How can FASD be prevented? Are there evidence-based pre-conception initiatives? I am going to focus specifically on school-based substance-use prevention programs, using an example to illustrate how we can move research in this area into practice.
   In 2008, the Public Health Agency of Canada published a summary of Canadian perspectives on FASD prevention, developed after consultation with Canadian experts in the field. This summary outlines four levels of prevention:

- The first level is raising general public awareness through broad strategies, including public policies and health-promotion activities that engage people at the community level. Examples of level one strategies would be information sheets, media campaigns, or booklets that are distributed to the general public.

- Level two strategies focus on women of childbearing age and their support networks. These strategies involve a collaborative discussion of alcohol use and its risks. Examples of level two strategies include programs that train physicians and other healthcare workers in substance-use prevention counseling.

- Level three prevention strategies include specialized perinatal programs that provide care and treatment for women who are using alcohol during their pregnancy.

Prevention of Fetal Alcohol Spectrum Disorder FASD: Who is Responsible?, First Edition. Edited by Sterling Clarren, Amy Salmon, Egon Jonsson.
© 2011 Wiley-VCH Verlag GmbH & Co. KGaA. Published 2011 by Wiley-VCH Verlag GmbH & Co. KGaA.

- Level four strategies involve long-term supports to enable new mothers to maintain whatever healthy changes they have already been able to make in their alcohol use during their pregnancy.

School-based substance-use prevention programs are pre-conception FASD initiatives that encompass both level one and level two strategies of prevention. School programs incorporate discussions about substance use and its risks, and provide children and youth with the knowledge and skills they need to resist substance use. The most effective programs incorporate three levels of knowledge: resistance skills training, which helps kids say no when they are in the vulnerable position of being encouraged by their peers to use substances; social and personal self-management skills, which help to support a child's self-esteem; and factual information about the risks of drug and alcohol use. There is strong evidence to support the effectiveness of school-based programs when knowledge in all three of these areas is included.

A review of school-based substance-use prevention programs can be found on the National Registry of Evidence-based Programs and Practices developed by the U.S. Department of Health and Human Services. This registry is a searchable database of evidence-based interventions for the prevention and treatment of both mental health and substance-use disorders across all ages. The registry regularly updates a report of evidence-based programs, which includes information about each intervention, its targeted outcomes, the research to support its effectiveness, and whether or not that intervention is at an appropriate stage of development for broad dissemination. The National Registry also rates the quality of the research to support the interventions. They do this using six indicators: the reliability and validity of the measures that were used in the research; intervention fidelity (was the program delivered in the way it was supposed to be delivered?); missing data and attrition (was there missing data or participant dropout that affected the results?); potential confounding factors; and the appropriateness of the analysis used. The registry asks independent reviewers to evaluate the quality of the research using these six indicators for every intervention that is available, and they assign a score between zero and four for each indicator, with the highest possible score being four.

Based on this evidence, and on an independent review of school-based substance-use prevention programs completed by a team of researchers at the University of Alberta, the Life Skills Training (LST) program developed by Dr Botvin at the Institute for Prevention Research at Cornell University has been found to be the most effective school-based substance-use prevention program available. The LST program has been evaluated in more than 30 scientific studies, most of which were randomized trials involving over 330 schools and 26 000 students in urban, suburban, and rural communities. Ratings of the quality of the research to support this intervention have consistently been between 3.9 and 4.0, which is the highest possible rating. Broad dissemination of the program began in 1995, and since then an estimated 50 000 teachers in 10 000 schools involving over 3 000 000 students in 32 countries have participated in the program. The LST program is an evidence-based generic program and, as mentioned, has been found by a number of different program providers to be highly effective with students from different geographic regions and different socioeconomic, racial and ethnic backgrounds. However, despite the overwhelming success of the program, it has never been evaluated with Canadian Aboriginal children and youth, and its effectiveness in this population is not known.

The Alexis Nakota Sioux Nation is a community of approximately 1500 people situated about 100 kilometers west of Edmonton. In 2005, the community invited researchers from the University of Alberta to adapt, deliver, and evaluate the effectiveness of the LST program in their community. The goals of the community were to review and adapt the program to ensure that it incorporated their language, visual images, and cultural teachings; to evaluate the effectiveness of the modified program; to make sure that the fidelity of the program was maintained after the adaptations were completed; and to restore and preserve their Isga culture. To achieve these goals, the Alexis Working Committee was established. This committee included community members as well as academic members from the University of Alberta. As a first step, terms of reference were developed that described the roles and responsibilities of each committee member. The committee successfully applied for funding to adapt, implement and evaluate the program, and a band council resolution and letters of community support were obtained. In addition to the working committee, an adaptations committee was established. The adaptations committee includes community members, school personnel and elders who attend each meeting.

Over a period of two years, the committees met on a regular basis and completed adaptations to the program, which included Alexis Nakota Sioux teachings, such as ceremonies, prayers, storytelling, and personal life stories, the Alexis Isga language, Isga artists' graphics and pictures, as well as drawings submitted by students who attend the Alexis Nakota Sioux Nation School.

Previous research has shown that cultural adaptations can significantly improve engagement and acceptability of a prevention intervention. Furthermore, I believe that there is an ethical imperative to ensure that interventions developed by one culture do not negatively impact the cultural values, competence, or language of another culture where the program will be delivered. Research has also shown that those who participate in culturally adaptive programs are able to relate more closely to the curricula and engage in the program. We know that culturally adaptive programs aid in the development of a stronger identity and cultural pride, which in turn function as protective factors against substance use. And a community that is involved in the adaptation and implementation of a prevention program is more likely to feel a sense of ownership and empowerment, both of which are critical first steps in creating social change.

The Alexis Nakota Sioux Nation School is attended by children from kindergarten to grade nine. During the 2008 school year, the first level of the three-year adapted program was successfully delivered to students at the school by a community program provider. After the first year of the program, pre- and post-program questionnaires showed positive changes in students' knowledge and attitudes towards drug and alcohol use and significant growth in their social skills. Talking circles, or focus groups, also showed ownership of and investment in the program, teaching approaches that correspond with the learning context, world views and relationships of the community, and participation of the community elders.

We were also able to document substantial growth in community capacity, using the Public Health Agency of Canada's Community Capacity Building tool. This tool measures nine areas of community capacity: community participation and leadership; the acquisition of community structures; external supports; asking why, which is getting to the root causes of why substance use occurs in the community in the first place; obtaining resources; community skills knowledge and learning; academic skills, knowledge and learning – there is definitely an academic component of capacity building that occurred; and linking with others in sense of community.

My summary and recommendations are as follows: Since highly effective evidence-based substance-use prevention programs for school-aged children and youth exist, these programs should be made available to all school-aged children, both Aboriginal and non-Aboriginal, as a part of their regular curriculum. Where appropriate, the programs should be adapted to incorporate the cultural beliefs, values, language and visual images of the community where the program will be delivered. And, to ensure community ownership of and investment in the program, adaptations and implementations should involve a community-based participatory approach.

4.2
Inventory of Primary Prevention Campaigns

Robin Thurmeier, *FASD Resources Researcher, Saskatchewan Prevention Institute*

We developed an inventory of FASD primary prevention resources across northwestern Canada in order to discover the scope of primary prevention activities and to explore the outcomes of those that have been evaluated. We completed an environmental scan to create an inventory of existing projects and to identify gaps and successes. For the purposes of our project, we used the primary prevention definition provided by the Canadian Center of Substance Abuse, which defines primary prevention as community efforts to protect health by increasing knowledge and awareness of a particular health problem.

Resources were included in our inventory if they had a focus on primary prevention, if they provided information about FASD, and if they were developed for use within northwestern Canada. The resources could be part of a larger awareness campaign strategy, or they could be produced independently of a strategy (for example, a one-off resource that organizations produced specifically for their communities). FASD stakeholders across northwestern Canada were contacted and asked to provide any resources they had developed and any evaluations done on those resources. We also searched the websites of relevant organizations across

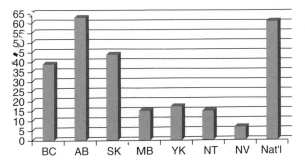

Figure 4.1   Resources Collected by Region.

Canada to find their current materials. In total, 262 resources were collected. Figure 4.1 shows the distribution across the provinces (Ontario resources are shown separately, but also included in the national bar).

We decided to include one campaign from Ontario in our inventory, the Be Safe campaign developed by Best Start. It included an evaluation component and was similar to many of the campaigns developed across northwestern Canada, such as This is Our Baby from the Yukon, and Alcohol and Pregnancy from British Columbia.

The inventory includes print resources, such as posters and brochures; multi-media resources, such as public service announcements videos and DVDs; and novelties, such as pins, coasters, bookmarks, and so on. The resources are used to inform their intended audience about FASD. Women-specific messages provided specific messages to women about how they can avoid alcohol abuse during pregnancy. Community and family-specific messages provide family and friends and community members with information about how to help prevent FASD. The key message across all of these resources is that alcohol consumption during pregnancy can harm the fetus. Targeted audiences included women, youth, friends, Aboriginal cultures, professionals, and the general public.

We found only four campaign evaluations. These were evaluations of the Born Free campaign from Alberta Children's Services, the Mother Kangaroo campaign from the Saskatchewan Prevention Institute, the With Child, Without Alcohol campaign from the Manitoba Liquor Control Commission, and the Be Safe campaign that I mentioned earlier. All of the evaluations showed an increase in awareness and knowledge about what FASD is, what causes FASD, and the ways FASD can be prevented. General awareness post-campaign was at least 90% across each of the campaigns that were evaluated. While print resources were the most numerous, multimedia resources were most often recalled by the public. The evaluations show that each campaign was successful in increasing awareness and knowledge of FASD; however, little is known about actual behavioral change. For example, the post-campaign evaluation of the Saskatchewan campaign showed that only 44% of respondents indicated that they had supported a woman's choice not to drink. There were only two questions in the entire survey asking if the respondent had supported past attempts to decrease drinking alcohol during pregnancy. While awareness campaigns generally do not contain a behavioral change component, this change is obviously a desired outcome of these campaigns. Many women continue to drink during pregnancy, and half of the pregnancies in Canada are still unplanned.

We are now looking at social marketing to address these behaviors. Social marketing may offer a tool for creating behavioral change, particularly in identifying and targeting groups at risk. Basford *et al.* [1] identified five target groups that could benefit from social marketing strategies being developed for them. These include women who may drink during pregnancy, women who might be pregnant but do not realize it, youth, partners and friends, and healthcare professionals. This framework also incorporates theory to help understand behavior, provides strategies for adopting new behaviors and reduces barriers to the desirable behavior, while providing opportunity for new behaviors and promoting the new behaviors as attractive alternatives.

Providing a framework to explore the reasons why people engage in harmful behaviors is key to creating effective campaigns. A behavioral change model needs to be employed to guide the creation of materials and interventions that will bring about the desired behavioral change, and to develop evaluation tools to better understand whether the intended outcomes are occurring. One model that we found to be effective, and which we recommend for future FASD campaigns, is the Protection Motivation Theory model. This model suggests that motivation to select positive behavior is maximized when the threat is viewed as particularly severe. The social, monetary and physical costs of making the change must be relatively small, and the people need to feel confident in their abilities to make the change.

Here are some recommendations on prevention and awareness campaigns:

1) An effective evaluation strategy is crucial, as it provides the tools for measuring outcomes, regular feedback to keep objectives on track, and a clear plan for future campaign development. It also provides other organizations with information helpful in developing and improving their campaigns. The evaluation process takes time to develop and implement, so it is advisable to begin prior to development of the campaign.

2) A behavioral change model should be incorporated into campaign design to guide the preventative strategies and to measure and explain any behavioral change that occurs. Each intended audience needs a targeted message with images and types of media that will engage them. A behavioral change model will help you understand what behavioral change is occurring, what specific groups need to know, how they can learn this information, and how they will move forward with a change. It also helps create a strong research-based precedent to assist in obtaining future funding and to ensure successful outcomes of future primary prevention campaigns.

3) Community engagement is important, as community partners and stakeholders can assist with campaign development and evaluation. Ensuring that you

have representation from each of your target groups will create a sense of ownership in the campaign and improve its chances of success, as they can help develop meaningful messages delivered by the most effective modes of communication for each group.

4.3
Primary Care Physician Perspective

June Bergman, *Associate Professor, Department of Family Medicine, Faculty of Medicine and Dentistry, University of Calgary*

Primary healthcare is the provision by clinicians of integrated, accessible healthcare services that address a large majority of personal healthcare needs and develops partnerships with patients within the context of family and community. Primary healthcare also has another dimension, one of looking at the determinants of health and the creation of community capacity. We know from the work of Barbara Starfield and others that a good, strong primary care system improves the health of the community, and is highly cost effective. Some 90% of all contacts with the healthcare system are in primary care, which means that primary care is the opportune setting in which to provide interventions to patients. However, we do not always take advantage of this opportunity.

Since the 1950s, primary care has been based on the following principles of family medicine: it is relationship-based, community-based and resourced in the community, and it has a strong focus on clinical excellence. One way to describe it is that primary care cares for the whole person as situated in the family and the community over time. Primary care is concerned about prevention, the identification of disease or risk factors, treating acute disease, supporting people, and opening doors to secondary and tertiary care.

Many organizations in Canada have created guidelines to identify and treat individuals who have FASD or are at risk of drinking during pregnancy. All are agreed that prevention is the area in which we should focus our efforts. The Canadian Task Force on the Periodic Health Exam has recommended that case finding, counseling and follow-up are effective. This is not a Level A recommendation because the evidence to support it is not available; but, as clinicians, we believe this to be a good recommendation. Other experts agree. A joint statement by the Canadian Pediatric Society and 17 co-signatories recommends prevention efforts that target women, their partners, their families and their communities before and during childbearing years. The College of Family Physicians recommends that primary care physicians be involved in screening for alcohol use during pregnancy, referral for diagnosis, follow-up and linking patients to community resources. In Alberta, a group called Toward Optimized Practice (TOP) has developed a clinical practice guideline on the prevention of FASD, most recently revised in 2005. This particular guideline divides prevention into three areas: Primary prevention advocates abstinence from alcohol during pregnancy in order to prevent FASD; secondary prevention tries to help women who drink while pregnant, in order to reduce harm to the fetus; and tertiary prevention looks at mitigating the harm to an affected individual.

What barriers do we face in providing effective screening for FASD? Little research has been done on barriers to screening specifically for FASD, but the literature on prevention and screening in general divides the issues into provider issues, system issues, and patient issues. The provider issues are likely obvious: a lack of training is a common one, although the TOP program tries to address this by helping primary care offices to implement quality-improvement activities. But training and knowledge is very often the least of the problems. Providers also face a lack of time, often due to business models of patient care that leave little time for screening. Clinicians know what they could do, but do not have the ability to do it at that particular time. Another provider issue is the uncertainty about where to get help if screening is done and a problem is found. Clinicians need to have contacts, to be able to draw upon a broad range of health professionals and skills. Providers also face personal discomfort in bringing this issue up with their patients, or in their ability to provide services in this area. System issues are short-ages of resources, such as qualified, public-funded counselors, or a lack of access to such resources. Patient issues include feeling stigmatized by the diagnosis and failing to comply with treatment because they lack understanding or are not con-vinced that it is the correct treatment.

Primary care reform is underway across Canada, and in recent years every province and territory has shifted the way they are providing primary care. Three provinces – Alberta, Ontario and Quebec – have moved into a partnership with physician networks, and the other provinces are in varying stages of the process. They have been more focused on a primary healthcare model looking at determi-nants of health and community development. All jurisdictions are looking at shifting their focus from responsibility for caring for individuals to responsibility for populations. They are looking more closely at who is receiving care and who is not. They are also thinking more about preventative screening – for example, a patient may have come in for her cold, but it may be an opportune time to do a cervical screen or mammogram as well. There is also a move to multidisciplinary teams that vary with the needs of the communities they serve. These can include nurses, occupational therapists, physiotherapists, dieticians, and so on. An impor-tant underpinning of each model is information management and technology, which provides a means of sharing information and improving the continuity of patient support. The underlying choice for people is another focus, and improving access is a strong indicator in all. Primarily, we are looking at ways of providing 24/7 access to care and of addressing the unattached element – that is, the many people in Canada who do not have a family doctor at present.

The new models take many different forms. There is *shared care*, where primary care physicians partner with specialists, other healthcare professionals, or other programs already in existence. There is *team-based care*, with improved access to mental health professionals. This approach can play an important role in FASD prevention, because a large part of the prevention we can do in primary care is to recognize families and individuals of chaos (that is, people who have high-risk behaviors). In my own primary care office, I have a behavioral therapist and I can get people in to see this person within a week. Some of models emphasize the colocation of teams, which is also helpful because we can learn so much from each other. Primary care offices are also now able to partner inside and outside of the health system in ways we never could before. For example, the primary care network that I am a part of is partnering directly with pediatricians in Calgary in the Kids in Care program. Kids are accepted into care in one of our chronic disease clinics, where they have access to pediatricians and ongoing care, but with the intention of moving them eventually to a primary care provider.

The role of primary care in FASD has several facets. First, our role is very much about prevention. New primary care models are giving us the ability to do more anticipatory counseling and early identification with primary, secondary, and tertiary prevention. In the area of treatment, we see people at a young age when they can be referred to specialists in order to receive early interventions. Our longitudinal relationships with patients enable us to support both individuals and families within the community. When an individual in a family has a problem, other family members often have their own issues and need support and coping techniques. Primary care also enables individuals to remain in their communities, as we are able to monitor them over the long term.

These are some of the strengths of primary care that can lead to successful partnerships in addressing any complex condition, but particularly FASD. First, primary care is good at maintaining continuous relationships with patients. This is a key benefit that primary care providers offer to the healthcare system. Primary care maintains a community focus and keeps people in the communities in which they have lived all their lives rather than institutionalizing them. Team-based primary care provides a wider range of skills and supports, and the multidisciplinary partnerships that we now have the organizational structure to enter into will provide some of the best intersectoral care in complex issues like FASD.

4.4
Mentoring Programs for At-Risk Mothers

Nancy Whitney, *Clinical Director, King County Parent–Child Assistance Program, University of Washington, US*

I am here to talk about mentoring programs for mothers at risk and, specifically, the Parent–Child Assistance Program (PCAP), which originated at the University of Washington in 1991. We talked yesterday about risky behaviors and the populations that are at most risk of having children with FAS. These are the mothers that we work with. The problem is maternal alcohol and drug use during pregnancy. It puts those children at risk for health effects that will last for the rest of their lives, and it puts them at risk for compromised home environments. Poverty, domestic violence, and untreated mental health problems are all factors that create a less than desirable home environment for children to grow up in. Without intervention, there is a very real possibility that these mothers will continue to have drug- and alcohol-affected children. These problems are very expensive to our society, both in actual dollars and, for lack of a better phrase, in injury to the soul. These families are hurting, and these problems are completely preventable.

PCAP started in 1991 as a federal-funded research program in Seattle. It has since acquired state funding for expansion into nine Washington counties and has been replicated all over the United States. Many sites here in Canada are based on the PCAP model, one of them being the First Steps program here in Edmonton. This program is evidence-based. I will talk about outcomes and how we measure whether or not we are doing a good job.

The primary goal of the program is to prevent the future births of children that are affected by drugs and alcohol. Simply put, not so easily done. This is an intensive three-year home visitation program. The staff who do this work are what we would call para-professionals – that is, we do not hire licensed social workers, we do not hire chemical-dependency professionals, and we do not hire nurses. We hire women who have some life experience that puts them a little closer to these clients and allows them to come to work with a little extra compassion for what these women face in their daily lives. We call it a *home-visitation program*. That is a bit of a misnomer, because in the very beginning of our work many of the clients do not have homes. The more accurate way to express it would be to say that we go where they are – if that is a street corner, a shelter, or a treatment center, that's where we go. I tell my clients, "We're going to stalk you for three years." And they believe that, eventually.

The enrollment criteria are very simple. A woman is eligible if she is pregnant or up to six months postpartum, has heavily used drugs or alcohol during the pregnancy, and is not successfully engaged with community service providers. This is a little subjective, so the way I explain it to social workers and people who recommend the program is that if you can give this woman a "to-do" list and she will do it, or an appointment card and she will keep the appointment, she is not a PCAP mom. A PCAP mom is the one who loses the card in the next five minutes, calls you several times to get the information again, and still does not show up.

Some basic characteristics of our clients are as follows. The average age is 26; most are not married; by the time we meet them, most have two children and are likely not to be caring for either of them. They have not completed high school; they are likely to be homeless; they are unemployed; they are on welfare as their main source of income; and they have been to jail at least once. As my boss, Dr Grant, is very fond of saying, these women are the children we are trying to prevent. For 90% of them, one or both parents were substance abusers. So a significant number of the moms that I work with are probably fetal alcohol-affected and have probably gone their entire lives without diagnosis or help. The majority have reported physical or sexual abuse, or both, during childhood. Many of them have been in foster care. What is rather scary to me is that although almost 90% of them were raised in substance-abusing households, only 25% were likely to have been removed. This means that a significant number of them stayed in those substance-abusing households for the duration of their childhood. Not surprisingly, 67% of them ran away from that household as a child.

At least half of them report at least some alcohol use during pregnancy. At least 25% of them report binge alcohol use, which we know is the most dangerous drinking pattern for FAS. They are also poly-substance abusers (methamphetamine 58%, cocaine 34%, heroin12%, marijuana 52%, tobacco 79%).

The PCAP intervention is a two-pronged approach. I have talked about the experience that the advocates bring to the job. The other important aspect of the advocate is that she is very well trained and closely supervised. We do not just throw these mentors out into the field. To do this work, they need a great deal of help and support and we make sure that they get that.

The advocates have two jobs. The first one is to work with the client and her family, which includes whoever is in the woman's circle. It may be her children; it may be her mother; it may be her boyfriend. We try to engage everyone in her circle in the process of her recovery, even if that means offering them services or connecting them to services in the community. The second job is to work with the community providers. You saw our earlier slide saying, "When case management isn't enough." That was the title of the original article. The reason it was called that is that these women had case managers, they had CPS [Child Protective Services] workers, they had welfare workers, they had probation officers, they had public health nurses, and still the problematic behavior continued. They were slipping through the cracks. So our job at PCAP is to work with those providers to keep an eye on what they are doing with her and asking her to do. If the chemical dependency counselor tells her to go to group three times a week and the social worker says to do visitation three times a week and they happen to be at the same time, these moms are not very good at advocating for themselves and saying, "I can't be at two places at once" or "How do I do this?" or "Can somebody try to switch the schedule?" So they pick one and they fail at the other. Our job is to keep an eye on those things and keep her on track. This is a comment from one of our advocates demonstrating where they come from:

> I know what it's like to be a single parent, homeless, and on welfare. I share a common ground with my clients as far as those things go. The difference is that I saw what the obstacles were and overcame them. I just kept moving ahead and learned that where there's a will, there's a way.

PCAP is a model of effective case management. We tailor the program to the individual. There is no curriculum that says that on visit one you do this and on visit two you do that—it is based on the individual woman's situation and needs. We promote competency in the individual. It is very much strength-based. We believe that the relationship between the advocate and client is the key to effective change. We actually believe, although we will never be able to measure it, that it might be that relationship—the first positive, unconditional relationship that they may have had in their lives—that is more crucial in change than any service that we may connect them to. Somebody standing behind them and saying, "You can do this, and I'm going to help you," is what we really think will make the biggest difference. It is very family-centered, community-based and multidisciplinary.

This is how we try to envision what we do. Mom is in the middle and the inner circle is everyone who is important to her and who we are going to try to engage in the process. An important part of this is what we do with the kids. PCAP moms are not the greatest parents, because they did not have the greatest parents. So when we are doing our home visitation, we are modeling parenting. We are sitting on the floor and talking to the kids, we are doing tummy time, we are encouraging bonding and attachment just by role modeling. We are also keeping an eye on those children. Is this child fetal alcohol-exposed? What are the developmental milestones we are going to look for and how are we going to get that child into early assessment and early intervention if it appropriate to do so? And then there are all the community providers on the outside.

PCAP does have a theoretical framework. The first of the three theories on which we base our model is Relational Theory, the idea that women must have a positive relationship in order to effect change. The second is Stages of Change: where is she in making those changes in her life? She may be at several different stages, depending on the problems. She may be in contemplation or action for chemical dependency, but she may be in pre-contemplation for domestic violence and family planning. And, finally, Harm Reduction. She is not going to get to the exact place we want her to be today, but we are going to keep working with her to make incremental changes and keep using motivational interviewing to move her along. These three theoretical foundations and our identified core components (which I did not bring today) are the basis and defining features of PCAP. If you want to call your organization PCAP, these are the things that you must base your model on. On the other hand, PCAP tries to be very responsive to the unique needs of its community. Within the state of Washington, we have 11 sites. They are in urban areas, in rural areas and on Native American reservations. And each team approaches their work as they need to in order to engage in that community.

Our formula for preventing alcohol- and drug-exposed births is to motivate women to stop drinking before and during pregnancy and to help women who cannot stop drinking to avoid becoming pregnant by using family planning.

We have a great deal of data on the outcomes of the program and have published three studies. Beyond that, we do ongoing program evaluation every six months and report that to our funder. Here are some of our three-year outcomes. Some 96% of our clients in the state of Washington have completed in-patient or out-patient treatment, or are in progress of treatment; 49% have been clean at least six months, and many of them more than six months at graduation. And 84% of them have been clean and sober at least six months during the program. We have numbers for people who go through the whole three years clean and sober, and for people who have two years clean and sober. They are excellent recovery rates.

One of the other outcomes that we keep an eye on is the family planning. About 7% of our clients are using family planning when they enroll in our program, and 68% are using it on exit. And 61% are choosing a reliable method, such as the pill or the patch. Only 12% of our clients have a subsequent substance-exposed birth. The reduced risks for subsequent alcohol and drug exposed births is 76% – that represents the women who are not going to have another exposed child, because they are either using reliable family planning or are clean and sober, or both.

Some other recovery-related outcomes are in employment, housing, and education. At graduation, 37% of clients have employment as their main source of income; and whereas 72% were on welfare when they started, only 37% are on welfare at the end. Also, 74% are in permanent housing and 72% have attended or are enrolled in a training or education program. I won't read them all, but these are very good outcomes. They show that over the three years these women really do start turning their lives around, from chaos to stability.

Outcomes translate to cost effectiveness. We can look at cost effectiveness on an individual basis, or we can look at it across a program. Here is an individual example. This mom had a warrant out that she forgot about and she got picked up. The offense was something like check forgery and they wanted to send her to prison for a year-and-a-half. She was clean and sober, she had custody of her child, and she had housing. If they had sent her to prison, it would have undone all of that and it would have cost us $18 000 to place her child in foster care for that time and $50 000 just for prison itself. We convinced the court to put her on home electronic monitoring instead, which would allow her to continue her treatment and continue to parent her child. The cost of electronic monitoring was $6500 per year. We saved the state of Washington over $62 000 by helping with that change.

A study by the Washington State Institute for Public Policy looked at more long-term cost savings for the kids down the road. They specifically looked at several evidence-based home visitation programs, including PCAP. They found that for every dollar spent on PCAP or similar programs, $2.27 was saved in the long run by keeping kids out of incarceration and other specialized services.

The big outcome, however, is in preventing future alcohol-exposed births. Without PCAP, 78 of the moms in a particular cohort were heavy drinkers and about 23 of them could have gone on to have another exposed pregnancy. By helping these women to stop drinking or to use family planning, or both, we reduced that by 66%, preventing about 15 alcohol-exposed births. Based on the estimated 4.7% to 21% incidence of FAS births among heavy drinkers, we think that PCAP prevented one to three cases of FAS. We talked before about the average lifetime cost of one kid with FAS being 1.5 million dollars. So, if we prevent just one mother from having another alcohol-exposed pregnancy then we have funded PCAP for 102 women.

PCAP does not achieve good outcomes because we do all the work ourselves. We have good policies and we have good support systems in our community. One thing that has been key for us is that Washington State has continually supported treatment for women. We have 153 beds in Washington where women can go for treatment for six months and take their children with them. Not having their children with them is the number one reason why women will say they cannot go to treatment. We took that excuse away, and that is why we have a 96% success rate engaging women in treatment.

At every three-year interview, we ask clients what they think about the program. Here are some quotes:

There were times when I felt like I was going to relapse and my advocate would be there for me and she would keep checking on me and I'd get through it. I learned so much about myself and how to be responsible again and being a good mother. It was all what she taught me and she changed my life.

I never thought about goals. They showed me the right direction. They showed me that I am responsible. That no matter who I am or what I do, I am somebody. It's never too late.

Pictures speak louder than anything. This is a "before" picture, and an "after" picture.

My recommendations are to support intensive case-management programs with the highest-risk mothers in the community, and to support specialized treatment centers for women where they can go and take their children with them.

PCAP Studies Cited

Ernst, C.C., Grant, T.M., Streissguth, A.P., and Sampson, P.D. (1999) Intervention with high-risk alcohol and drug-abusing mothers: II. Three-year findings from the Seattle model of paraprofessional advocacy. *J. Community Psychol.*, **27** (1), 19–38.

Grant, T., Ernst, C.C., Pagalilauan, G., and Streissguth, A.P. (2003) Post-program follow-up effects of paraprofessional intervention with high-risk women who abused alcohol and drugs during pregnancy. *J. Community Psychol.*, **31** (3), 211–222.

Grant, T., Ernst, C., Streissguth, A., and Stark, K. (2005) Preventing alcohol and drug exposed births in Washington State: Intervention findings from three Parent-Child Assistance Program sites. *Am. J. Drug Alcohol Abuse*, **31** (3), 471–490.

4.5
Strength and Support: A Women's Perspective

Amy Salmon, *Managing Director, Canada Northwest FASD Research Network; Clinical Assistant Professor, School of Population and Public Health, Faculty of Medicine, University of British Columbia*

My presentation is going to encourage us to shift our focus from FASD prevention as a children's health issue – and a health issue that extends for those children across their lives – to consider what it means to address FASD prevention from a women's health perspective. I by no means want to suggest that we look only at children's health or only at women's health in order to do good FASD-prevention work. Rather, I want to try to balance our conversation by noting that we talk a great deal about mothers' drinking behavior when we talk about FASD, but women's health often slips away from the conversation. I am going to focus on some of the structural factors that sometimes frustrate our ability to address FASD prevention more broadly as a women's health issue. Nancy Poole will then present some of the solutions to these frustrating challenges that have been put in place across Canada. Specifically, we will focus on some of the work of the Canada Northwest FASD Research Network.

In Canada, our approach to FASD prevention is largely centered on children's health. When we look more broadly at care for women during pregnancy, which is of course crucial to FASD-prevention work, we tend to think about such care from a social determinants health framework. We do that because it is an evidence-based approach and alcohol does seem to have a greater teratogenic potential in the presence of what are sometimes called "permissive or provocative cofactors." Most broadly, we talk about low socioeconomic status as one of those indications.

We think about the health of women in pregnancy because we assume that healthy women have healthy babies. But what produces health for women? In addition to biological factors and genetic endowment, we look at social determinants of health. In the report "What Determines Health?"–which many of us use to guide our work–the Public Health Agency of Canada has enumerated social determinants of health to include income and social status, social support networks, education, employment and working conditions, social environments, personal health practices, healthy child development, culture, and gender. All of these factors are important when we think about FASD prevention. However, it is important to note that social determinants of health have been very unevenly supported by governments across Canada in the development of policy and programs. In one study that looked at this very closely, Jim Frankish and colleagues at the University of British Columbia surveyed all of the health regions in Canada to examine how nonmedical (or social) determinants of health are being addressed. They found that we have invested a great deal in child development and personal health practices–and by personal health practices we mean specific actions that people take to make themselves healthier. The majority of health regions report making those investments, both within their systems and through intersectoral activities that include partners outside of the healthcare system. However, culture, gender, employment, and working conditions, which are of course closely linked to income and social status, have received the least attention in most regions. This is a problem for us in FASD prevention, because we recognize very clearly that culture, gender, income, social status, and the potential for engaging meaningfully in employment, are very important in supporting not only women's health but also the health of their children and families across the life course.

We know that women who give birth to children with FASD are the ones most likely to have their own health and well-being compromised by addictions and mental health problems, including diagnosed psychiatric disorders, very high stress levels, depression and anxiety, and extensive experiences of trauma, grief, and loss. We know that these women's lives are impacted by violence, by isolation, by poverty, and by a lack of social support and care before, during and after their pregnancy. The complexity of these issues demands a coordinated response and approach to care, and the Parent-Child Assistance Program (PCAP) models give us an example of how we can do that when we have a strong infrastructure to make that possible.

Unfortunately, women who require such care are often bounced around programs and systems, and many of the services that respond to these issues remain soiled. We see a great deal of this with women who are at risk for having a child with FASD. A woman goes to an addictions treatment center to try to address her substance use, and the addictions treatment center says, "Sorry, we also note that you have a bipolar one diagnosis, so you're going to have to go over to mental health services before we can treat you for addiction." Mental health services says, "Sorry you have to be clean and sober before you can come to mental health services." In the meantime, she is getting beaten up daily by her partner at home and she needs somewhere safe to go. When she goes to the transition house, they say, "We'll be glad to take you if you're not using substances and you get some treatment for your bipolar disorder." Eventually, these women are bounced out of the systems entirely and we lose many opportunities to provide them with the care they need.

We have talked a great deal about shame and blame, and have acknowledged that the lives of birth mothers and children with FASD are imbued with shame and blame at a fundamental level. Shame comes from many places, including women's knowing that they should not drink when they are pregnant, and yet lacking the support they need to keep from doing what we often refer to as "hurting your baby" – as though this is something they do on purpose. Blame often comes from a woman's acknowledgment that her children have disabilities or are experiencing problems at school or in the community that are attributable to her substance use. When we think about what this means for prevention, we have to think about the fact that most of our prevention approaches have remained grounded in blame and shame – not just on an interpersonal level in interactions between women and individual service providers, but also at a societal level. These approaches to FASD prevention have been shown repeatedly to be ineffective at reducing drinking among the highest-risk groups, and result in many missed opportunities for providing supportive care.

I have the tremendous honor of being able to do my research in Vancouver's Downtown Eastside, where I work with women who are teaching me a great deal about what it means to do good FASD-prevention work at the primary, secondary, and tertiary levels. One of the things that I have learned is that FASD as a diagnosis is different from other kinds of diagnoses, because it is rooted very much in shame and blame.

Here is an example from one study. Super Woman is a young woman who is raising her child, aged about seven years. The mother managed to keep her child with her, largely as a result of her engagement in a mentoring program. She had exited the sex trade, she had good housing, she made sure that the daughter had the supports that she needed, and that she as a mom had the supports she needed. Now her daughter, who had a diagnosis of fetal alcohol syndrome, was having problems at school. So this mother went to the school, as we are all supposed to do as parents of children with disability, to do advocacy work. She talked to me about how frustrated she felt after this experience. She said:

I was the one advocating to get my daughter all of these supports. I'm the one who put her on all the wait lists and signed her up and filled out all the paper work and advocated for myself. And now she's having problems, the principal at the school is telling me that the problems are stemming from home. And I told him, "No, there's stuff going on at school, too. I'll take my blame or my responsibility for part of it, but there's stuff going on at school." And he said, "No, I don't think that is the case."

These mother-blaming messages not only reinforce the shame, blame, stigma, and discrimination toward substance-using pregnant women, but often operate to exclude women from exactly the kinds of care they need. Social isolation and marginalization decrease timely access to supportive care, as we have seen documented across a wide range of sites. In the context of my research, one woman described her interaction with service providers in trying to get this supportive care:

"It's like I have to beg and, if it's not begging for things that I or my kids need, I have to fall on my face before they recognize that I have problems that I need to face. That's the frustrating thing. It makes life a lot harder."

We have systems for responding to crisis, but we do not have systems that are able to work with women in a preventive way to keep them from "falling on their face," or that tell women they do not have to demean themselves or "beg" in order to get the help that they need. We see this not only in social services, but also in primary care settings. In a recent study that we did on access to primary care for women who use drugs in the Downtown Eastside, one participant explained, "When you don't get health care, you don't get a sense of belonging, you don't get a sense of your importance."

If women are coping with feelings of marginalization and exclusion by using substances, we can see the implications for FASD prevention. Mothers also see it. Again and again through research, mothers have shown us that social support is critical to having a healthy pregnancy; and interventions that increase social support – like those that have been described within the PCAP model – reduce the likelihood of future substance-exposed pregnancy. We also see this documented in evaluations that Nancy Poole has made of the Sheway program, and in evaluations of the Breaking the Cycle program in Toronto. In a study at Sheway which examined the importance of social support, women were asked, "Why did you get help from Sheway, and what was meaningful to you about it?" One woman responded:

"Because they took me for who I was and they didn't care that I used and they didn't care that I used when I was pregnant. They just wanted to make sure that I was fed and had somewhere to go. I honestly think that if it wasn't for this place, my children wouldn't have survived my pregnancy."

A very clear articulation of the need for a sense of belonging and importance.

Unfortunately, we continue to find that while we have very good examples of stand-alone programs that can work with women on an individual level, that work is more often than not made impossible – or at least very frustrating – by a lack of system coordination and cohesion. This further increases isolation and frustrates our efforts to provide care to women when they need it. I'll show you some examples of the situation in British Columbia, which is a relatively well-resourced province. These images are from a mapping study that we carried out with the Canada Northwest FASD Research Network. The study looked at the availability of specific types of services that could be engaged in FASD-prevention work, and are a part of that coordinated system of care that women require. On each of these maps of British Columbia, the white dots represent places in the province that are densely enough populated that we would expect to find services there. In Figure 4.2, the blue dots are the locations of addiction treatment services that are prepared to enroll women in treatment during pregnancy. You will see that many of the white dots do not have blue dots. What this means in the life of an individual

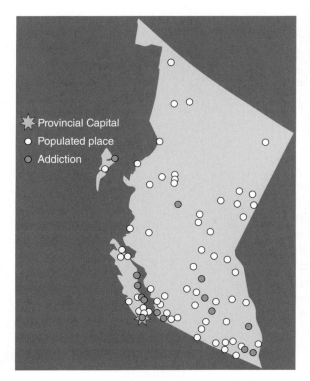

Figure 4.2 Map locating addictions treatment programs for women in British Columbia (2008). Poole, N. and Salmon, A. (March 10, 2007). *FASD Prevention from a Women's Health Determinants Perspective:* *The Work of the Network Action Team of the Canada Northwest FASD Research Network.* Presentation to the the Canada Northwest FASD Partnership, Vancouver, BC.

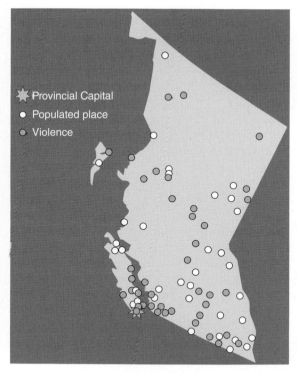

Figure 4.3 Map locating transition houses for women in British Columbia (2008). Poole, N. and Salmon, A. (March 10, 2007). *FASD Prevention from a Women's Health Determinants Perspective: The Work of the* *Network Action Team of the Canada Northwest FASD Research Network.* Presentation to the the Canada Northwest FASD Partnership, Vancouver, BC.

woman is that, if she is thinking about going for treatment – and that's what we all tell her she should do – going for treatment means going hundreds of kilometers away from her community – if there's a bed – and always leaving her children behind unless she ends up in one of the fewer than 20 beds in the Peardonville House treatment center in Abbottsford.

The purple dots in Figure 4.3 are the locations of transition houses at the community level in British Columbia. Again, we see a lot of white dots, but no purple dots. If we were to map solely those transition houses prepared to admit pregnant women who are using substances, most of those purple dots would disappear. Figure 4.4 shows the locations of pregnancy outreach programs that are prepared to serve pregnant substance-using women and work with them on their substance use as part as a healthier pregnancy. Again, you will see that there are many communities that do not have pregnancy outreach programs, do not have addictions treatment services, and do not have anti-violence services for women. While we are very keen to blame and shame women for not getting the care that they need

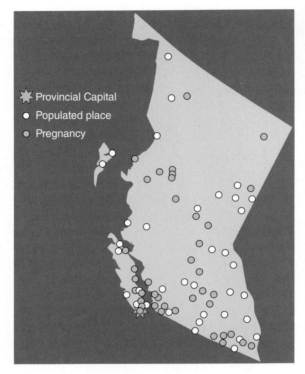

Figure 4.4 Map locating Pregnancy Outreach Programs in British Columbia (2008). Poole, N. and Salmon, A. (March 10, 2007). *FASD Prevention from a Women's Health Determinants Perspective: The Work of the* *Network Action Team of the Canada Northwest FASD Research Network.* Presentation to the the Canada Northwest FASD Partnership, Vancouver, BC.

when they need it, we also must think about the fact that we have not built systems that are ready for women to access help when they need it most urgently .

4.5.1
Recommendations

Evidence tells us that, within services, the most important aspects of service provision are to take a welcoming, supportive, nonjudgmental approach that addresses the fear, shame, blame, stigma, misinformation, and discrimination that substance-using pregnant women encounter on a daily basis; to meet women where they are; and to help women with related harms. Between services, intersectoral collaboration is critical and note that in order to have intersectoral collaboration within our communities we need multiple sectors at work. This requires collaborative efforts – not simply knowing where the other services are, but cross-training, development of program mandates and policies for working with women in a positive way, and providing support to enable staff to do the collaboration with other agencies that is required. The evidence tells us that collaboration is especially important between primary care, maternity care, addictions treatment, mental health services, child welfare authorities, anti-violence services, and income and employment supports.

Increasing system capacity for FASD prevention requires the recognition that FASD is not only a children's health issue but also a women's health issue. It requires responses to maternal substance use that are meaningful, effective, compassionate and, in particular, recognize the root causes of women's substance use and are willing to work on those with women, when they need it and in a way that works. This requires increased systems capacity for interagency co-operation that is wrapped around the mother, child, and family unit.

References

1 Basford, D.L., Thorpe, K., William, R., and Cardwell, K. (2004) *State of evidence: Fetal alcohol spectrum disorder (FASD) prevention.* Alberta Centre for Child, Family & Community Research, Lethbridge, AB.

Appendices

Abbreviations

95% CI	95% confidence interval
AEP	alcohol-exposed pregnancy
AMSTAR	Assessment of Multiple Systematic Reviews
AO	assessment only
AR-CARES	Arkansas Center for Addictions Research, Education and Services
ARND	alcohol-related neurodevelopmental disorder
ARBD	alcohol-related birth defect
ASI	Addiction Severity Index
ASPEN	Adolescent Substance Prevention Education Network
BAC	blood alcohol content
BALANCE	Birth Control and Alcohol Awareness; Negotiating Choices Effectively
BI	brief intervention
CCT	controlled clinical trial
CDC	Centers for Disease Control
CPG	clinical practice guidelines
DDP	Drinking During Pregnancy Questionnaire
EPHPP	Effective Public Health Practice Project
EtOH	ethyl alcohol
FAS	fetal alcohol syndrome
FASD	fetal alcohol spectrum disorder
FASTRAC	Fetal Alcohol Spectrum Teaching and Research Awareness Campaign
g	gram
IGR	intrauterine growth retardation
IQR	interquartile range
ITS	interrupted time series
ITT	intention-to-treat
kg	kilogram
max	maximum
MDI	mental development index

Prevention of Fetal Alcohol Spectrum Disorder FASD: Who is Responsible?, First Edition. Edited by Sterling Clarren, Amy Salmon, Egon Jonsson.
© 2011 Wiley-VCH Verlag GmbH & Co. KGaA. Published 2011 by Wiley-VCH Verlag GmbH & Co. KGaA.

MI	motivational interview
mo	month
NA	not applicable
NHMRC	National Health and Medical Research Council
NICE	National Institute for Health and Clinical Excellence
NICU	neonatal intensive care unit
NR	not reported
NSVD	normal spontaneous vaginal delivery
OR	odds ratio
PALS	Positive Adolescent Life Skills
PCAP	Parent–Child Assistance Program
PDI	psychomotor development index
pFAS	partial fetal alcohol syndrome
PHFE-WIC	Public Health Foundation Enterprises Management Solutions Special Supplemental Nutrition Program for Women, Infants and Children
PHP	Pregnancy and Health Program
PHRED	Public Health Research Education and Development Program
PICOD	population, intervention, outcomes and design
PNCC	Prenatal Care Coordination Program
POSIT	Problem-Oriented Screening Instrument for Teenagers
PPWI	Pregnant and Postpartum Women and their Infants
RCT	randomized controlled trial
RR	risk ratio
SD	standard deviation
SR	systematic review
T-ACE	Tolerance, Annoyed, Cut down, Eye-opener
TOA	time to outcome assessment
TWEAK	Tolerance, Worried, Eye-opener, Amnesia, and K/Cut down
UK	United Kingdom
USA	United States of America
wk	week
WMD	weighted mean difference
yr	year

Glossary

Allocation: The process by which an individual is assigned to an intervention group or a control group in a randomized controlled trial. Ideally, the invetigators do not know which comparison group individual patients have been placed in.

Before-and-after study: A nonexperimental study design where data are collected before and after an intervention is implemented. A separate control group is not used; rather, the participants act as their own controls, with outcomes compared to previous baseline data.

Bias: A systematic deviation from the truth. In studies, it refers to systematic errors in measurement or assessment that cause either an overestimation or underestimation of the results.

Blinding: A research strategy in which people involved in a study (whether researchers, participants or other persons) are prevented from knowing certain information about the study process. Blinding is used to prevent conscious as well as subconscious bias that can be introduced by knowing which intervention group the participants belong to.

Confidence interval: A measure of the uncertainty around the main finding of a statistical analysis. This means that if someone were to keep repeating a study in other samples from the same population, 95% of the confidence intervals from those studies would contain the true value of the unknown quantity. In general, a higher degree of confidence will require a larger interval. Confidence intervals are smaller when estimates are based on larger sample sizes.

Control: In clinical trials, a participant who is compared with an individual that received the intervention under study. The control participant may have received usual care, no intervention, or another active intervention.

Controlled clinical trial: A planned experiment in which participants are allocated to an intervention or a control group using a quasi-random or nonrandom methods, and the outcomes are compared between the groups.

Confounding variable/confounder: In medical research and epidemiology, a variable that is associated with the exposure or intervention under investigation, and can cause or prevent the outcome that is being examined. Unless these variables are measured as part of the research, their effects cannot be distinguished from those of the exposure(s) or intervention(s) being studied.

Fetal Alcohol Spectrum Disorders: The range of harms that can result from prenatal alcohol exposure, including vision and hearing problems, slow growth, and brain damage that results in lifelong problems with attention, memory, reasoning, and judgment.

Immediate outcomes: Immediate events, occurrences or conditions that are the intended results of an intervention. They constitute the first-level effect of a preventive intervention. Examples of immediate outcomes are changes in knowledge, attitudes, intentions, perceptions, and awareness.

Indicated prevention: Interventions (such as alcoholism treatment) that target individuals who have alcohol-related problems or a history of alcohol-exposed pregnancies.

Individual study: See *Primary study*.

Intermediate outcomes: Intermediate events, occurrences or conditions expressed as behavioral changes that are expected to follow from the achievement of one or more immediate outcomes.

Interrupted time series: A research design in which a single group of participants is tested or observed at multiple time points (at least three times), before and after an intervention. The design attempts to detect whether the intervention has had an effect significantly greater than the underlying trend.

Interrupted time series study: A type of study in which a single group of participants is tested at least three times before and three times after an intervention or exposure to an event.

Intervention integrity: The degree to which a replicated intervention (program, model or strategy) is implemented according to specification.

Meta-analysis: The use of statistical techniques in a systematic review to integrate the results of included studies.

MESH: The Medical Subject Headings (MESH) comprise the National Library of Medicine's controlled vocabulary used for indexing articles and cataloging books in the life sciences.

Methodological quality: The extent to which the design and conduct of a study are likely to have prevented systematic errors (bias). Variation in methodological quality can explain variation in the results of studies included in a systematic review. More rigorously designed (higher quality) studies are more likely to yield results that are closer to the 'truth'.

p-value (e.g., p < 0.05): A statistical term for the probability that the results of a particular study (e.g., an observed mean difference) could have been produced by chance in the absence of a real difference [1]. By scientific convention, p-values of <0.05 or <0.01 indicate a low probability that the difference is by chance and are used as a guideline for determining when an observed difference can be considered real.

Primary study: Original research in which data are collected. The term primary study is sometimes used to distinguish it from a *secondary study* (re-analysis of previously collected data), *meta-analysis,* and other ways of combining studies (such as economic analysis and decision analysis). Also called an *individual study.*

Primary disabilities: Inherent functional problems directly caused by alcohol exposure *in utero.* They can include mental retardation, learning disabilities, sensory impairments, and speech and language difficulties.

Prospective analytical cohort study: A type of observational study in which a group of participants (a cohort) that have been exposed to a characteristic of interest (e.g., a preventive intervention) are followed over a period of time to assess outcomes [2]. Comparisons are made with a group of individuals that are not exposed to the intervention of interest.

Randomized clinical trial: A planned experiment in which participants are assigned to intervention or control groups using a random method. Comparisons between the groups are made for the outcomes of interest.

Retrospective analytical cohort study: A type of observational study in which a group of participants (a cohort) is assembled based on their previous exposure to a characteristic of interest (e.g., a preventive intervention). Comparisons are made with a group of individuals that were not exposed to the intervention of interest in the past.

Risk ratio: A measure of the risk of a certain undesirable outcome in an intervention group compared to the risk of the same outcome in a control group. A risk ratio of 1 indicates no difference between comparison groups. A risk ratio of <1 indicates that the intervention was effective in reducing the risk of an undesirable outcome.

Secondary disabilities: Functional problems that are acquired as individuals develop, such as mental illness, criminal activity, inappropriate sexual behavior, alcohol or drug abuse, and difficulty obtaining and maintaining employment.

Selective prevention: Preventive interventions (e.g., counseling, referral to specialized treatment) that target groups or subsets of the population who may already have alcohol-use problems or are at a higher risk of developing alcohol-use problems than the general population, or both.

Statistically significant: A result that is unlikely to have happened by chance. The usual threshold for a determination of statistical significance is a probability of less than 0.05 that the result would have occurred by chance.

Systematic review: A review of a clearly formulated question that uses systematic and explicit methods to identify, select, and critically appraise relevant research, and to collect and analyze data from the studies that are included in the review. Statistical methods (meta-analysis) may or may not be used to analyze and summarize the results of the included studies [1].

Thematic analysis: A method of synthesizing findings from a number of studies, in which key themes in the studies are identified and the evidence is then summarized within these themes or categories.

Ultimate outcomes: The highest-level outcomes that can be reasonably attributed to a policy, program or initiative, and are the consequences of one or more intermediate outcomes having been achieved. Ultimate outcomes usually represent the raison d'être of a policy, program or initiative. They are long-term outcomes that represent a change of state in a target population.

Universal prevention: Interventions and programs (e.g., social marketing interventions, educational, and legal/system activities) that are targeted and delivered to whole populations. Each member of the population is considered to have the same level of risk [3].

References

1 The Cochrane Collaboration (2010) Glossary of Cochrane Collaboration and research terms. Available at: http://www2.cochrane.org/resources/glossary.htm (accessed 23 August 2010).

2 Elliott, L., Coleman, K., Suebwongpat, A., and Norris, S. (2008) Fetal Alcohol Spectrum Disorders (FASD): Systematic reviews of prevention, diagnosis and management. Health Services Assessment Collaboration Report, 1 (9), i-535.

3 Institute of Medicine (1996) *Fetal Alcohol Syndrome: Diagnosis, Epidemiology, Prevention, and Treatment.* National Academy Press, Washington, DC.

Index

Prevention of Fetal Alcohol Spectrum Disorder FASD: Who is Responsible?, First Edition. Edited by Sterling Clarren, Amy Salmon, Egon Jonsson.
© 2011 Wiley-VCH Verlag GmbH & Co. KGaA. Published 2011 by Wiley-VCH Verlag GmbH & Co. KGaA.

A very clear articulation of the need for a sense of belonging and importance. Unfortunately, we continue to find that while we have very good examples of stand-alone programs that can work with women on an individual level, that work is more often than not made impossible—or at least very frustrating—by a lack of system coordination and cohesion. This further increases isolation and frustrates our efforts to provide care to women when they need it. I'll show you some examples of the situation in British Columbia, which is a relatively well-resourced province. These images are from a mapping study that we carried out with the Canada Northwest FASD Research Network. The study looked at the availability of specific types of services that could be engaged in FASD-prevention work, and are a part of that coordinated system of care that women require. On each of these maps of British Columbia, the white dots represent places in the province that are densely enough populated that we would expect to find services there. In Figure 4.2, the blue dots are the locations of addiction treatment services that are prepared to enroll women in treatment during pregnancy. You will see that many of the white dots do not have blue dots. What this means in the life of an individual

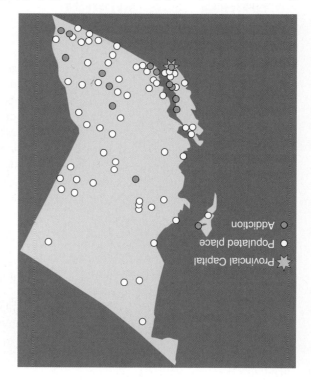

Figure 4.2 Map locating addictions treatment programs for women in British Columbia (2008). Poole, N. and Salmon, A. (March 10, 2007). *FASD Prevention from a Women's Health Determinants Perspective:*

The Work of the Network Action Team of the Canada Northwest FASD Research Network. Presentation to the the Canada Northwest FASD Partnership, Vancouver, BC.

I was the one advocating to get my daughter all of these supports. I'm the one who put her on all the wait lists and signed her up and filled out all the paper work and advocated for myself. And now she's having problems, the principal at the school is telling me that the problems are stemming from home. And I told him, "No, there's stuff going on at school, too. I'll take my blame or my responsibility for part of it, but there's stuff going on at school." And he said, "No, I don't think that is the case."

These mother-blaming messages not only reinforce the shame, blame, stigma, and discrimination toward substance-using pregnant women, but often operate to exclude women from exactly the kinds of care they need. Social isolation and marginalization decrease timely access to supportive care, as we have seen documented across a wide range of sites. In the context of my research, one woman described her interaction with service providers in trying to get this supportive care:

"It's like I have to beg and, if it's not begging for things that I or my kids need, I have to fall on my face before they recognize that I have problems that I need to face. That's the frustrating thing. It makes life a lot harder."

We have systems for responding to crisis, but we do not have systems that are able to work with women in a preventive way to keep them from "falling on their face," or that tell women they do not have to demean themselves or "beg" in order to get the help that they need. We see this not only in social services, but also in primary care settings. In a recent study that we did on access to primary care for women who use drugs in the Downtown Eastside, one participant explained, "When you don't get health care, you don't get a sense of belonging, you don't get a sense of your importance."

If women are coping with feelings of marginalization and exclusion by using substances, we can see the implications for FASD prevention. Mothers also see it. Again and again through research, mothers have shown us that social support is critical to having a healthy pregnancy; and interventions that increase social support—like those that have been described within the PCAP model—reduce the likelihood of future substance-exposed pregnancy. We also see this documented in evaluations that Nancy Poole has made of the Sheway program, and in evaluations of the Breaking the Cycle program in Toronto. In a study at Sheway which examined the importance of social support, women were asked, "Why did you get help from Sheway, and what was meaningful to you about it?" One woman responded:

"Because they took me for who I was and they didn't care that I used and they didn't care that I used when I was pregnant. They just wanted to make sure that I was fed and had somewhere to go. I honestly think that if it wasn't for this place, my children wouldn't have survived my pregnancy."